AF711764

Workbook for

Fordney's Medical Insurance

Workbook for

Fordney's Medical Insurance

Fifteenth Edition

Linda M. Smith, CPC, CPC-I, CEMC, CMBS
Training and Consulting
MedOffice Resources
Greene, New York

ELSEVIER

WORKBOOK FOR FORDNEY'S MEDICAL INSURANCE,
FIFTEENTH EDITION

ISBN: 978-0-323-59441-7

International Standard Book Number: 978-0-323-59441-7

Publishing Director: Kristin Wilhelm
Senior Content Strategist: Linda Woodard
Senior Content Development Manager: Ellen Wurm-Cutter
Senior Content Development Specialist: Maria Broeker
Publishing Services Manager: Shereen Jameel
Project Manager: Aparna Venkatachalam

Printed in the United States of America

Last digit is the print number: 9 8 7 6 5 4 3 2 1

ELSEVIER

3251 Riverport Lane
St. Louis, Missouri 63043

Contributors

CONTRIBUTORS

Rachael D'Andrea, MS, RHIA, CPHQ, CDIP, CHTS-TR
Professor, Health Information Management
Lake Sumter State College
Leesburg, Florida

Professor, Health Information Management and Health Care Administration
Charter Oak State College
New Britain, Connecticut

Cheryl Fassett, CPC, CPB, CPPM, CPC-I
Educator
Practice Manager
Riverside Associates in Anesthesia, PC
Binghamton, New York

Nanette Sayles, EdD, RHIA, CCS, CHPS, CHDA, CPHI, CPHIMS, FAHIMA
Associate Professor, Health Information Management
East Central College
Union, Missouri

Contents

Instruction Guide to the Workbook

LEARNING OBJECTIVES

***The student will be able to*:**

- Define and spell key terms and key abbreviations for each chapter.
- Answer review questions for each chapter of *Fordney's Medical Insurance*.
- Complete assignments to enhance and develop better critical thinking skills.
- Define abbreviations as they appear on a patient record.
- Abstract subjective and objective data from patient records.
- Review documentation on patient records.
- Code professional services properly, using the *Current Procedural Terminology* (CPT) Code Book.
- Select diagnostic code numbers, using the *International Classification of Diseases*, Tenth Revision, Clinical Modifications (ICD-10-CM).
- Locate errors on insurance claims before submission to insurance companies.
- Locate errors on returned insurance claims.
- Carry out collection procedures on delinquent accounts.
- Execute financial management procedures for tracing managed care plans.
- Extract information necessary to complete insurance claim forms from patient records and billing statements/ledger cards.
- Post payments, adjustments, and balances to patients' statements/ledger cards when submitting insurance claims.
- Compute mathematic calculations for Medicare and TRICARE cases.
- Analyze insurance claims for errors in both hospital inpatient and outpatient settings.
- Answer questions about the insurance verification process using patients' health insurance cards.
- Study case scenarios and explain how these violate security and confidentiality and give solutions to prevent the breaches.
- List important activities in each stage of the life cycle of an insurance claim.
- Prepare a cover letter, résumé, job application, and follow-up letter to search for employment.
- Access the Internet and visit websites to research and/or obtain data.

INSTRUCTIONS TO THE STUDENT

The 15th edition of *Workbook for Fordney's Medical Insurance* has been prepared for those who use the textbook, *Fordney's Medical Insurance*. It is designed to assist the learner in a practical approach to doing insurance billing and coding.

The key terms and key abbreviations are repeated for quick reference when studying. Each chapter's outline serves as a lecture guide to use for note taking. The review questions in the form of short answer, true/false, multiple choice, and matching are presented to reinforce learning of key concepts for each topic.

Some assignments give students hands-on experience in completing claim forms using National Uniform Claim Committee (NUCC) guidelines. Insurance claim forms and other sample documents that are easily removable are included for practice.

Current procedural and diagnostic code exercises are used throughout to facilitate and enhance coding skills for submitting a claim or making an itemized billing statement.

Self-study assignments encompass important points from each chapter and allow you to study at your own pace.

Critical thinking assignments require skills that help prepare you for real-world scenarios encountered in insurance billing.

KEY TERMS AND KEY ABBREVIATIONS

Key terms and key abbreviations are presented for each chapter, and definitions may be located in the glossary at the end of *Fordney's Medical Insurance*. It is suggested that you make up 3- by 5-inch index cards for each term or abbreviation and write in the definitions as you encounter them while reading each chapter in the *Fordney's Medical Insurance*. Doing this will reinforce your knowledge and help you learn the words and abbreviations. Your instructor may wish to select certain words for you to study for pop quizzes.

NOTE TAKING

Taking notes is an important key to success in studying and learning. Note taking helps an individual pay attention during class and retain information. Each chapter has a study outline for organizational purposes, and the outline may be used as a guide for writing down key points during lectures or when studying or reviewing from *Fordney's Medical Insurance* for tests. Use file cards, notepads, notebooks, computers, or tablets for taking notes. Underline or highlight important words or phrases. To improve the usefulness of notes, try the following format:

1. Using a tablet note-taking app, notepad sheet, or file card, draw a margin 3 inches from the left.
2. Use the left side for topic headings and the right side for notes.
3. Skip a few lines when the topic changes.
4. Write numbers or letters to indicate sub-ideas under a heading.
5. Be brief; do not write down every word except when emphasizing a quotation, rule, or law. Write notes in your own words because that is what you will understand.
6. Use abbreviations that you know how to translate.
7. Listen carefully to the lecture.
8. After the lecture, reread your notes. Highlight the word(s) on the left side of the page to identify the topic of the notes on the right.
9. For study purposes, cover the right side and see if you can explain to yourself or someone else the topic or word.
10. Remember: learning is by doing, and doing is up to you. So take notes for better understanding.

REVIEW QUESTION ASSIGNMENTS

Review questions have been designed to encompass important points for each chapter to assist you in studying insurance billing and coding theory.

SIMULATION ASSIGNMENTS

Assume that you have been hired as an insurance billing specialist and that you are working in a clinic setting for an incorporated group of medical doctors, other allied health specialists, and a podiatrist. You will be asked to complete various assignments. These doctors will be on the staff of a nearby hospital. Appendix A details this clinic's policies and procedures, which you must read completely before beginning the competency-based assignments. Within each chapter, the simulation assignments progress from easy to more complex. Some assignments are given with critical thinking problems, which the instructor may use for class discussion.

Always read the assignment entirely before starting.

MEDICAL TERMINOLOGY AND ABBREVIATIONS

A list of abbreviations is provided in Appendix A to help you learn how to abstract and read physicians' notes. Decode any abbreviations that you do not understand or that are unfamiliar to you. To reinforce learning these abbreviations, write their meanings on the assignment pages. If you do not have a background in medical terminology, it may be wise to use a good medical dictionary as a reference or, better yet, enroll in a terminology course to master that skill.

PATIENT RECORDS

Patient records, financial accounting records (ledgers), and encounter forms are presented, so the learner may have the tools needed to extract information to complete claim forms.

Patient records have been abbreviated because of space and page constraints. The records contain pertinent data for each type of case, but it has been necessary to omit a lengthy physical examination. Because detailed documentation is encouraged in medical practices, the records all appear typewritten rather than in handwritten notes. The physician's signature appears after each dated entry on the record.

All the materials included in the assignments have been altered to prevent identification of the cases or parties involved. The names and addresses are fictitious, and no reference to any person living or dead is intended. No evaluation of medical practice or medical advice is to be inferred from the patient records, nor is any recommendation made toward alternative treatment methods or prescribed medications.

FINANCIAL RECORDS

Financial accounting record statements (ledgers) are included for practice in posting, totaling fees, and properly recording appropriate information when an insurance claim is submitted. Refer to Appendix A to obtain information about the Mock Fee Schedule and the physicians' fees for posting to the statements.

CMS-1500 CLAIM FORM

If you have access to a computer, use the practice management software that accompanies the *Workbook* to complete each assignment and print it out for evaluation. To complete the CMS-1500 claim form properly for each type of program, refer to the section in Chapter 14 of *Fordney's Medical Insurance* that describes in detail the correct information to be put in each block.

Do's and don'ts for claim completion and NUCC guidelines are mentioned in Chapter 14. If you do not have access to a computer, type or neatly write in the information on the insurance form as you abstract it from the patient record.

PERFORMANCE EVALUATION CHECKLIST

The 15th edition features a competency-based format for each assignment indicating performance objectives to let you know what is to be accomplished. The task (job assignment), conditions (elements needed to perform and complete the task), and standards (time management), as well as directions for the specific task, are included.

A two-part performance evaluation checklist used when completing a CMS-1500 claim form is depicted in Figures I.1 and I.2. Reproduce these sheets only for the assignments that involve completing the CMS-1500 claim form. Your instructor will give you the number of points to be assigned for each step.

STUDENT REFERENCE NOTEBOOK

A student reference notebook is recommended so that you can access information quickly to help you complete the *Workbook* assignments. Before beginning the assignments, tear out Appendix A and place it in a three-ring binder with the chapter indexes. Appendix A includes the clinic policies and guidelines, data about the clinic staff, medical and laboratory abbreviations, and the Mock Fee Schedule used while working as an insurance billing specialist for the College Clinic.

Besides these suggestions, you may wish to either tear out or make photocopies of other sections of *Fordney's Medical Insurance* for your personal use. In addition, your instructor may give you handouts from time to time, pertaining to regional insurance program policies and procedures, to place in your notebook.

TESTS

Tests appear at the end of the *Workbook* to provide a complete, competency-based educational program.

REFERENCE MATERIAL

To do the assignments in this *Workbook* and gain expertise in coding and insurance claims completion, an individual must have access to the books listed here. Addresses for obtaining these materials are given in parentheses. Additional books and booklets on these topics, as well as on Medicaid, Medicare, TRICARE, and more, can be found at bookstores or online retailers.

Dictionary

Dorland's Illustrated Medical Dictionary, 32nd edition, Elsevier, 2012 (6277 Sea Harbor Drive, Orlando, FL 32821-9989; 1-800-545-2522).

Code Books

Current Procedural Terminology, American Medical Association, published annually (515 North State Street, Chicago, IL 60610; 1-800-621-8335).

International Classification of Diseases, Tenth Revision, Clinical Modification, Elsevier, published annually (6277 Sea Harbor Drive, Orlando, FL 32821-9989; 1-800-545-2522).

Word Book

Sloane's Medical Word Book, 5th edition, by Ellen Drake, CMT, FAAMT, Elsevier (6277 Sea Harbor Drive, Orlando, FL 32821-9989; 1-800-545-2522).

Pharmaceutical Book

Optional publications for drug names and descriptions might be either drug books used by nurses (e.g., *Mosby's Gen RX*, Elsevier, published annually [3251 Riverport Lane, St. Louis, MO 63043; 1-800-325-4177; www.elsevier.com]) or ones used by physicians (e.g., *Physician's Desk Reference* [PDR], Medical Economics Company, published annually [5 Paragon Drive, Montvale, NJ, 07645; 1-800-432-4570]).

PERFORMANCE EVALUATION CHECKLIST

Assignment No. ____________

Name: ____ Date: ____________________________

Performance Objective

Task: Given access to all necessary equipment and information, the student will complete a CMS-1500 health insurance claim form.

Standards: Claim Productivity Management
Time __________ minutes
Note: Time element may be given by instructor.

Directions: See assignment.

NOTE TIME BEGAN __________ **NOTE TIME COMPLETED** __________

PROCEDURE STEPS	ASSIGNED POINTS	STEP PERFORMED SATISFACTORY	COMMENTS
1. Assembled CMS-1500 claim form, patient record, E/M code slip, ledger card, computer, pen or pencil, and code books.	__________	__________	__________
2. Posted ledger card correctly.	__________	__________	__________
3. Proofread form for spelling and typographical errors while form remained on computer screen.	__________	__________	__________
4. Points earned for correct completion of CMS-1500 block-by-block data.	__________	__________	__________

Figure I-1

PERFORMANCE EVALUATION CHECKLIST

BLOCK	INCORRECT	MISSING	NOT NEEDED	REMARKS	BLOCK	INCORRECT	MISSING	NOT NEEDED	REMARKS
					18				
1A					19				
2					20				
3					21				
4									
5					22				
6					23				
7					24A				
8					24B				
					24C				
9					24D				
9A									
9B									
9C					24E				
9D									
					24F				
10A					24G				
10B					24H, 24I				
10C					24J				
10D									
11					25, 26				
11A					27				
11B					28				
11C					29				
11D									
12					30				
13									
14					31				
15									
16					32				
17									
17A					33				
					Reference Initials				

TOTAL POINTS EARNED: ________ TOTAL POINTS POSSIBLE: ________

Evaluator's signature ____________________ NEED TO REPEAT: ________

Figure I-2

EMPLOYEE INSURANCE PROCEDURAL MANUAL

If you currently work in a health care office, you may custom design an insurance manual for your organization's practice as you complete insurance claims in this *Workbook*. Obtain a three-ring binder with indexes and label them "Group Plans," "Private Plans," "Medicaid," "Medicare," "Managed Care Plans," "State Disability," "TRICARE," and "Workers' Compensation." If many of your patients have group plans, complete an insurance data or fact sheet for each plan and organize them alphabetically by group plan (Figure I.3).

An insurance manual with fact sheets listing benefits can keep you up to date on policy changes and ensure maximum reimbursement. Fact sheets can be prepared from information obtained when patients bring in their benefit booklets. Obtain and insert a list of the procedures that must be performed as an outpatient and those that must have second opinions for each of the insurance plans.

As you complete the assignments in this *Workbook*, place them in the insurance manual as examples of completed claims for each particular program.

INSURANCE DATA

1. Employer's name ______________________
2. Address ______________________ Telephone Number ______________________
3. Insurance Company Contact Person ______________________
4. Insurance Carrier ______________________
5. Address ______________________ Telephone Number to Call for Benefits ______________________
6. Group Policy Number ______________________
7. Group Account Manager ______________________ Telephone Number ______________________
8. **Insurance Coverage:**
   Annual Deductible ______________________ Patient Copayment Percentage ______________________
   Noncovered Procedures ______________________
   Maximum Benefits ______________________
9. **Diagnostic Coverage:**
   Limited Benefits ______________________
   Maximum Benefits ______________________
   Noncovered Procedures ______________________
10. **Major Medical:**
    Annual Deductible ______________________ Patient Copayment Percentage ______________________
    Limited Benefits ______________________
    Maximum Benefits ______________________
    Noncovered Procedures ______________________

Mandatory Outpatient Surgeries ______________________

Second Surgical Opinions ______________________

Preadmission Certification Yes ______ No ______ Authorized Labs ______________________

Payment Plan:

UCR ______________ Schedule of Benefits ______________ CPT ______________ RVS ______________

Send claims to: ______________________

____

Date Entered ______________________ Date Updated ______________________

Figure I-3

1 Role of an Insurance Billing Specialist

Linda M. Smith

KEY TERMS

Your instructor may wish to select some specific words pertinent to this chapter for a test. For definitions of the terms, further study, and/or reference, the words, phrases, and abbreviations may be found in the glossary at the end of the Textbook. *Key terms for this chapter follow.*

American Medical Association
cash flow
claims assistance professional
claims examiner
cycle
electronic mail
errors and omissions insurance
ethics
etiquette
facility billing
independent contractor
insurance billing specialist
list service
medical billing representative
professional billing
reimbursement specialist
respondeat superior
revenue
self-pay patient
senior billing representative

KEY ABBREVIATIONS

See how many abbreviations and acronyms you can translate and then use this as a handy reference list. Definitions for the key abbreviations are located near the back of the Textbook *in the glossary.*

AAMA ______________________________
____
____
AMA ______________________________
ASHD ______________________________
CAP ______________________________
e-mail ______________________________
listserv ______________________________
MSO ______________________________
NPP ______________________________

PERFORMANCE OBJECTIVES

The student will be able to:

- Define and spell the key terms and key abbreviations for this chapter, given the information from the *Textbook* glossary, within a reasonable time period and with enough accuracy to obtain a satisfactory evaluation.
- Answer the fill-in-the-blank, multiple choice, and true/false review questions after reading the chapter, with enough accuracy to obtain a satisfactory evaluation.
- Use critical thinking to write one or two grammatically correct paragraphs with sufficient information to obtain a satisfactory evaluation.
- Visit websites and site-search information via the Evolve website at http://evolve.elsevier.com/Smith/Fordneys/, with sufficient information to obtain a satisfactory evaluation.

STUDY OUTLINE

Background of Insurance Claims, Coding, and Billing
Role of the Insurance Billing Specialist
- Job Responsibilities
- Educational and Training Requirements
- Career Advantages
- Self-Employment or Independent Contracting
- Flexible Hours
- Disabled Workers
- Qualifications and Attributes
- Skills
- Personal Image
- Behavior

Medical Etiquette
Professional Ethics
Scope of Practice and Liability
- Employer Liability
- Employee Liability
- Independent Contractor Liability
- Claims Assistant Professional Liability

Future Challenges

ASSIGNMENT 1.1 REVIEW QUESTIONS

Part I Fill in the Blank

Review the objectives, key terms, and chapter information before completing the following review questions.

1. Name some of the settings where facility billing is used.

   a. ______________________________

   b. ______________________________

   c. ______________________________

   d. ______________________________

   e. ______________________________

2. Name some of the various types of providers who use professional billing.

   a. ______________________________

   b. ______________________________

   c. ______________________________

   d. ______________________________

   e. ______________________________

3. Name examples of non-physician practitioners (NPPs).

   a. ______________________________

   b. ______________________________

   c. ______________________________

   d. ______________________________

   e. ______________________________

   f. ______________________________

   g. ______________________________

   h. ______________________________

4. Name several job titles associated with medical billing personnel in both small and large health care organizations.

   a. ______________________________

   b. ______________________________

   c. ______________________________

5. List some of the responsibilities and duties an insurance billing specialist might perform generally, as well as when acting as a collection manager. Refer to the section on "Job Responsibilities" in Fig. 1.1 of the text.

   a. ______________________________

   b. ______________________________

   c. ______________________________

   d. ______________________________

   e. ______________________________

   f. ______________________________

   g. ______________________________

6. List the duties of a claims-assistance professional.

   a. ______________________________

   b. ______________________________

   c. ______________________________

7. Insurance claims must be promptly submitted within ____________ business days to ensure continuous cash flow.

8. Define *cash flow*.

   ____

9. An individual who takes a patient to a private area before their visit with the provider to discuss the practice's financial policies and review the patient's insurance coverage.

   ____

10. Reasons for a medical practice's large accounts receivable are:

    a. ______________________________

    b. ______________________________

    c. ______________________________

    d. ______________________________

11. Skills required for an insurance billing specialist are:

    a. ______________________________

    b. ______________________________

    c. ______________________________

    d. ______________________________

    e. ______________________________

f. ______________________________

g. ______________________________

h. ______________________________

i. ______________________________

j. ______________________________

12. Standards of conduct by which an insurance billing specialist determines the propriety of his or her behavior in a relationship are known as ______________.

13. Complete these statements with either the word *illegal* or *unethical.*
    a. To make critical remarks about another health care organization or physician is ______________________.
    b. To report incorrect information to a Medicare fiscal intermediary is ______________________.

14. To treat a patient with a lack of courtesy is ________. When a physician is legally responsible for an employee's conduct during employment, it is known as ________.

15. A claims assistance professional neglects to submit an insurance claim to a Medicare supplemental insurance carrier within the proper time limit. What type of insurance is needed for protection against this loss for the client?

____

Part II Multiple Choice

Choose the best answer.

16. Two billing components are facility billing and professional billing. Professional billing is done for:
    a. hospitals.
    b. skilled nursing facilities.
    c. ambulatory surgical centers.
    d. physicians.

17. *Physician extenders* are health care personnel trained to provide medical care under the direct or indirect supervision of a physician, are also referred to as:
    a. independent contractors.
    b. claims assistance professionals (CAPs).
    c. non-physician practitioners (NPPs).
    d. insurance billing specialists.

18. The individual responsible for documenting the patient's clinical notes and assigning a diagnosis code and procedure code for medical services rendered is a/an:
    a. physician.
    b. insurance biller.
    c. office manager.
    d. financial accounting clerk.

19. Insurance payers that require the provider to submit insurance claims for the patient are:
    a. federal and state programs.
    b. private insurance plans.
    c. managed care programs.
    d. health care insurance plans.

20. Facility billing is charging for services done by:
    a. hospitals.
    b. physicians.
    c. ambulatory surgical centers.
    d. both a and c.

Part III True/False

Write "T" or "F" in the blank to indicate whether you think the statement is true or false.

_______ 21. Insurance billing specialists have a well-defined scope of practice.

_______ 22. If you knowingly submit a false claim or allow such a claim to be submitted, you can be liable for a civil violation.

_______ 23. It is the coder's responsibility to inform administration or his or her immediate supervisor if unethical or illegal coding practices are occurring.

_______ 24. A claims assistant professional (CAP) can interpret insurance policies for patients.

_______ 25. Independent contractors are covered under the health care organization's professional liability insurance whom they provide services to.

CRITICAL THINKING

To enhance your critical thinking skills, problems will be interspersed throughout the *Workbook*. Thinking is the goal of instruction and a student's responsibility. When trying to solve a problem by critical thinking, it is desirable to have more than one solution and to take time to think out answers. Remember that an answer may be changed when additional information is provided in a classroom setting.

ASSIGNMENT 1.2 CRITICAL THINKING

Performance Objective

Task: Describe why you are training to become an insurance billing specialist.

Conditions: Use one or two sheets of white typing paper and pen or pencil.

Standards: Time: ________________ minutes

Accuracy: ________________

(Note: The time element and accuracy criteria may be given by your instructor.)

Directions: Write one or two paragraphs describing why you are training to become an insurance billing specialist. Or, if enrolled in a class that is part of a medical assisting course, explain why you are motivated to seek a career as a medical assistant. Make sure grammar, punctuation, and spelling are correct.

ASSIGNMENT 1.3 VISIT WEBSITES

Performance Objective

Task: Access the Internet and visit several websites.

Conditions: Use a computer with printer and/or pen or pencil to make notes.

Standards: Time: ________________ minutes

Accuracy: ________________

(Note: The time element and accuracy criteria may be given by your instructor.)

Directions: Use a computer and use a browser to access the Internet. Go to some search engines to locate job opportunities.

1. Access the Internet and find one of the web search engines (Yahoo, Google, Bing). Begin a web search (e.g., key in "insurance billers") to search for information about insurance billers. List three to five websites found. Go to one or more of those resources and list the benefits that those sites might have for a student in locating job opportunities or networking with others for professional growth and knowledge. Bring the website addresses to share with the class.

2. Site-search information on standards of ethical coding by visiting the website of the American Health Information Management Association (AHIMA). Download and print a hard copy of this code of ethics developed by the AHIMA. Next, obtain information on the eHealth code of ethics, and respond to the following:

   A. Write a brief definition for each of the following terms: health information, health products, and health services.

   health information: ____

   health products: ____

   health services: ____

   B. State the eight guiding principles of organizations and individuals who provide health information over the Internet.

   ____

   ____

ASSIGNMENT 1.4 COMPOSE EMAIL MESSAGES

Performance Objective

Task: Compose brief messages for electronic mail transmission after reading each scenario.

Conditions: List of scenarios, one sheet of 8½- × 11-inch plain typing paper, and a computer or a pen.

Standards: Time: ________________ minutes

Accuracy: ________________

(Note: The time element and accuracy criteria may be given by your instructor.)

Directions: Read each scenario. Compose polite, effective, and brief messages that, on the job, would be transmitted via e-mail. Use the guidelines for e-mail presented on the Evolve website. Be sure to list a descriptive subject line as the first item in each composition. Single-space the message. Insert a short signature at the end of the message to include your name and affiliation, and create an e-mail address for yourself if you do not have one. Print hard copies of e-mail messages for Scenarios 1 through 5 to give to your instructor. After the instructor has returned your work, either make the necessary corrections and place your work in a three-ring notebook for future reference or, if you received a high score, place it in your portfolio for use when applying for a job.

Scenario 1:

Ask an insurance biller, Mary Davis, in a satellite office to locate and fax you a copy of the billing done on account number 43500 for services rendered to Margarita Sylva on March 2, 20xx. Explain that you must telephone the patient about her account. Mary Davis' e-mail address is mdavis@aal.com.

Scenario 2:

Patient Ellen Worth was recently hospitalized; her hospital number is 20-9870-11. Compose an e-mail message to the medical record department at College Hospital (collegehospmedrecords@rrv.net) for her final diagnosis and the assigned diagnostic code needed to complete the insurance claim form.

Scenario 3:

You are working for a billing service and receive an encounter form that is missing the information about the patient's professional service received on August 2, 20xx. The patient's account number is 45098. You have the diagnosis data. Compose an e-mail message to Dr. Mason (pmason@email.mc.com) explaining what you must obtain to complete the billing portion of the insurance claim form.

Scenario 4:

A new patient, John Phillips, has e-mailed your office to ask what the outstanding balance is on his account. The account number is 42990. You look up the financial record and note the service was for an office visit on June 14, 20xx. The charge was $106.11. Compose an e-mail response to Mr. Phillips, whose e-mail address is jphillips@hotmail.com.

Scenario 5:

You are having difficulty deciding whether the codes 13101, 13102, and 13132 with modifier 51 selected for a case are appropriate. Compose an e-mail message that will be posted on the American Academy of Professional Coders (AAPC)'s list service (listserv) (www.aapc.com) asking for comments. The case involves a 12-year-old boy who fell against a bicycle, lacerating the left side of his chest to the pectoralis muscle through a 12-cm gaping wound. He also sustained a 5-cm laceration to his left cheek. Complex repairs were required for these two wounds and totaled 17 cm. Find out whether modifier 51 should be appended to the second code or to the third code.

For each message, check for concise composition, single-spaced message, closing signature, and accuracy and effectiveness of message in terms of scenario presented. E-mail may contain abbreviations. On the job, a biller would compose a message quickly, so the instructor might want to award additional points for the speed with which this assignment is done.

2 Privacy, Security, and HIPAA

Cheryl Fassett

KEY TERMS

Your instructor may wish to select some specific words pertinent to this chapter for a test. For definitions of the terms, further study, and/or reference, the words, phrases, and abbreviations may be found in the glossary at the end of the Textbook. *Key terms for this chapter follow.*

American Recovery and Reinvestment Act
authorization
authorization form
breach of confidential communication
business associate
clearinghouse
confidential communication
confidentiality
consent
covered entity
designated record sets
disclosure
electronic media
health care organization
Health Information Technology for Economic and Clinical Health Act
HIPAA Omnibus Rule
Incidental use and disclosure
individually identifiable health information
Minimum Necessary Rule
mitigation
National Provider Identifier
nonprivileged information
Notice of Privacy Practices
Patient Protection and Affordable Care Act
portability
preexisting condition
privacy
privacy officer, privacy official
privileged information
protected health information
psychotherapy notes
security officer
Security Rule
transaction
use

KEY ABBREVIATIONS

See how many abbreviations and acronyms you can translate, and then use this as a handy reference list. Definitions for the key abbreviations are located near the back of the Textbook *in the glossary.*

ARRA ______________________

DHHS ______________________

EIN ______________________

ePHI ______________________

FBI ______________________

FTP ______________________

HIPAA ______________________

HITECH ______________________

IIHI ______________________

NPI ______________________

NPP ______________________

OCR ______________________

OIG ______________________

P&P ______________________

PHI ______________________

PO ______________________

PPACA ______________________

TPO ______________________

PERFORMANCE OBJECTIVES

The student will be able to:

- Define and spell the key terms and key abbreviations for this chapter, given the information from the Textbook glossary, within a reasonable time period and with enough accuracy to obtain a satisfactory evaluation.
- Answer the fill in the blank, multiple choice, and true/false review questions after reading the chapter, with enough accuracy to obtain a satisfactory evaluation.
- Decide when a situation is an incidental disclosure, HIPAA violation, or neither, with sufficient information to obtain a satisfactory evaluation.
- Visit websites and site-search information via the Evolve website, with sufficient information to obtain a satisfactory evaluation.

STUDY OUTLINE

Health Information Portability and Accountability Act
- Title I: Health Insurance Reform
- Title II: Administrative Simplification
- Defining HIPAA Roles, Relationships, and Key Terms

Transaction and Code Set Regulations

National Identifiers

The Privacy Rule: Confidentiality and Protected Health Information
- Privileged and Nonprivileged Information
- Patients' Rights
- Obligations of the Health Care Organization

The Security Rule: Administrative, Physical, and Technical Safeguards

Health Information Technology for Economic and Clinical Health Act
- Business Associates
- Notification of Breach
- HIPAA Compliance Audits
- Increased Penalties for Noncompliance With the Provisions of HIPAA
- HIPAA Omnibus Rule
- Consequences of Noncompliance With HIPAA and the HITECH Act

Application to the Health Care Setting
- Organization and Staff Responsibilities in Protecting Patient Rights

Best Practices to Avoid Common HIPAA Violations

ASSIGNMENT 2.1 REVIEW QUESTIONS

Part I Fill in the Blank

Review the objectives, key terms, and chapter information before completing the following review questions.

1. What is the primary purpose of HIPAA Title I: Insurance Reform?

   ____

   ____

2. The focus on the health care practice setting and reduction of administrative costs and burdens are the goals of which part of HIPAA?

   ____

3. An independent organization that receives insurance claims from the physician's office, performs edits, and transmits claims to insurance carriers is known as a/an

   ____.

4. Name the standard code sets used for the following:

   a. Drugs and supplies ______________________________

   b. Inpatient procedures ______________________________

   c. Diagnosis coding ______________________________

5. Under HIPAA guidelines, a health care coverage carrier, such as Blue Cross/Blue Shield, that transmits health information in electronic form in connection with a transaction is called a/an ______________________________.

6. Dr. John Doe contracts with an outside billing company to manage claims and accounts receivable. Under HIPAA guidelines, the billing company is considered a/an ________________ of the provider.

7. An individual designated to assist the provider by putting compliance policies and procedures in place and training office staff is known as a/an ______________ under HIPAA guidelines.

8. If you give, release, or transfer information to another entity, it is known as

   ____.

9. Define *protected health information* (PHI).

   ____

   ____

   ____

10. Unauthorized release of a patient's health information is called ________________.

11. A confidential communication related to the patient's treatment and progress that may be disclosed only with the patient's permission is known as

____.

12. Under HIPAA, exceptions to the right of privacy are those records involving

a. ____

b. ____

c. ____

d. ____

e. ____

f. ____

g. ____

h. ____

i. ____

13. At a patient's first visit under HIPAA guidelines, the document that must be given so the patient acknowledges the provider's confidentiality of his or her PHI is the

____.

14. If a breach of privacy is discovered, the health care provider is required to take affirmative action to respond to the breach and alleviate the severity of it. This is known as

____.

15. Name the three main sections of the HIPAA Security Rule for protecting electronic health information.

a. ____

b. ____

c. ____

16. Name the three specific areas of significant change that resulted from the Health Information Technology for Economic and Clinical Health (HITECH) Act.

a. ____

b. ____

c. ____

Part II Multiple Choice

Choose the best answer.

17. HIPAA transaction standards apply to the following, which are called *covered entities*:
    a. health care third-party payers.
    b. health care providers.
    c. health care clearinghouses.
    d. all of the above.

18. Enforcement of the privacy standards of HIPAA is the responsibility of the:
    a. Health Care Fraud and Abuse Control Program (HCFAP).
    b. National Committee on Vital and Health Statistics (NCVHS).
    c. Office for Civil Rights (OCR).
    d. Federal Bureau of Investigation (FBI).

19. Verbal or written agreement that gives approval to some action, situation, or statement is called:
    a. authorization.
    b. consent.
    c. disclosure.
    d. release.

20. An individual's formal written permission to use or disclose his or her personally identifiable health information for purposes other than treatment, payment, or health care operations is called:
    a. authorization.
    b. disclosure.
    c. release.
    d. consent.

21. The Notice of Privacy Practices (NPP) document is given to patients:
    a. at the first visit to the practice.
    b. at every visit to the practice.
    c. on an annual basis.
    d. only on request of the patient.

22. Privacy regulations allow patients the right to obtain a copy of PHI:
    a. under all circumstances.
    b. if they have a court order.
    c. only if the health care provider has determined that it would be appropriate and would not endanger the patient or any other person.
    d. only if the patient can pay the associated fee for the copies.

23. Under HIPAA, patient sign-in sheets:
    a. are never permissible.
    b. are permissible.
    c. are permissible but limit the information that is requested.
    d. are permissible but require the practice to give the patient a number to be used when calling the patient.

24. Which section of the HIPAA Security Rule recommends unique usernames and passwords to log on to any computer with access to PHI?
    a. Administrative safeguards
    b. Technical safeguards
    c. Physical safeguards

25. Which section of the HIPAA Security Rule recommends use of screensavers that will activate after 1 to 60 minutes of inactivity?
    a. Administrative safeguards
    b. Technical safeguards
    c. Physical safeguards

26. Under HITECH, if a breach occurs, the covered entity:
    a. does not have to notify the affected party.
    b. only has to notify the affected party if they feel it is reasonable.
    c. must notify the affected party no later than 30 calendar days after the discovery of the breach.
    d. must notify the affected party no later than 60 calendar days after the discovery of the breach.

27. The HIPAA Omnibus Rule enhanced:
    a. patients' privacy rights.
    b. patients' rights to restrict immunization records to schools.
    c. health care providers' rights limiting access to patient records.
    d. business associates' rights to use and disclose patient records.

28. Measurable solutions that have been taken, based on accepted standards, and are periodically monitored to demonstrate that an office is in compliance with HIPAA privacy rules are referred to as:
    a. reasonable safeguards.
    b. privacy safeguards.
    c. security safeguards.
    d. standards.

29. A person or organization that performs a function for a covered entity but is not employed by them is a/an:
    a. business associate.
    b. clearinghouse.
    c. provider.
    d. employee.

30. Health information that does not identify the patient is called:
    a. confidential communication.
    b. nonprivileged information.
    c. de-identified health information.
    d. protected health information.

Part III True/False

Write "T" or "F" in the blank to indicate whether you think the statement is true or false.

_______ 31. Individually identifiable health information (IIHI) is any part of a person's health data (e.g., demographic information, address, date of birth) obtained from the patient that is created or received by a covered entity.

_______ 32. HIPAA requirements protect disclosure of PHI outside of the organization but do not protect against internal use of health information.

_______ 33. Under HIPAA, patients may request confidential communications and may restrict certain disclosures of PHI.

_______ 34. It is not necessary to turn documents over or lock them in a secure drawer if you are only leaving your desk for a few moments.

_______ 35. Deleting files or formatting the hard drive is sufficient to keep electronic protected health information from being accessed.

_______ 36. Under HIPAA privacy regulations, patients do not have the right to access psychotherapy notes.

_______ 37. The HITECH Act requires that business associates comply with the HIPAA Security Rule in the same manner that a covered entity would.

_______ 38. Under HITECH, civil penalties for HIPAA violations are $100 for each violation with a maximum penalty of $25,000 for all violations of the same provision in a calendar year.

_______ 39. The Federal Register publishes regulations pertaining to health care regulations.

_______ 40. The penalty for violating HIPAA and HITECH can be $100 to $50,000 or more per violation.

ASSIGNMENT 2.2 CRITICAL THINKING: INCIDENTAL DISCLOSURE VERSUS HIPAA VIOLATION

Performance Objective

Task: Make a decision using your best judgment after reading each case study regarding whether it should be considered an incidental disclosure, a HIPAA violation, or neither.

Conditions: Use pen or pencil.

Standards: Time: _______________ minutes

Accuracy: _______________

(Note: The time element and accuracy criteria may be given by your instructor.)

Directions: Read through each case study. Use your best judgment and circle whether you think it is an incidental disclosure issue (ID), a HIPAA violation (V), or neither (N). Briefly explain the answer that you selected.

Scenarios

1. Dr. Practon's office sign-in sheets ask patients to fill in their names, appointment times, and physicians' names.

   ID V N

   Explain:

   ____

   ____

2. It is Monday morning and you are inundated with work that needs to be done. You receive a telephone call and give patient information without confirming who is on the line.

   ID V N

   Explain:

   ____

   ____

3. You send a fax, but accidentally you switch the last two digits of the fax number and the patient's billing information is received in the wrong location.

   ID V N

   Explain:

   ____

   ____

4. You are in a high-traffic area where patients might overhear PHI, and you are careful to keep your voice down.

   ID V N

   Explain:

   ____

   ____

5. It is 10:30 AM, and you go on a coffee break, leaving two patients' charts on the checkout counter.

   ID V N

   Explain:

   ____

   ____

6. In the reception room, a patient, Martha Havasi, overhears your telephone conversation, even though you spoke quietly and shut the glass window.

   ID V N

   Explain:

   ____

   ____

7. You telephone a patient, Alex Massey, to remind him of tomorrow's appointment and leave a voicemail message on his answering machine.

   ID V N

   Explain:

   ____

   ____

8. Three patients near the reception area of the office overhear you telling another staff member that Daisy Dotson is scheduled for a Pap smear tomorrow at 4:00 PM.

   ID V N

   Explain:

   ____

   ____

9. You telephone a patient, Janet Hudson. She is not home, so you leave a message on her answering machine that her breast cancer biopsy results came back negative.

   ID V N

   Explain:

   ____

   ____

10. You call out Fran O'Donnell's complete name in the waiting room where other patients are sitting.

    ID V N

    Explain:

    ____

    ____

11. You do not close the glass window to the reception room when talking on the telephone with your sister.

ID V N

Explain:

___

___

12. The office nurse tells a patient, Hugo Wells, his test results in front of his relatives in a treatment area.

ID V N

Explain:

___

___

13. You leave Katy Zontag's medical chart open at the receptionist's counter.

ID V N

Explain:

___

___

14. You telephone a patient, José Ramirez, and leave your name, the physician's name, and your telephone number on his answering machine.

ID V N

Explain:

___

___

15. A patient, Kim Lee, is in the examination room and overhears a conversation concerning blood test results of another patient in an adjoining room.

ID V N

Explain:

___

___

16. While waiting in the reception room, a patient, Xavier Gomez, overhears a receptionist talking with another patient on the telephone about a colonoscopy appointment.

ID V N

Explain:

___

___

17. Betty Burton, a patient who is being weighed on the office scale by the medical assistant, overhears a conversation between an insurance billing specialist and an insurance company representative in which the billing specialist is trying to obtain preauthorization for another patient's medical procedure.

ID V N

Explain:

___

___

18. In a restaurant, a waitress overhears an insurance biller talking to a friend and telling her about a famous actress who visited her physician's office yesterday.

ID V N

Explain:

___

___

___

___

ASSIGNMENT 2.3 VISIT WEBSITES

Performance Objective

Task: Access the Internet and visit several websites.

Conditions: Use a computer with printer and/or pen or pencil to make notes.

Standards: Time: _______________ minutes

Accuracy: _______________

(Note: The time element and accuracy criteria may be given by your instructor.)

Directions: Use a computer and use a browser to access the Internet. Go to some search engines to locate information.

1. Site-search information on patient confidentiality by visiting the website of the American Medical Association (www.ama-assn.org). At top of menu, click on Resources/Legal Issues and then click the link physician/hospital engagement issues. Site-search information on patient confidentiality in health care by visiting the Google search engine. Key in *patient confidentiality in health care*. Locate an article and print a hard copy to share and discuss with the class.

2. Site-search information of settled HIPAA investigations by visiting the website for the Department of Human Services/Office of Civil Rights (https://www.hhs.gov/hipaa/for-professionals/index.html). Print out a press release to share and discuss with the class.

3 Compliance, Fraud, and Abuse

Cheryl Fassett

KEY TERMS

Your instructor may wish to select some specific words pertinent to this chapter for a test. For definitions of the terms, further study, and/or reference, the words, phrases, and abbreviations may be found in the glossary at the end of the Textbook. *Key terms for this chapter follow.*

abuse
assumption coding
auditing
Civil False Claims Act
Civil Monetary Penalty
Clinical Laboratory Improvement Amendments
clustering
compliance
compliance plan
Comprehensive Error Rate Testing
corrective action plan
cost reports
Criminal False Claims Act
DRG creep
embezzlement
Emergency Medical Treatment and Labor Act
Federal Deposit Insurance Corporation
fraud
Fraud Enforcement and Recovery Act
Health Care Fraud Prevention and Enforcement Action Team
Health Care Fraud and Abuse Control
medical necessity
Medicare Administrative Contractor
Medicare Integrity Program
monitoring
Occupational Safety and Health Administration
Office of Inspector General
Operation Restore Trust
patient dumping
phantom bills
qui tam
Recovery Audit Contractor
Self-Disclosure Protocol
upcoding
Zone Program Integrity Contractor

KEY ABBREVIATIONS

See how many abbreviations and acronyms you can translate and then use this as a handy reference list. Definitions for the key abbreviations are located near the back of the Textbook *in the glossary.*

CERT ____________________

CLIA ____________________

CMP ____________________

CMS ____________________

DHHS ____________________

DOJ ____________________

EMTALA ____________________

FCA ____________________

FDIC ____________________

FERA ____________________

HCFAC ____________________

HEAT ____________________

MAC ____________________

MIP ____________________

OCR ____________________

OIG ____________________

ORT ____________________

OSHA ____________________

RAC ____________________

SDP ____________________

ZPIC ____________________

PERFORMANCE OBJECTIVES

The student will be able to:

- Define and spell the key terms and key abbreviations for this chapter, given the information from the *Textbook* glossary, within a reasonable time period and with enough accuracy to obtain a satisfactory evaluation.
- Answer the fill-in-the-blank, multiple choice, and true/false review questions after reading the chapter, with enough accuracy to obtain a satisfactory evaluation.
- Make decisions after reading scenarios regarding whether the situations are considered fraud, abuse, or neither, with sufficient information to obtain a satisfactory evaluation.
- Visit websites and site-search information via the Evolve website, with sufficient information to obtain a satisfactory evaluation.

STUDY OUTLINE

Compliance Defined
Fraud and Abuse Laws
- Defining Fraud and Abuse Roles, Responsibilities, and Key Terms
- Criminal False Claims Act (18 US Code §287)
- Civil False Claims Act (31 US Code §3729-3733)
- Qui Tam Provision
- Exclusion Statute (42 US Code §1320a-7)
- Stark Laws (42 US Code §1395nn)
- Anti-Kickback Statute (42 US Code §1320a-7b[b])
- Civil Monetary Penalties Law (41 US Code §1320a-7a)
- Safe Harbors
- Operation Restore Trust
- Additional Laws and Compliance
- Compliance Audits and Oversight
- Special Alerts, Bulletins, and Guidance Documents

Compliance Programs
- Increased Productivity and Decreased Penalties With Compliance Plan
- Seven Basic Components of a Compliance Plan
  - *Written Policies, Procedures, and Standards of Conduct*
  - *Compliance Program Oversight*
  - *Training and Education*
  - *Open Lines of Communication*
  - *Auditing, Monitoring, and Disclosure*
  - *Consistent Discipline*
  - *Corrective Actions*

OIG Compliance Program Guidelines
- Individual and Small Group Practices
- Third-Party Medical Billing Companies
- Hospitals

Compliance as a Career
What to Expect From Your Health Care Organization

ASSIGNMENT 3.1 REVIEW QUESTIONS

Part I Fill in the Blank

Review the objectives, key terms, and chapter information before completing the following review questions.

1. *Compliance* is the process of

____

____

2. What is the first step health insurance specialists should take toward achieving compliance so they do not violate laws, which may result in penalties or fines?

____

3. Indicate whether each of the following situations is one of fraud or abuse.

   a. Under the FCA, billing a claim for services not medically necessary ____________

   b. Changing a figure on an insurance claim form to get increased payment ____________

   c. Dismissing the copayment owed by a Medicare patient ____________

   d. Neglecting to refund an overpayment to the patient ____________

   e. Billing for a complex fracture when the patient suffered a simple break ____________

4. The OIG publication that lists guidelines for compliance programs is the

____

5. CLIA certifies ______________________________.

6. The law that prohibits self-referrals is the ______________________________.

7. The term for providing appropriate care for the diagnosis is ____________________.

8. Accepting a gift for referring a patient to a specific physical therapy group is a

____

9. According to the Affordable Care Act, the seven steps required for an effective compliance program are:

   1) ______________________________

   2) ______________________________

   3) ______________________________

   4) ______________________________

   5) ______________________________

   6) ______________________________

   7) ______________________________

10. The statute that requires the OIG to exclude individuals, providers, and health care organizations from participating in federal health care programs if they are found guilty of fraud or abuse is ______________________________.

Part II Multiple Choice

Choose the best answer.

11. One of the agencies charged with enforcing laws that regulate the health care industry is the:
    a. Drug Enforcement Agency (DEA).
    b. Office of Inspector General (OIG).
    c. National Committee on Vital and Health Statistics (NCVHS).
    d. Department of Internal Affairs (DIA).

12. Stealing money that has been entrusted in one's care is referred to as:
    a. fraud.
    b. abuse
    c. embezzlement.
    d. obstruction.

13. Under the Criminal False Claims Act, fines and imprisonment penalties for making a false claim in connection with payment for health care benefits can be imposed on:
    a. the physician who provided the services.
    b. the health care billing specialist who prepared the claim.
    c. the health care administrator who oversees the practice or organization.
    d. anyone who knowingly and willfully participated in the scheme.

14. The FCA provision that allows a private citizen to bring civil action for a violation on behalf of the federal government and share in any money recovered is referred to as:
    a. minimum necessary.
    b. qui tam.
    c. privileged information.
    d. exclusion statute.

15. The initiative that established hotlines for the public to report issues that might indicate fraud, abuse, or waste is:
    a. Operation Restore Trust (ORT).
    b. Civil Monetary Penalty (CMP).
    c. Health Care Fraud Prevention and Enforcement Action Team (HEAT).
    d. Recovery Audit Contractor (RAC).

16. Health care providers who determine that they have submitted false claims should resolve the issue by seeking the Department of Health and Human Services (HHS) and OIG guidance established in 2006 and referred to as:
    a. Operation Restore Trust.
    b. Stark I and II.
    c. Self-Disclosure Protocol.
    d. Safe Harbor.

17. The OIG recommends that health care staff should attend trainings in "general" compliance:
    a. as part of their initial orientation.
    b. at least annually.
    c. every 6 months.
    d. every 6 years.

18. When faced with the discovery of an offense or an error, health insurance specialists should immediately report concerns:
    a. using the established chain of command outlined in their compliance plan.
    b. to the OIG through their telephone hotline.
    c. to the OIG through their e-mail address directly to the HHS.
    d. directly to the HHS.

19. Compliance is the responsibility of:
    a. physicians.
    b. coders.
    c. everyone.
    d. the compliance officer.

20. The following are parts of a well-rounded compliance program except:
    a. policies and procedures.
    b. staff education.
    c. open lines of communication.
    d. practice management software.

21. The OIG has published compliance guidelines for all of the following except:
    a. hospitals.
    b. private physician groups.
    c. patients.
    d. billing companies.

22. The law that states that emergency rooms must evaluate and stabilize patients regardless of ability to pay is called:
    a. EMTALA.
    b. The Stark Law.
    c. Anti-Kickback Statute.
    d. False Claims Act.

23. Fraudulent claims may include:
    a. multiple modifiers.
    b. unbundled codes.
    c. more than one diagnosis code.
    d. place of service codes.

24. Penalties of noncompliance may include:
    a. jail time.
    b. monetary penalties.
    c. termination.
    d. all of the above.

25. The purpose of an RAC audit is to:
    a. recoup overpayments.
    b. determine if a provider is clinically sound.
    c. investigate discrimination.
    d. all of the above.

Part III True/False

Write "T" or "F" in the blank to indicate whether you think the statement is true or false.

_______ 26. Every compliance program should include a method for employees to report issues anonymously.

_______ 27. To submit an insurance claim for medical services that were not medically necessary is a violation of the FCA.

_______ 28. Organizations who hire or contract with individuals who have been convicted of a misdemeanor or criminal offense and are on the OIG's list of excluded individuals may be subject to civil monetary penalties.

_______ 29. In the federal health care program, accepting discounts, rebates, or other types of reductions in price is encouraged.

_______ 30. Recovery audit contractors are highly motivated to find claim errors, as they are paid a percentage of the money they recover.

_______ 31. If fraud and abuse are detected, Zone Program Integrity Contractors (ZPICs) report to the Department of Justice (DOJ) for further investigation.

_______ 32. In the event of an OIG audit, the presence of an OIG compliance program will prevent any penalties and fines from being imposed.

_______ 33. Disciplinary standards for situations involving misconduct may result in termination of employment.

_______ 34. Private medical groups are exempt from CMS fraud audits.

_______ 35. In a qui tam lawsuit, the whistleblower shares in penalty money.

_______ 36. Reporting multiple codes instead of one combination code is an example of up-coding.

_______ 37. A coding or billing specialist cannot be found guilty of fraud.

_______ 38. It is fraudulent to always adjust off deductibles and coinsurance.

_______ 39. If a health care organization receives an overpayment from a third-party payer, it is compliant to apply the amount to another patient's balance.

_______ 40. When a patient is transferred from one hospital to another, it is fraudulent for the first hospital to bill for a discharge.

ASSIGNMENT 3.2 CRITICAL THINKING: FRAUD VERSUS ABUSE

Performance Objective

Task: Make a decision after reading each case study regarding whether it is considered fraud, abuse, or neither.

Conditions: Use pen or pencil.

Standards: Time: ________________ minutes

Accuracy: ________________

(Note: The time element and accuracy criteria may be given by your instructor.)

Directions: Read through each scenario and circle whether it is a fraud (F) issue, practice of abuse (A), or neither (N). To distinguish the difference between fraud and abuse situations, remember that under the Medicare program, abuse relates to incidents or practices that are inconsistent with accepted sound business practices, whereas fraud is intentional deception that an individual knows, or should know, to be false, and the individual knows the deception could result in some unauthorized benefit to himself or herself or to some other person(s). Briefly explain the answer you selected.

Scenarios

1. Dr. Pedro Atrics has a friend whose child needs elective surgery. He agrees to perform the surgery and bill as an "insurance only" case.

   F A N

   Explain:

   ____

   ____

2. A patient, Carl Skinner, calls the office repeatedly about his prescriptions. When seen in the office the next time, Dr. Input bills a higher level of evaluation and management service to allow for the additional time.

   F A N

   Explain:

   ____

   ____

3. Dr. Skeleton sets a simple fracture and puts a cast on Mr. Davis. He bills for a complex fracture.

   F A N

   Explain:

   ____

   ____

4. A patient, Maria Gomez, asks a friendly staff member to change the dates on the insurance claim form. The medical assistant complies with the request.

   F A N

   Explain:

   ____

   ____

5. A patient, Roberto Loren, asks the physician to restate a diagnosis so the insurance company will pay because payment would be denied based on the present statement. The physician complies with the request.

F A N

Explain:

____

____

6. Dr. Rumsey sees a patient twice on the same day but bills as though the patient was seen on two different dates.

F A N

Explain:

____

____

7. A Medicare patient, Joan O'Connor, is seen by Dr. Practon, and the insurance claim shows a charge to the Medicare fiscal intermediary at a fee schedule rate higher than and different from that of non-Medicare patients.

F A N

Explain:

____

____

8. A patient, Hazel Plunkett, receives a service that is not medically necessary to the extent rendered, and an insurance claim is submitted.

F A N

Explain:

____

____

9. A patient, Sun Cho, paid for services that were subsequently declared not medically necessary, and Dr. Cardi failed to refund the payment to the patient.

F A N

Explain:

____

____

10. Dr. Ulibarri tells the insurance biller not to collect the deductible and copayments from Mrs. Gerry Coleman.

F A N

Explain:

____

____

ASSIGNMENT 3.3 VISIT WEBSITES

Performance Objective

Task: Access the Internet and visit several websites.

Conditions: Use a computer with printer and/or pen or pencil to make notes.

Standards: Time: ________________ minutes

Accuracy: ________________

(Note: The time element and accuracy criteria may be given by your instructor.)

Directions: Use a computer and use a browser to access the Internet. Go to some search engines to locate information.

1. Site-search for information on fraud and abuse by visiting one or more of the federal websites. See what you can discover and either print out or take notes and bring back information to share with the class for discussion.

2. Search the AAPC site (http://www.aapc.com) for their Code of Ethics. How will this support your health care organization's compliance goals?

4 Basics of Health Insurance

Cheryl Fassett

KEY TERMS

Your instructor may wish to select some words pertinent to this chapter for a test. For definitions of the terms, further study, and/or reference, the words, phrases, and abbreviations may be found in the glossary at the end of the Textbook. *Key terms for this chapter follow.*

accounts receivable management
assignment
cancelable
Civilian Health and Medical Program of the Department of Veterans Affairs
claim
coinsurance
competitive medical plan
conditionally renewable
Consumer Directed Health Plan
contract
coordination of benefits
copayment (copay)
daysheet
deductible
disability income insurance
emancipated minor
Exchanges
exclusions
exclusive provider organization
expressed contract
foundation for medical care
guaranteed renewable
guarantor
health maintenance organization
implied contract
Indemnity Health Insurance
independent or individual practice association
major medical
mandated benefits
Maternal and Child Health Program
Medicaid
medically necessary
Medicare
Medicare/Medicaid
noncancelable policy
nonparticipating health care organization or provider
optionally renewable
participating health care organization or provider
point-of-service plan
preauthorization
precertification
predetermination
preexisting conditions
preferred provider organization
premium
running balance
State Children's Health Insurance Program
State Disability Insurance
TRICARE
unemployment compensation disability
Veterans Health Administration (CHAMPVA)
Veterans Affairs outpatient clinic
workers' compensation insurance

KEY ABBREVIATIONS

See how many abbreviations and acronyms you can translate and then use this as a handy reference list. Definitions for the key abbreviations are located near the back of the Textbook *in the glossary.*

ACA ____________________

A/R ____________________

CDHP ____________________

CHAMPVA ____________________

CMP ____________________

COB ____________________

COBRA ____________________

DOS ____________________

EPO ____________________

FMC ____________________

FSA ____________________

HCERA ____________________

HDHP ____________________

HMO ____________________

HRA ____________________

HSA ____________________

IPA ____________________

MCHP ____________________

Medi-Medi ____________________

MSA ____________________

nonpar ____________________

NPP ____________________

par ____________________

PMS ____________________

POS plan ____________________

PPACA ____________________

PPO ____________________

ROA ____________________

SCHIP ____________________

SDHP ____________________

SDI ____________________

SHOP ____________________

SOF ____________________

UCD ____________________

VA ____________________

WC ____________________

PERFORMANCE OBJECTIVES

The student will be able to:

- Define and spell the key terms and key abbreviations for this chapter, given the information from the *Textbook* glossary, within a reasonable time period and with enough accuracy to obtain a satisfactory evaluation.
- Answer the fill in the blank, multiple choice, and true/false review questions after reading the chapter, with enough accuracy to obtain a satisfactory evaluation.
- Arrange 18 administrative processing steps of an insurance claim in proper sequence, given data from the textbook, within a reasonable time period and with enough accuracy to obtain a satisfactory evaluation.
- Use critical thinking to explain some of the differences in insurance key terms, given data from the textbook, within a reasonable time period and with enough accuracy to obtain a satisfactory evaluation.
- Prepare a financial accounting record, given data from the textbook, within a reasonable time period and with enough accuracy to obtain a satisfactory evaluation.
- Abstract data from some insurance identification cards, given data from the textbook, within a reasonable time period and with enough accuracy to obtain a satisfactory evaluation.

STUDY OUTLINE

History of Health Insurance in the United States
Health Care Reform
- Individual Mandate
- Health Benefit Exchanges

Legal Principles of Insurance
- Insurance Contracts

Health Care Organization–Patient Contracts and Financial Obligation
- Implied or Expressed Contracts

The Insurance Policy
- Policy Application
- Policy Renewal Provisions
- Policy Terms
- Coordination of Benefits
- Case Management Requirements

Choice of Health Insurance
Conversion Privilege
Types of Health Insurance Coverage
- Examples of Insurance Billing Exception

Handling and Processing Insurance Claims
Life Cycle of an Insurance Claim
Keeping Up to Date

ASSIGNMENT 4.1 REVIEW QUESTIONS

Part I Fill in the Blank

Review the objectives, key terms, glossary definitions to key terms, chapter information, and figures before completing the following review questions.

1. A/an ______________ is a legally enforceable agreement or contract.

2. An individual promising to pay for medical services rendered is known as a/an ______________________________.

3. List five health insurance policy renewal provisions.

   a. ______________________________

   b. ______________________________

   c. ______________________________

   d. ______________________________

   e. ______________________________

4. Insurance reimbursement or payment is also called ______________________.

5. Name two examples of services that are typically excluded in general health insurance policies.

   a. ______________________________

   b. ______________________________

6. Under PPACA, health plans must allow employees to keep their children on their plans until the children are ______________ years old.

7. The act of determining whether treatment is covered under an individual's health insurance policy is called ______________________________.

8. The procedure to obtain permission for a procedure before it is done, to determine whether the insurance program agrees it is medically necessary, is termed ______________________________.

9. Determining the maximum dollar amount the insurance company will pay for a procedure before it is done is known as ______________________.

10. Name two ways an individual may obtain health insurance.

    a. ______________________________

    b. ______________________________

11. List four methods a health care organization may use to submit insurance claims to insurance companies.

   a. ______________________________

   b. ______________________________

   c. ______________________________

   d. ______________________________

12. A document signed by the insured directing the insurance company to pay benefits directly to the health care organization is known as a/an ____________________.

13. A patient service slip personalized to the health care organization and used as a communications/billing tool during routing of the patient, can also be referred to as the following terms.

   a. ______________________________

   b. ______________________________

   c. ______________________________

   d. ______________________________

   e. ______________________________

   f. ______________________________

14. For electronic access to computer data, computerized signatures may consist of the following verification or access methods:

   a. ______________________________

   b. ______________________________

   c. ______________________________

   d. ______________________________

   e. ______________________________

   f. ______________________________

   g. ______________________________

15. A method of making an automatic deposit of funds from the payer into the provider's bank account and used in place of a mailed paper check is referred to as

   ______________________________.

Part II Mix and Match

16. Match the following insurance terms in the right column with their descriptions, and fill in the blank with the appropriate letter.

_______ An insurance company considering benefits payable by another carrier in determining its own liability

_______ Transfer of one's right to collect an amount payable under an insurance contract

_______ Time that must elapse before benefits for sickness or accident become payable

_______ Acts for insurance company or insured in settlement of claims

_______ Periodic payment to keep insurance policy in force

_______ Amount insured person must pay before policy will pay

_______ Time period in which a claim must be filed

_______ Certain illnesses or injuries listed in a policy that the insurance company will not cover

_______ Insurance company that carries the insurance

_______ One who belongs to an insurance plan

a. Adjuster
b. Assignment
c. Carrier
d. Coordination of benefits (COB)
e. Deductible
f. Exclusions
g. Premium
h. Subscriber
i. Time limit
j. Waiting period

Part III Multiple Choice

Choose the best answer.

17. When a patient goes to a health care organization seeking medical services, the health care organization accepts the patient and agrees to render treatment, and both parties agree. This contract is known as a/an:
    a. expressed contract.
    b. agreed contract.
    c. implied contract.
    d. written contract.

18. The process of checking and confirming that a patient is covered under an insurance plan is known as:
    a. precertification.
    b. eligibility verification.
    c. COB.
    d. predetermination.

19. A provision that allows the policyholder the right to refuse to renew the insurance policy on a premium due date is called:
    a. conditionally renewable.
    b. guaranteed renewable.
    c. optionally renewable.
    d. noncancelable.

20. A provision in a health insurance policy in which two insurance carriers work together for payment so that there is no duplication of benefits paid between the primary insurance carrier and the secondary insurance carrier is called:
    a. copayment.
    b. coinsurance.
    c. COB.
    d. cost-share rider.

21. A type of tax-free savings account that allows individuals and their employers to set aside money to pay for health care expenses is known as:
    a. a health savings account.
    b. a medical savings account.
    c. a flexible spending account.
    d. all of the above.

22. Time limits for filing insurance claims to a commercial carrier may have a range of:
    a. 10 days from the date medical service is received to 1 year.
    b. 30 days from the date of service to 1½ years.
    c. 60 days from the date of service.
    d. no time limit.

Part IV True/False

Write "T" or "F" in the blank to indicate whether you think the statement is true or false.

_______ 23. If a health care organization belongs to a preferred provider organization (PPO) and does not follow his or her contract with the PPO, the patient is liable for the bill.

_______ 24. The birthday rule is a change in the order of determination of COB regarding primary and secondary insurance carriers for dependent children.

_______ 25. The Consolidated Omnibus Budget Reconciliation Act of 1985 (COBRA) mandates that when an employee is laid off from a company, the group health insurance coverage must continue at group rates for up to 18 months.

_______ 26. A group policy usually provides better benefits; however, the premiums are generally higher than an individual contract would be.

_______ 27. A signature stamp is acceptable by all insurances as proof of the provider's signature on a CMS-1500 claim form.

ASSIGNMENT 4.2 CRITICAL THINKING: ADMINISTRATIVE SEQUENCE OF PROCESSING AN INSURANCE CLAIM

Performance Objective

Task: Number from 1 to 18 the proper sequence of processing an insurance claim.

Conditions: Use given data and pen or pencil.

Standards: Time: _______________ minutes

Accuracy: _______________

(Note: The time element and accuracy criteria may be given by your instructor.)

Directions: Arrange the listed steps 1 through 18 in proper sequence by placing the correct number to the left of the statement. (Note: Each medical practice has its own order of the way office procedures are carried out; thus, these steps may vary slightly from practice to practice.)

_______ Bank deposit made and unpaid claims followed up

_______ Patient's financial account is pulled

_______ Insurance information (obtained and verified)

_______ Payer processing/payment received with explanation of benefits (EOB) document

_______ Patient's financial data posted and patient checkout

_______ Patient appointment and preregistration

_______ CMS-1500 paper claim forms submitted

_______ Provider's signature is obtained

_______ Electronic (Health Insurance Portability and Accountability Act [HIPAA] X12 837) claims transmitted

_______ Insurance claims preparation

_______ HIPAA Notice of Privacy is reviewed and signed

_______ Balance due statement mailed to patient

_______ Track pending insurance claims

_______ All required patient's signatures are obtained

_______ Assignment of benefits

_______ Medical services performed and encounter form completed

_______ Insurance identification card photocopied

_______ Full payment received and financial records retained

ASSIGNMENT 4.3 CRITICAL THINKING: DIFFERENCES IN INSURANCE KEY TERMS

Performance Objective

Task: Describe and/or explain your response to five questions.

Conditions: Use one or two sheets of white paper and pen or pencil.

Standards: Time: ________________ minutes

Accuracy: ________________

(Note: The time element and accuracy criteria may be given by your instructor.)

Directions: Respond verbally or in writing to these questions or statements.

1. Explain the difference between the following:

Blanket contract ____

Individual contract ____

2. Explain the difference between a participating health care organization and a nonparticipating health care organization for the following:

Commercial insurance company or managed care plan participating health care organization:

____

Commercial insurance company or managed care plan nonparticipating health care organization:

____

Medicare participating health care organization:

____

Medicare nonparticipating health care organization:

____

3. State the difference between the following:

Implied contract: ____

Expressed contract: ____

4. Explain the birthday law (rule) and when it is used.

____

ASSIGNMENT 4.4 ABSTRACT DATA FROM AN INSURANCE IDENTIFICATION CARD

Performance Objective

Task: Answer questions in reference to an insurance identification card for Case A.

Conditions: Use an insurance identification card (Fig. 4.1), the questions presented, and pen or pencil.

Standards: Time: ________________ minutes

Accuracy: ________________

(Note: The time element and accuracy criteria may be given by your instructor.)

Directions: An identification card provides much of the information needed to establish a patient's insurance coverage. You have photocopied the front and back sides of three patients' cards and placed copies in their patient records, returning the originals to the patients. Answer the questions by abstracting or obtaining the data from the cards.

CASE A

1. Name of patient covered by the policy. ________________________________
2. Provide the insurance policy's effective date. ________________________________
3. List the telephone number for preauthorization. ________________________________
4. State name and address of insurance company. ________________________________
5. List the telephone number to call for provider access. ________________________________
6. Name the type of insurance plan. ________________________________
7. List the insurance identification number (e.g., subscriber, certificate, or member numbers) ________________ ________________________________.
8. Furnish the group number. ________________ Plan or coverage code. ______________
9. State the copay requirements. ________________________________
10. Does the card indicate the patient has hospital coverage? ________________________________

Blue Cross of California*

CALIFORNIA CARE HEALTH PLANS

Type of Insurance: **PRUDENT BUYER PLAN** ®'

GROUP: C54G28

PPO ®

XDS - 564 - 00 - 9044

EFFECTIVE DATE: 05-01-95

PLAN CODE: 5031B

LINDA L FIELD

PLAN 040: MEDICAL - WELLPOINT PHARMACY

CLAIMS & INQUIRIES: P.O. BOX 9072 OXNARD CA 93031-9072

CUSTOMER SERVICE: 1-800-627-8797

COPAY $20 OFFICE

This is your employer health plan Identification Card. Present it to the provider of health care when you or your eligible dependents receive services. See your certificate(s) or booklet(s) for a description of your benefits, terms, conditions, limitations, and exclusions of coverage. When submitting inquiries always include your member number from the face of this card. Possession or use of this card does not guarantee payment.

Wellpoint Pharmacy	(800) 700-2541
BlueCard Provider Access	(800) 810-BLUE

FOR BLUE CROSS AND BLUE SHIELD PROVIDERS NATIONWIDE:
Please submit claims to your local Blue Cross and/or Blue Shield plan. To ensure prompt claims processing, please include the three-digit alpha prefix that precedes the patient's identification number listed on the front of this card.

TO THE PROVIDER:
For pre-authorization or Pre-Service Review call: (800) 274-7767

* An Independent License of the Blue Cross Association.

® Registered Mark of the Blue Cross Association.

®' Registered Mark of WellPoint Health Networks Inc.

Hospital coverage: Yes

Fig. 4.1

ASSIGNMENT 4.5 ABSTRACT DATA FROM AN INSURANCE IDENTIFICATION CARD

Performance Objective

Task: Answer questions in reference to the insurance identification card for Case B.

Conditions: Use an insurance identification card (Fig. 4.2), the questions presented, and pen or pencil.

Standards: Time: ___________ minutes

Accuracy: ___________

(Note: The time element and accuracy criteria may be given by your instructor.)

CASE B

1. Name of patient covered by the policy. ___________
2. Provide the insurance policy's effective date. ___________
3. List the telephone number for preauthorization. ___________
4. State name of insurance company. ___________
5. List the telephone number to call for patient benefits and eligibility. ___________
6. Name the type of insurance plan. ___________
7. List the insurance identification number (e.g., subscriber, certificate, or member numbers). ___________

   ____
8. Furnish the group number. ___________ Plan or coverage code. ___________
9. State the copay requirements, if any. ___________
10. List the Blue Shield website. ___________

Blue Shield of California
An Independent Member of the Blue Shield Association

Preferred Plan

PPO

SUBSCRIBER NAME:

M T FORDHAM

EFFECTIVE DATE:

010120XX

SUBSCRIBER ID NUMBER

AJC557469969

GROUP NUMBER

00P1901

PLAN CODE

542

CUSTOMER SERVICE

(800) 331-2001

07/16/20XX

Use Blue Shield of California Preferred Physicians and Hospitals to receive maximum benefits.

Carry the Blue Shield Identification Card with you at all times and present it whenever you or one of your covered dependents receives medical services. Read your employee booklet/Health Services Agreement which summarizes the benefits, provisions, limitations and exclusions of your plan. Your health plan may require prior notification of any hospitalization and notification, within one business day, of an emergency admission. Review of selected procedures may be required before some services are performed. To receive hospital pre-admission and pre-service reviews, call 1-800-343-1691. Your failure to call may result in a reduction of benefits.

For questions, including those related to benefits, and eligibility, call the customer service number listed on the front of this card.

The PPO logo on the front of this ID Card identifies you to preferred providers outside the state of California as a member of the Blue Card PPO Program.

When you are outside of California call 1-800-810-2583 to locate the nearest PPO Provider. Remember, any services you receive are subject to the policies and provisions of your group plan.

ID-23200-PPO REVERSE

www.blueshieldca.com

Fig. 4.2

ASSIGNMENT 4.6 ABSTRACT DATA FROM AN INSURANCE IDENTIFICATION CARD

Performance Objective

Task: Answer questions in reference to the insurance identification card for Case C.

Conditions: Use an insurance identification card (Fig. 4.3), the questions presented, and pen or pencil.

Standards: Time: ___________ minutes

Accuracy: ___________

(Note: The time element and accuracy criteria may be given by your instructor.)

CASE C

1. Name of patient covered by the policy. ___________
2. Provide the insurance policy's effective date, if there is one. ___________
3. List the number to call for out-of-network preauthorization. ___________
4. State name and address of insurance company. ___________
5. List the telephone number to call for member inquiries. ___________
6. Name the type of insurance plan. ___________
7. List the insurance identification number (e.g., subscriber, certificate, or member numbers). ___________
8. Furnish the group number. ___________
9. State the copay requirements, if any. ___________
10. Who is the patient's primary care physician? ___________

UNITEDhealthcare

LINDA L. FLORES
Member # 52170-5172

CALMAT

Group # 176422
COPAY: Office Visit $10 ER $50
Urgent $35

Electronic Claims Payor ID 87726

Call 800-842-5751 for Member Inquiries

POS PCP Plan
WITH RX D - UHC
and MH/CD
PCP: G. LOMAN
805-643-9973

MTH

This identification card is not proof of membership nor does it guarantee coverage. Persons with coverage that remains in force are entitled to benefits under the terms and conditions of this group health benefit plan as detailed in your benefit description.

IMPORTANT MEMBER INFORMATION
In non-emergencies, call your Primary Care Physician to receive the highest level of benefits. If you have an emergency and are admitted to a hospital, you are required to call your Primary Care Physician within two working days.
For out of network services that require authorization, call the Member Inquiries 800 number on the front of this card.

Claim Address: P.O. Box 30990, Salt Lake City, UT 84130-0990

Fig. 4.3

5 The Blue Plans, Private Insurance, and Managed Care Plans

Linda M. Smith

KEY TERMS

Your instructor may wish to select some words pertinent to this chapter for a test. For definitions of the terms, further study, and/or reference, the words, phrases, and abbreviations may be found in the glossary at the end of the Textbook. *Key terms for this chapter follow.*

ancillary services
Blue Cross/Blue Shield Association
buffing
capitation
churning
coinsurance
copayment
deductible
direct referral
disenrollment
exclusive provider organization
fee-for-service
formal referral
gatekeeper
group practice model
health maintenance organization
indemnity insurance plan
independent (or individual) practice association
managed care
participating physician
per capita
physician provider group
point-of-service plan
preferred provider organization
prepaid group practice model
primary care physician
private health insurance
self-referral
staff model
stop-loss
tertiary care
traditional insurance plan
turfing
utilization review
verbal referral
withhold

KEY ABBREVIATIONS

See how many abbreviations and acronyms you can translate and then use this as a handy reference list. Definitions for the key abbreviations are located near the back of the Textbook *in the glossary.*

BCBSA ____________________

copay ____________________

____

EPO ____________________

____

____

____

HMO ____________________

IPA ____________________

MCO ____________________

NCQA ____________________

PCP ____________________

POS ____________________

PPG ____________________

PPO ____________________

____

QISMC ____________________

UR ____________________

PERFORMANCE OBJECTIVES

The student will be able to:

- Define and spell the key terms and key abbreviations for this chapter, given the information from the *Textbook* glossary, within a reasonable time period and with enough accuracy to obtain a satisfactory evaluation.
- After reading the chapter, answer the fill in the blank, multiple choice, and true/false review questions with enough accuracy to obtain a satisfactory evaluation.
- Complete treatment authorization forms of managed care plans, given completed new patient information forms, within a reasonable time period and with enough accuracy to obtain a satisfactory evaluation.

STUDY OUTLINE

Private Health Insurance
- Blue Cross and Blue Shield Plans
- Fee-for-Service Plans

Managed Care

Managed Care Systems
- Health Maintenance Organizations
- Preferred Provider Organizations
- Exclusive Provider Organizations
- Point-of-Service Plans
- Physician Provider Groups
- Triple-Option Health Plans
- Provider-Sponsored Organization
- Consumer Directed Health Plans

Medical Review
- Quality Improvement System for Managed Care
- Utilization Review of Management

Management of Plans
- Contracts

Plan Administration
- Patient Information Letter
- Preauthorization or Prior Approval
- Diagnostic Tests
- Managed Care Guide

Financial Management
- Payment
- Statement of Remittance
- Accounting
- Fee-for-Service
- Year-End Evaluation
- Bankruptcy

ASSIGNMENT 5.1 REVIEW QUESTIONS

Part I Fill in the Blank

Review the objectives, key terms, glossary definitions of key terms, figures, and chapter information before completing the following review questions.

1. An insurance plan requires the insured to pay a fixed monthly premium. The insurance that will pay the health care organization for services each time the service is rendered is referred to as

   ____.

2. A group of techniques used by insurance companies to reduce the cost of providing health care while improving access to care and the quality of care is referred to as

   ____.

3. What type of medical insurance provides coverage of health services for a prepaid fixed annual fee and requires enrollees to seek services through a panel of providers contracted with the insurance company? ______________________.

4. A not-for-profit organization that has built a set of standards to which health plans attest that they have met key elements required by state and federal laws allowing them to participate in managed care programs is called ______________________.

5. In a managed care setting, a primary care physician who controls patient access to specialists and diagnostic testing services is known as a/an ______________________.

6. Name four types of health maintenance organization (HMO) models.

   a. ____

   b. ____

   c. ____

   d. ____

7. If a physician or hospital in a managed care plan is paid a fixed, per capita amount for each patient enrolled, regardless of the type and number of services rendered, this is a payment system known as

   ____.

8. A health benefit program in which enrollees may choose any physician or hospital for services but obtain a higher level of benefits if preferred providers are used is known as a/an ______________________.

9. HMOs and preferred provider organizations (PPOs) consisting of a network of physicians and hospitals that provide an insurance company or employer with discounts on their services are referred to collectively as a/an ______________________.

10. To control health care costs, the process of reviewing and establishing medical necessity for services and providers' use of medical care resources is termed ______________________

    ____.

11. Explain the meaning of a "stop-loss" provision that might appear in a managed care contract.

____

____

12. When a certain percentage of the monthly capitation payment or a percentage of the allowable charges to physicians is set aside to operate a managed care plan, it is known as a/an

____.

Part II Multiple Choice

Choose the best answer.

13. A specified dollar amount that the patient must pay annually before an insurance plan begins covering health care costs is called:
a. coinsurance.
b. copayment.
c. deductible.
d. withhold.

14. A type of managed care plan regulated under insurance statutes that combines features of HMOs and PPOs and requires that employers agree not to contract with any other plan is known as a/an:
a. independent practice association (IPA).
b. exclusive provider organization (EPO).
c. physician provider group (PPG).
d. point-of-service (POS) plan.

15. Which of the following is a term used in utilization review when the sickest high-cost patients are transferred to other physicians?
a. Churning
b. Turfing
c. Buffing
d. Carving

16. Medical services that are not included in a managed care contract's capitation rate but that may be contracted for separately are referred to as:
a. carve outs.
b. stop-loss limits.
c. payment mechanisms.
d. copayments.

17. When the primary care physician informs the patient and telephones the referring physician that the patient is being referred for an appointment, it is called a:
a. direct referral.
b. formal referral.
c. self-referral.
d. verbal referral.

18. Plan-specified facilities listed in managed care plan contracts where patients are required to have laboratory and radiology tests performed are called:
a. hospital facilities.
b. medical facilities.
c. network facilities.
d. outside facilities.

19. A type of payment model in which the patient pays a monthly or annual fee to the physician is known as:
a. capitation.
b. cash only practice.
c. concierge medicine.
d. copayment.

20. A value-based reimbursement model in which providers receive performance-based incentives to share cost savings combined with disincentives to share the excess costs of health care delivery is called:
a. shared risk.
b. shared savings.
c. one-sided risk.
d. full risk.

Part III True/False

Write "T" or "F" in the blank to indicate whether you think the statement is true or false.

_________ 21. Private health insurances are government-sponsored programs.

_________ 22. Blue Cross plans provide health care coverage for hospital expenses.

_________ 23. All managed care plans are alike.

_________ 24. A provider-sponsored organization is a managed care plan that can be owned and operated by a hospital rather than an insurance company.

_________ 25. Consumer-driven health plans (CDHP) are referred to as low deductible plans.

_________ 26. The Quality Improvement System for Managed Care (QISMC) provides oversight and ensures accountability of managed care programs.

_________ 27. Obtaining preapproval for services always ensures payment of a claim by the insurance company.

_________ 28. Value-based reimbursement programs reward health care providers with incentive payments for the quality of care they provide.

_________ 29. When a health care organization agrees to accept a single negotiated fee to deliver all medical services related a patient's hip replacement surgery, it is referred to as *pay for performance.*

ASSIGNMENT 5.2 OBTAIN AUTHORIZATION FOR A CONSULTATION FROM A MANAGED CARE PLAN

Performance Objective

Task: Complete a treatment authorization form to obtain permission for an office consultation for a patient covered by a managed care plan.

Conditions: Use a treatment authorization form (Fig. 5.1), a new patient information form (Fig. 5.2), a computer, and a printer.

Standards: Time: ________________ minutes

Accuracy: ________________

(Note: The time element and accuracy criteria may be given by your instructor.)

Directions: Complete a treatment authorization form (see Fig. 5.1) for Mrs. Cohn's managed care plan to obtain permission for the office consultation and date it August 2 of the current year. To obtain information, refer to the New Patient Information form completed by Mrs. Cohn when she came into the office for her visit with Dr. Practon (see Fig. 5.2). Dr. Practon's Family Health Plan provider number is FHP C01402X.

Scenario: Meriweather B. Cohn's primary care physician, Dr. Gerald Practon, took her clinical history. Physical examination revealed a normal blood pressure (120/80); however, abnormal heart sounds were heard, and a diagnosis of a heart murmur was made. Dr. Practon decided to make a semiurgent request to refer Mrs. Cohn for a cardiac consultation (other service) to Dr. Victor M. Salazar, whose office is located at 20 Excalibur Street, Woodland Hills, XY 12345, and whose office telephone number is 555-625-7344. Dr. Salazar will take a detailed history, perform a detailed examination, and make low-complexity medical decisions to evaluate Mrs. Cohn's heart murmur.

After the instructor has returned your work to you, either make the necessary corrections and place your work in a three-ring notebook for future reference or, if you receive a high score, place it in your portfolio for reference when applying for a job.

FHP® HEALTH CARE

IPA TREATMENT AUTHORIZATION FORM

____ Referral
____ Participating
____ Nonparticipating
____ Commercial
____ Senior

For Billing Instructions, Patient and Nonaffiliated Providers, and Consultants please see reverse side for instructions

THIS PORTION COMPLETED BY PHYSICIAN

Patient Name ______________________ Date ____/____/____

M ____ F ____ Age ____ FHP # ______________ Home Phone ______________

Address ______________________

Primary Care MD______________ Primary Care MD's FHP # ______________

Referring MD ______________ Referring MD's FHP # ______________

Referred To ______________ Address ______________

______________ Office Phone ______________

Type of Service: ☐ In-Patient ☐ Out-Patient Services ☐ Initial Visit ☐ Return Visit ☐ Other

Clinical History and Findings ______________________

Diagnosis ______________________

ICD-10-CM CODE

Evaluation and Treatment to Date ______________________

Procedure ______________________

RVS CPT-4 CODE

Reason for Referral/Consultation/Procedure ______________________

Accident: ☐ Yes ☐ No Where Occurred: ☐ Home ☐ Work ☐ Auto ☐ Other

☐ Urgent ☐ Semi-Urgent ☐ Elective

Facility to be Used: ______________ Estimated Length of Stay ______________

☐ Office ☐ Out-Patient ☐ In-Patient

THIS PORTION COMPLETED BY FHP UR

THIS AUTHORIZATION GOOD FOR 60 DAYS ONLY

Type of Contract: ☐ Capitation ☐ Fee For Service ☐ Per Diem

Projected Cost of Procedure ______________ Projected Cost of Facility ______________

HMO Verification: Effective ______________ Group # ______________

Benefits: Co-Pay Per Visit ______________ Hospital ______________

Limitations: ______________________

____ Authorized	Date ____	Initials ____	Reason ____	Authorization #____
____ Deferred	Date ____	Initials ____	Reason ____	
____ Denied	Date ____	Initials ____	Reason ____	
____ Modified	Date ____	Initials ____	Reason ____	

WHITE – UR Copy CANARY – Hospital Copy PINK – Physician Copy GOLDENROD – Claims Copy

Fig. 5.1

Welcome To Our Office

NEW PATIENT INFORMATION

DATE 8-2-20xx

PATIENT'S NAME (PLEASE PRINT)	S.S. #	MARITAL STATUS	SEX	BIRTH DATE	AGE	RELIGION (optional)
Meriweather B. Cohn	430-XX-0261	S [X]M W D SEP	M [X]F	11-14-65		

STREET ADDRESS PERMANENT TEMPORARY	CITY AND STATE	ZIP CODE	HOME PHONE #
267 Blake Street	Woodland Hills XY	12345	555-263-0911

PATIENT'S OR PARENT'S EMPLOYER	OCCUPATION (INDICATE IF STUDENT)	HOW LONG EMPLOYED	BUS. PHONE # EXT #
Sun Corporation	sales representative	5 yrs	555-263-0099

EMPLOYER'S STREET ADDRESS	CITY AND STATE	ZIP CODE
74 Rain Street	Woodland Hills XY	12345

DRUG ALLERGIES, IF ANY	
Penicillin	

SPOUSE OR PARENT'S NAME	S.S. #	BIRTH DATE
Starkweather L. Cohn	273-XX-9961	7-9-63

SPOUSE OR PARENT'S EMPLOYER	OCCUPATION (INDICATE IF STUDENT)	HOW LONG EMPLOYED	BUS. PHONE #
B & L Stormdrain Co.	accountant	10 yrs	555-421-0091

EMPLOYER'S STREET ADDRESS	CITY AND STATE	ZIP CODE
20 South Wind Road	Woodland Hills XY	12345

*SPOUSE'S STREET ADDRESS, IF DIVORCED OR SEPARATED	CITY AND STATE	ZIP CODE	HOME PHONE #

PLEASE READ: ALL CHARGES ARE DUE AT THE TIME OF SERVICES. IF HOSPITALIZATION IS INDICATED, THE PATIENT IS RESPONSIBLE FOR FURNISHING INSURANCE CLAIM FORMS TO THE OFFICE PRIOR TO HOSPITALIZATION.

PERSON RESPONSIBLE FOR PAYMENT, IF NOT ABOVE	STREET ADDRESS, CITY, STATE	ZIP CODE	HOME PHONE #

BLUE SHIELD (GIVE NAME OF POLICYHOLDER)	EFFECTIVE DATE	CERTIFICATE #	GROUP #	COVERAGE CODE
☐				

OTHER (WRITE IN NAME OF INSURANCE COMPANY)	EFFECTIVE DATE	POLICY #
☐ FHP Healthcare	1-1-8X	FHP # A4932
OTHER (WRITE IN NAME OF INSURANCE COMPANY)	EFFECTIVE DATE	POLICY #
☐		

MEDICARE (PLEASE GIVE NUMBER)	RAILROAD RETIREMENT (PLEASE GIVE NUMBER)
☐	☐

MEDICAID	EFFECTIVE DATE	PROGRAM #	COUNTY #	CASE #	ACCOUNT #
☐					

INDUSTRIAL	WERE YOU INJURED ON THE JOB?	DATE OF INJURY	INDUSTRIAL CLAIM #
☐	☐ YES [X] NO		

ACCIDENT	WAS AN AUTOMOBILE INVOLVED?	DATE OF ACCIDENT	NAME OF ATTORNEY
☐	☐ YES [X] NO		

WERE X-RAYS TAKEN OF THIS INJURY OR PROBLEM?	IF YES, WHERE WERE X-RAYS TAKEN? (HOSPITAL, ETC)	DATE X-RAYS TAKEN
☐ YES [X] NO		

HAS ANY MEMBER OF YOUR IMMEDIATE FAMILY BEEN TREATED BY OUR PHYSICIAN(S) BEFORE? INCLUDE NAME OF PHYSICIAN AND FAMILY MEMBER

No

REFERRED BY	STREET ADDRESS, CITY, STATE	ZIP CODE	PHONE #
BREEZIE N. CLOUD	521 N. Wind Rd, Woodland Hills XY	12345	555-721-9641

ALL PROFESSIONAL SERVICES RENDERED ARE CHARGED TO THE PATIENT. NECESSARY FORMS WILL BE COMPLETED TO HELP EXPEDITE INSURANCE CARRIER PAYMENTS. HOWEVER, THE PATIENT IS RESPONSIBLE FOR ALL FEES, REGARDLESS OF INSURANCE COVERAGE. IT IS ALSO CUSTOMARY TO PAY FOR SERVICES WHEN RENDERED UNLESS OTHER ARRANGEMENTS HAVE BEEN MADE IN ADVANCE WITH OUR OFFICE BOOKKEEPER.

INSURANCE AUTHORIZATION AND ASSIGNMENT

Name of Policy Holder Meriweather B. Cohn HC Number ______

I request that payment of authorized Medicare/Other Insurance company benefits be made either to me or on my behalf to College Clinic for any services furnished me by that party who accepts assignment/physician. Regulations pertaining to Medicare assignment of benefits apply.

I authorize any holder of medical or other information about me to release to the Social Security Administration and Health Care Financing Administration or its intermediaries or carrier or any other insurance company any information needed for this or a related Medicare/Other Insurance company claim.

I understand my signature requests that payment be made and authorizes release of medical information necessary to pay the claim. If item 9 of the HCFA-1500 claim form is completed, my signature authorizes releasing of the information to the insurer or agency shown. In Medicare/Other Insurance company assigned cases, the physician or supplier agrees to accept the charge determination of the Medicare/Other Insurance company as the full charge, and the patient is responsible only for the deductible, coinsurance, and noncovered services. Coinsurance and the deductible are based upon the charge determination of the Medicare/Other Insurance company.

Signature Meriweather B. Cohn Date 8-2-20XX

NEW PATIENT INFORMATION

Fig. 5.2

ASSIGNMENT 5.3 OBTAIN AUTHORIZATION FOR PHYSICAL THERAPY FROM A MANAGED CARE PLAN

Performance Objective

Task:	Complete a treatment authorization form to obtain permission for physical therapy for a patient covered by a managed care plan.
Conditions:	Use a treatment authorization form (Fig. 5.3), computer, and printer.
Standards:	Time: _________________ minutes
	Accuracy: _________________
	(Note: The time element and accuracy criteria may be given by your instructor.)

Directions: Complete the treatment authorization form for this patient (see Fig. 5.3), date it July 7 of the current year, and submit it to the managed care plan. Refer to Fig. 5.2 in the *Textbook* for visual guidance.

Scenario: Mrs. Rosario Jimenez comes into Dr. Gerald Practon's office complaining of neck pain. Mrs. Jimenez is a member of the managed care program HealthNet, and Dr. Practon is her primary care physician. Mrs. Jimenez lives at 350 South Carib Street, Woodland Hills, XY 12345-0003. Her telephone number is 555-450-9987, and she was born April 6, 1960. Her plan identification number is JIM40896, and the effective date is January 1, 20xx. After taking a history, completing a physical examination, and taking and reviewing radiographs, Dr. Practon makes a diagnosis of cervical radiculitis. He gives Mrs. Jimenez a prescription for some medication and says it is necessary to order outpatient physical therapy (one area, for 15 minutes; therapeutic exercises to develop strength, motion, and flexibility) twice a week for 6 weeks at College Hospital. Authorization must be obtained for this treatment. Dr. Practon's HealthNet provider number is HN C01402X.

After the instructor has returned your work to you, either make the necessary corrections and place your work in a three-ring notebook for future reference or, if you receive a high score, place it in your portfolio for reference when applying for a job.

College Clinic
4567 Broad Avenue
Woodland Hills, XY 12345-0001
Telephone No. (555) 487-8976
Fax No. (555) 487-8976

MANAGED CARE PLAN AUTHORIZATION REQUEST

❑ Health Net ❑ Met Life
❑ Pacificare ❑ Travelers
❑ Secure Horizons ❑ Pru Care
❑ Other

Member/Group No.

TO BE COMPLETED BY PRIMARY CARE PHYSICIAN OR OUTSIDE PROVIDER

Patient Name_______________ Date_______________

❑ Male ❑ Female Birthdate_______________ Home Telephone Number _______________

Address _______________

Primary Care Physician_______________ NPI_______________

Referring Physician _______________ NPI_______________

Referred to _______________ NPI_______________

Address _______________ Telephone No. _______________

Diagnosis Code _______________ Diagnosis_______________

Diagnosis Code _______________ Diagnosis_______________

Treatment Plan _______________

Authorization Requested for: ❑ Consult Only ❑ Treatment Only ❑ Consult/Treatment
❑ Consult/Procedure/Surgery ❑ Diagnostic Tests

Procedure Code: _______________ Description: _______________

Procedure Code: _______________ Description: _______________

Place of Service ❑ Office ❑ Outpatient ❑ Inpatient ❑ Other Number of Visits: _______________

Facility: _______________ Length of Stay: _______________

Physician's Signature: _______________

TO BE COMPLETED BY PRIMARY CARE PHYSICIAN

PCP Recommendations: _______________ PCP Initials: _______________

Date Eligibility Checked: _______________

TO BE COMPLETED BY UTILIZATION MANAGEMENT

Authorized: _______________ Auth. No: _______________ Not Authorized _______________

Deferred: _______________ Modified: _______________

Effective Date: _______________ Expiration Date: _______________ No. of Visits: _______________

Fig. 5.3

ASSIGNMENT 5.4 OBTAIN AUTHORIZATION FOR DIAGNOSTIC ARTHROSCOPY FROM A MANAGED CARE PLAN

Performance Objective

Task: Complete a treatment authorization form to obtain permission for diagnostic arthroscopy with debridement for a patient covered by a managed care plan.

Conditions: Use a treatment authorization form (Fig. 5.4), computer, and printer.

Standards: Time: ________________ minutes

Accuracy: ________________

(Note: The time element and accuracy criteria may be given by your instructor.)

Directions: Complete the treatment authorization form for this patient (see Fig. 5.4), date it August 12 of the current year, and submit it to the managed care plan. Refer to Fig. 5.2 in the *Textbook* for visual guidance.

Scenario: Daniel Chan has been referred by his primary care physician, Dr. Gerald Practon, to an orthopedic surgeon, Dr. Raymond Skeleton. Both physicians are members of his managed care plan, Metropolitan Life. The patient comes into Dr. Skeleton's office complaining of pain, swelling, and crepitus of the right knee. The patient is having difficulty walking but indicates no recent injury to the knee.

Mr. Chan lives at 226 West Olive Avenue, Woodland Hills, XY 12345-0001, and his telephone number is 555-540-6700. His plan identification number is FTW90876, effective February 1, 20xx, and he was born February 23, 1971.

After taking a history, completing a physical examination, and taking and reviewing radiographs, Dr. Skeleton suspects the patient has a tear of the medial meniscus and may require débridement of articular cartilage. This procedure will be performed on an outpatient basis at College Hospital. Authorization must be obtained for the surgical arthroscopy with débridement of articular cartilage. Dr. Practon's Metropolitan Life provider number is ML C01402X and Dr. Skeleton's Metropolitan Life provider number is ML C4561X.

After the instructor has returned your work to you, either make the necessary corrections and place your work in a three-ring notebook for future reference or, if you received a high score, place it in your portfolio for reference when applying for a job.

College Clinic
4567 Broad Avenue
Woodland Hills, XY 12345-0001
Telephone No. (555) 487-8976
Fax No. (555) 487-8976

MANAGED CARE PLAN AUTHORIZATION REQUEST

☐ Health Net	☐ Met Life
☐ Pacificare	☐ Travelers
☐ Secure Horizons	☐ Pru Care
☐ Other	

Member/Group No.

TO BE COMPLETED BY PRIMARY CARE PHYSICIAN OR OUTSIDE PROVIDER

Patient Name__________ Date__________

☐ Male ☐ Female Birthdate__________ Home Telephone Number __________

Address __________

Primary Care Physician__________ NPI__________

Referring Physician __________ NPI__________

Referred to __________ NPI__________

Address __________ Telephone No. __________

Diagnosis Code __________ Diagnosis__________

Diagnosis Code __________ Diagnosis__________

Treatment Plan __________

Authorization Requested for: ☐ Consult Only ☐ Treatment Only ☐ Consult/Treatment ☐ Consult/Procedure/Surgery ☐ Diagnostic Tests

Procedure Code: __________ Description: __________

Procedure Code: __________ Description: __________

Place of Service ☐ Office ☐ Outpatient ☐ Inpatient ☐ Other Number of Visits: __________

Facility: __________ Length of Stay: __________

Physician's Signature: __________

TO BE COMPLETED BY PRIMARY CARE PHYSICIAN

PCP Recommendations: __________ PCP Initials: __________

Date Eligibility Checked: __________

TO BE COMPLETED BY UTILIZATION MANAGEMENT

Authorized: __________ Auth. No: __________ Not Authorized __________

Deferred: __________ Modified: __________

Effective Date: __________ Expiration Date: __________ No. of Visits: __________

Fig. 5.4

ASSIGNMENT 5.5 OBTAIN AUTHORIZATION FOR CONSULTATION FROM A MANAGED CARE PLAN

Performance Objective

Task: Complete a treatment authorization form to obtain permission for consultation for a patient from a managed care plan.

Conditions: Use a treatment authorization form (Fig. 5.5), computer, and printer.

Standards: Time: ________________ minutes

Accuracy: ________________

(Note: The time element and accuracy criteria may be given by your instructor.)

Directions: Complete the treatment authorization form for this patient (see Fig. 5.5), date it September 3 of the current year, and submit it to the managed care plan. Refer to Fig. 5.2 in the *Textbook* for visual guidance.

Scenario: Frederico Fellini, with a history of getting up four times during the night with a slow urinary stream, was seen by his primary care physician, Dr. Gerald Practon. An intravenous pyelogram yielded negative results except for distention of the urinary bladder. Physical examination of the prostate showed an enlargement. The preliminary diagnosis is benign prostatic hypertrophy (BPH).

The patient will be referred to Dr. Douglas Lee, a urologist, for consultation (Level 4) and cystoscopy. Transurethral resection of the prostate is possible at a future date. Dr. Lee's address is 4300 Cyber Street, Woodland Hills, XY 12345, and his office telephone number is 555-675-3322. His National Provider Identifier (NPI) is 55026717XX.

Dr. Practon's managed care contract is with PruCare, identification number PC C01402X, of which this patient is a member.

Mr. Fellini lives at 476 Miner Street, Woodland Hills, XY 12345, and his telephone number is 555-679-0098. His PruCare plan identification number is VRG87655, effective January 1, 20xx. His birth date is May 24, 1944.

After the instructor has returned your work to you, either make the necessary corrections and place your work in a three-ring notebook for future reference or, if you received a high score, place it in your portfolio for reference when applying for a job.

College Clinic
4567 Broad Avenue
Woodland Hills, XY 12345-0001
Telephone No. (555) 487-8976
Fax No. (555) 487-8976

MANAGED CARE PLAN AUTHORIZATION REQUEST

❑ Health Net ❑ Pacificare ❑ Secure Horizons ❑ Other ❑ Met Life ❑ Travelers ❑ Pru Care

Member/Group No.

TO BE COMPLETED BY PRIMARY CARE PHYSICIAN OR OUTSIDE PROVIDER

Patient Name__________ Date__________

❑ Male ❑ Female Birthdate__________ Home Telephone Number __________

Address __________

Primary Care Physician__________ NPI__________

Referring Physician __________ NPI__________

Referred to __________ NPI__________

Address __________ Telephone No. __________

Diagnosis Code __________ Diagnosis__________

Diagnosis Code __________ Diagnosis__________

Treatment Plan __________

Authorization Requested for: ❑ Consult Only ❑ Treatment Only ❑ Consult/Treatment ❑ Consult/Procedure/Surgery ❑ Diagnostic Tests

Procedure Code: __________ Description: __________

Procedure Code: __________ Description: __________

Place of Service ❑ Office ❑ Outpatient ❑ Inpatient ❑ Other Number of Visits: __________

Facility: __________ Length of Stay: __________

Physician's Signature: __________

TO BE COMPLETED BY PRIMARY CARE PHYSICIAN

PCP Recommendations: __________ PCP Initials: __________

Date Eligibility Checked: __________

TO BE COMPLETED BY UTILIZATION MANAGEMENT

Authorized: __________ Auth. No: __________ Not Authorized __________

Deferred: __________ Modified: __________

Effective Date: __________ Expiration Date: __________ No. of Visits: __________

Fig. 5.5

ASSIGNMENT 5.6 OBTAIN AUTHORIZATION FOR DIAGNOSTIC BODY SCAN FROM A MANAGED CARE PLAN

Performance Objective

Task: Complete a treatment authorization form to obtain permission for diagnostic complete body bone scan and mammogram for a patient covered by a managed care plan.

Conditions: Use a treatment authorization form (Fig. 5.6), computer, and printer.

Standards: Time: _________________ minutes

Accuracy: _________________

(Note: The time element and accuracy criteria may be given by your instructor.)

Directions: Complete the treatment authorization form for this patient (see Fig. 5.6), date it October 23 of the current year, and submit it to the managed care plan. Refer to Fig. 5.2 in the *Textbook* for visual guidance.

Scenario: A patient, Debbie Dye, sees her primary care physician, Dr. Gerald Practon, for complaint of midback pain. She underwent a lumpectomy 2 years ago for a malignant neoplasm of the lower left breast; thus she has a history of breast cancer. She has been referred by Dr. Practon (PacifiCare identification number PC C01402X) to Dr. Donald Patos, an oncologist, for a complete workup. He finds that her complaint of midback pain warrants the need to refer her to XYZ Radiology for bilateral diagnostic mammography and a complete body bone scan.

Dr. Patos' address is 4466 East Canter Drive, Woodland Hills, XY 12345, and his office telephone number is 555-980-5566. Dr. Patos' PacifiCare identification number is PC 5673X. His NPI is 6520101678XX.

Ms. Dye lives at 6700 Flora Road, Woodland Hills, XY 12345, and her telephone number is 555-433-6755. Her PacifiCare plan identification number is SR45380, effective January 1, 20xx. Her birth date is August 6, 1952.

XYZ Radiology's address is 4767 Broad Avenue, Woodland Hills, XY 12345-0001, and the office telephone number is 555-486-9162.

After the instructor has returned your work to you, either make the necessary corrections and place your work in a three-ring notebook for future reference or, if you received a high score, place it in your portfolio for reference when applying for a job.

College Clinic
4567 Broad Avenue
Woodland Hills, XY 12345-0001
Telephone No. (555) 487-8976
Fax No. (555) 487-8976

MANAGED CARE PLAN AUTHORIZATION REQUEST

❑ Health Net ❑ Met Life
❑ Pacificare ❑ Travelers
❑ Secure Horizons ❑ Pru Care
❑ Other

Member/Group No.

TO BE COMPLETED BY PRIMARY CARE PHYSICIAN OR OUTSIDE PROVIDER

Patient Name__________ Date__________

❑ Male ❑ Female Birthdate__________ Home Telephone Number __________

Address __________

Primary Care Physician__________ NPI__________

Referring Physician __________ NPI__________

Referred to __________ NPI__________

Address __________ Telephone No. __________

Diagnosis Code __________ Diagnosis__________

Diagnosis Code __________ Diagnosis__________

Treatment Plan __________

Authorization Requested for: ❑ Consult Only ❑ Treatment Only ❑ Consult/Treatment
❑ Consult/Procedure/Surgery ❑ Diagnostic Tests

Procedure Code: __________ Description: __________

Procedure Code: __________ Description: __________

Place of Service ❑ Office ❑ Outpatient ❑ Inpatient ❑ Other Number of Visits: __________

Facility: __________ Length of Stay: __________

Physician's Signature: __________

TO BE COMPLETED BY PRIMARY CARE PHYSICIAN

PCP Recommendations: __________ PCP Initials: __________

Date Eligibility Checked: __________

TO BE COMPLETED BY UTILIZATION MANAGEMENT

Authorized: __________ Auth. No: __________ Not Authorized __________

Deferred: __________ Modified: __________

Effective Date: __________ Expiration Date: __________ No. of Visits: __________

Fig. 5.6

6 Medicare

Linda M. Smith

KEY TERMS

Your instructor may wish to select some words pertinent to this chapter for a test. For definitions of the terms, further study, and/or reference, the words, phrases, and abbreviations may be found in the glossary at the end of the Textbook. *Key terms for this chapter follow.*

adjudication
adjustment
Advance Beneficiary Notice of Noncoverage
Advanced Alternative Payment Model
approved charges
assignment
beneficiaries
benefit period
Centers for Medicare and Medicaid Services
Correct Coding Initiative
crossover claim
disabled
donut hole
durable medical equipment
end-stage renal disease
formulary
hospice
hospital insurance
jurisdiction
limiting charge
Local Coverage Determination
medical necessity
Medicaid
Medicare
Medicare administrative contractor
Medicare Access and CHIP Reauthorization Act of 2015
Medicare Advantage Plan
Medicare Beneficiary Identifier
Medicare Claims Processing Manual—Internet Only Manual
Medicare Improvements for Patients and Providers Act
Medicare/Medicaid
Medicare Part A
Medicare Part B
Medicare Part C
Medicare Part D
Medicare secondary payer
Medicare Summary Notice
Medigap
Merit-based Incentive Payment System
National Coverage Determination
national health insurance
national provider identifier
nonparticipating provider
nursing facility
participating provider
premium
prepayment screen
prospective payment system
Quality Improvement Organization
Recovery Audit Contractor Initiative
remittance advice
resource-based relative value scale
respite care
Supplemental Security Income
value-based programs

KEY ABBREVIATIONS

See how many abbreviations and acronyms you can translate and then use this as a handy reference list. Definitions for the key abbreviations are located near the back of the Text-book *in the glossary.*

ABN ____________________

APM ____________________

CCI ____________________

____

CMS ____________________

DC ____________________

DHHS ____________________

DME ____________________

ERA ____________________

ESRD ____________________

GPCIs ____________________

ICU ____________________

LCDs ____________________

LGHP ____________________

MA Plan ________________

MAC ________________

MACRA ________________

MBI ________________

Medi-Medi ________________

MIPAA ________________

MIPS ________________

MG ________________

MMA ________________

MSA ________________

MSN ________________

MSP ________________

NCDs ________________

NF ________________

nonpar ________________

NPI ________________

par ________________

PFFS plan ________________

PPS ________________

PSO ________________

QIO ________________

RA ________________

RAC Initiative ________________

RBRVS ________________

SSI ________________

PERFORMANCE OBJECTIVES

The student will be able to:

- Define and spell the key terms and key abbreviations for this chapter, given the information from the *Textbook* glossary, within a reasonable time period and with enough accuracy to obtain a satisfactory evaluation.
- After reading the chapter, answer the fill in the blank, multiple choice, and true/false review questions, with enough accuracy to obtain a satisfactory evaluation.
- Compute mathematical calculations, given Medicare problem situations, within a reasonable time period and with enough accuracy to obtain a satisfactory evaluation.
- Complete an ABN form.

STUDY OUTLINE

Background

Policies and Regulations
- Eligibility Requirements
- Medicare Enrollment
- Health Insurance Card
- Benefits

Additional Insurance Programs
- Medicare/Medicaid
- Medicare/Medigap
- Medicare Secondary Payer
- Automobile or Liability Insurance Coverage

Utilization and Quality Control
- Quality Improvement Organizations
- Medicare Billing Compliance Issues

Program Fundamentals
- Provider
- Prior Authorization
- National and Local Coverage Determinations
- Prepayment Screens

Medicare Reimbursement
- Medicare Fee Schedule
- Prospective Payment System
- Value-Based Programs
- Medicare Improvements for Patients and Providers Act
- Medicare Access and CHIIP Reauthorization Act of 2015

Claim Submission
- Medicare Administrative Contractors
- Provider Identification Numbers

After Claim Submission
- Remittance Advice
- Medicare Summary Notice
- Posting Payments
- Medicare Overpayments

ASSIGNMENT 6.1 REVIEW QUESTIONS

Part I Fill in the Blank

Review the objectives, key terms, glossary definitions of key terms, chapter information, and figures before completing the following review questions.

1. Medicare is administered by the federal agency ______________________________.

2. Medicare Part A is ______________________________ coverage, and Medicare Part B is ______________________________ coverage.

3. A program designed to provide pain relief, symptom management, and supportive services to terminally ill individuals and their families is known as ______________________________.

4. An individual becomes eligible for Medicare Parts A and B at age ______________.

5. The program of income support for low-income, aged, blind, and disabled persons established by the Social Security Act is called a/an ______________________________.

6. An individual who is not a citizen of the United States is called a/an ____________.

7. Patients who are entitled to received Medicare benefits are referred to as ______________________________.

8. The number that will replace social security numbers on Medicare insurance cards is referred to as the ______________________________.

9. Define a Medicare Part A hospital benefit period.

____

____

____

10. Short-term inpatient medical care for terminally ill individuals to give temporary relief to the caregiver is known as ______________________________.

11. The frequency of Pap tests for Medicare patients is ______________________________, and that for mammograms is ______________________________.

12. Medicare coverage plans offered by private insurance companies to Medicare beneficiaries are known as ______________________________.

13. ______________________________ is a temporary limit on what a Medicare drug plan will cover.

14. A list of covered drugs kept by each Medicare drug plan is called a/an ______________________________.

15. A document by Medicare explaining the decision made on a claim for services that were paid is called a/an ______________________________

16. Some third-party payers offer policies that fall under guidelines issued by the federal government and may cover prescription costs, Medicare deductibles, and copayments; these secondary or supplemental policies are known as ______________________ ____________________ insurance policies.

17. The amount that a nonparticipating provider can charge the Medicare beneficiary is referred to as ____ ______________________________.

18. If a Medicare beneficiary is injured in an automobile accident, the physician submits the claim form to ____.

Part II Multiple Choice

Choose the best answer.

19. The fee that Medicare decides a medical service is worth, is referred to as the:
    a. reasonable charge for services.
    b. assigned amount.
    c. approved amount.
    d. paid amount.

20. Physicians who are nonparticipating with the Medicare program are only allowed to bill the limiting charge to the patient, which is:
    a. the provider's usual fee.
    b. 80% of the provider's fee schedule.
    c. 20% of the Medicare fee schedule allowed amount.
    d. 115% of the Medicare fee schedule allowed amount.

21. National Coverage Determinations are coverage guidelines that are mandated:
    a. at the federal level.
    b. at the Medicare contractor level.
    c. at the Medicare Advantage Plan level.
    d. by Recovery Audit Contractors Initiative.

22. A decision by a Medicare administrative contractor (MAC) whether to cover (pay) a particular medical service on a contractor-wide basis in accordance with whether it is reasonable and necessary is known as a/an:
    a. Local Coverage Determination.
    b. Correct Coding Initiative edit.
    c. prepayment screen.
    d. redetermination process.

23. A Medicare prepayment screen which would suspend a claim for the excision of an appendix performed by an audiologist would be referred to as:
    a. diagnosis to procedure edits.
    b. procedure to procedure edits.
    c. procedure to specialty code edits.
    d. procedure to place of service edits.

24. The resource-based relative value scale establishes fees, taking into account:
    a. physician's specialty, work value, and overhead expense.
    b. work value, overhead expense, and malpractice expense.
    c. work value, physician's specialty, and malpractice expense.
    d. physician's specialty, overhead expense, and malpractice expense.

25. The prospective payment system is a method of reimbursement to:
    a. physicians.
    b. ambulance services.
    c. hospitals.
    d. pharmacies.

26. The number of Medicare administrative contractors that currently process claims for DME suppliers is:
    a. 1.
    b. 4.
    c. 12.
    d. 50.

27. The 10-digit identification number required on a claim form to identify a service provider is the:
    a. SSN.
    b. MBI.
    c. NPI.
    d. PIP.

28. According to regulations, a Medicare patient must be billed for a copayment:
    a. at least once before a balance is adjusted off as uncollectible.
    b. at least two times before a balance is adjusted off as uncollectible.
    c. at least three times before a balance is adjusted off as uncollectible.
    d. no more than four times before a balance is adjusted off as uncollectible.

Part III True/False

Write "T" or "F" in the blank to indicate whether you think the statement is true or false.

_______ 29. All patients who have a Medicare health insurance card have Part A hospital and Part B medical coverage.

_______ 30. Prescription drug plans refer to the drugs in their formularies by tier numbers.

_______ 31. Nonparticipating physicians may decide on a case-by-case basis whether to accept assignment when providing medical services to Medicare patients.

_______ 32. Medicare's Correct Coding Initiative was implemented by the Centers for Medicare and Medicaid Services to identify procedures that are usually described by a single code or are inherent to another procedure.

_______ 33. A Medicare/Medigap claim is not called a crossover claim.

_______ 34. A Medicare preventive health benefit is an annual mammogram screening.

_______ 35. Medicare patients must pay for diabetes screening.

_______ 36. Obesity screening and counseling are Medicare preventive health benefits.

_______ 37. Pneumococcal pneumonia vaccine may be administered annually to Medicare patients.

_______ 38. Glaucoma screening is a covered screening for Medicare patients when performed every 6 months.

ASSIGNMENT 6.2 CALCULATE MATHEMATICAL PROBLEMS

Performance Objective

Task: Calculate and insert the correct amounts for nine Medicare scenarios.

Conditions: Use a pen or pencil and the description of the problem.

Standards: Time: ________________ minutes

Accuracy: ________________

(Note: The time element and accuracy criteria may be given by your instructor.)

Directions: Submitting insurance claims, particularly Medicare claims, involves a bit of arithmetic. Several problems are given here so that you will gain experience with situations encountered daily in your work. The Medicare deductible is always subtracted from the allowed amount first before mathematical computations continue.

Problem 1: Mr. Doolittle has Medicare Parts A and B coverage. He was well during the entire past year. On January 1, Mr. Doolittle is rushed to the hospital, where Dr. Input performs an emergency gastric resection. The hospital bills Medicare under the Part A coverage, and under the Part B coverage, the physician bills $450 for surgical services. The doctor agrees to accept assignment. The patient has not met any of his deductible for 2017 which is $183. Complete the following statements by putting in the correct amounts.

Original Bill

a. Medicare allows $400. Medicare payment: ________________

b. Patient owes Dr. Input: ________________

c. Dr. Input's courtesy adjustment: ________________

Mathematical computations:

Problem 2: Mrs. James has Medicare Parts A and B coverage. She met her deductible when she was ill in March of this year. On November 1, Dr. Caesar performs a bilateral salpingo-oophorectomy. The hospital bills Medicare under the Part A coverage, and under Part B coverage, the physician bills $300 for surgical services. The doctor agrees to accept a Medicare assignment.

Original Bill

a. Medicare allows $275. Medicare payment: ________________

b. Patient owes Dr. Caesar: ________________

c. Dr. Caesar's courtesy adjustment: ________________

Mathematical computations for surgeon:

The assistant surgeon charged Mrs. James $60 (the Medicare limiting charge) and does not accept assignment. After receiving her check from Medicare, Mrs. James sends the surgeon his $60. Medicare has allowed $55 for the fee.

a. How much of the money was from Mrs. James' private funds? $ ____________

b. How much did Medicare pay? ______________

Mathematical computations:

Problem 3: You work for Dr. Coccidioides. He does not accept assignment. He is treating Mr. Robinson for allergies. Mr. Robinson has Medicare Part A. You send in a bill to Medicare for the $135 that Mr. Robinson owes you. What portion of the bill will Medicare pay?

Problem 4: In June, Mr. Fay has an illness that incurs $89 in medical bills. He asks you to bill Medicare, and the physician does not accept assignment. He has paid the deductible at another physician's office.

a. If Medicare allows the entire amount of your fees, the Medicare check to the patient is $____________ (which comes to you).

b. The patient's part of the bill to you is____________.

Mathematical computations:

Problem 5: Mr. Iba, a Medicare patient with a Medigap insurance policy, is seen for an office visit, and the fee is $80. The Medicare-approved amount is $54.44. The patient has met his deductible for the year.

a. The Medicare payment check is $ ______________________.
b. After the claim is submitted to the Medigap insurance, the Medigap payment check is $ ______________________.
c. To zero out the balance, the Medicare courtesy adjustment is ______________.

Mathematical computations:

Problem 6: Mrs. Smith, a Medicare patient, had surgery, and the participating physician's fee is $1250. This patient is working part-time, and her employer group health plan (primary insurance) allowed $1100, applied $500 to the deductible, and paid 80% of $600.

a. Amount paid by this plan: $____________________

b. The spouse's employer group health plan (secondary insurance) is billed for the balance, which is $____________________. This program also has a $500 deductible. This plan pays 100% of the fee billed, minus the deductible.

c. The spouse's employer group plan makes a payment of ____________________.

You send copies of the remittance advice from the two group health plans and submit a claim to Medicare (the third insurance) for $1250. The balance at this point is $ ________________.

Mathematical computations:

Problem 7: Beverly James has Medicare Part B coverage. She has $242 in medical bills and has met $100 of the $183 (2017 deductible). Dr. Practon agrees to accept assignment.

Original Bill

a. Medicare allows $200. Medicare payment: ______________________________

b. Beverly James owes Dr. Practon: ______________________________

c. Dr. Practon's courtesy adjustment: ______________________________

Mathematical computations:

Problem 8: Oliver Mills has Medicare Part B coverage. He fell at home and suffered a sprain and Dr. Skeleton treated him. His medical bill totaled $370, and he has met $60 of the $183 (2017 deductible). Dr. Skeleton agrees to accept assignment.

Original Bill

a. Medicare allows $280. Medicare payment: ______

b. Oliver Mills owes Dr. Skeleton: ______

c. Dr. Skeleton's courtesy adjustment: ______

Mathematical computations:

Problem 9: Maria Sanchez has Medicare Part B coverage. She has $565 in medical bills at Dr. Cardi's office and met $45 of the $183 (2017 deductible) at another physician's office. Dr. Cardi agrees to accept assignment.

Original Bill

a. Medicare allows $480. Medicare payment: ______

b. Maria Sanchez owes Dr. Cardi: ______

c. Dr. Cardi's courtesy adjustment: ______

Mathematical computations:

ASSIGNMENT 6.3 COMPLETE A MEDICARE ADVANCE BENEFICIARY NOTICE OF NONCOVERAGE

Performance Objective

Task: Complete Medicare ABN.

Conditions: Use the ABN form (Fig. 6.1)

Standards: ABN Completion Productivity Measurement

Time: _______________ minutes

Accuracy: _______________

(Note: The time element and accuracy criteria may be given by your instructor.)

Directions:

1. Complete an ABN form using the information provided below.

2. Patient: Raymond Fay (Medicare ID # A887661235A)
   a. Procedure performed: nystagmus test (CPT 92531) is a noncovered service and requires that an ABN be on file.
   b. The estimated cost of the nystagmus test is $26.00.
   c. After review of the ABN with the patient, the patient would like to proceed with the test and understands that they may be responsible for payment of the service.
   d. Provider of Services: Concha Antrum, MD; College Clinic; 4567 Broad Ave., Woodland Hills, XY 12345

A. Notifier:

B. Patient Name: **C. Identification Number:**

Advance Beneficiary Notice of Noncoverage (ABN)

NOTE: If Medicare doesn't pay for **D.** ____________ below, you may have to pay.

Medicare does not pay for everything, even some care that you or your health care provider have good reason to think you need. We expect Medicare may not pay for the **D.** ____________ below.

D.	E. Reason Medicare May Not Pay:	F. Estimated Cost

WHAT YOU NEED TO DO NOW:

- Read this notice, so you can make an informed decision about your care.
- Ask us any questions that you may have after you finish reading.
- Choose an option below about whether to receive the **D.** ____________ listed above.

  Note: If you choose Option 1 or 2, we may help you to use any other insurance that you might have, but Medicare cannot require us to do this.

G. OPTIONS: Check only one box. We cannot choose a box for you.

☐ **OPTION 1.** I want the **D.** ____________ listed above. You may ask to be paid now, but I also want Medicare billed for an official decision on payment, which is sent to me on a Medicare Summary Notice (MSN). I understand that if Medicare doesn't pay, I am responsible for payment, but **I can appeal to Medicare** by following the directions on the MSN. If Medicare does pay, you will refund any payments I made to you, less co-pays or deductibles.

☐ **OPTION 2.** I want the **D.** ____________ listed above, but do not bill Medicare. You may ask to be paid now as I am responsible for payment. **I cannot appeal if Medicare is not billed.**

☐ **OPTION 3.** I don't want the **D.** ____________ listed above. I understand with this choice I am **not** responsible for payment, and **I cannot appeal to see if Medicare would pay.**

H. Additional Information:

This notice gives our opinion, not an official Medicare decision. If you have other questions on this notice or Medicare billing, call **1-800-MEDICARE** (1-800-633-4227/**TTY:** 1-877-486-2048).

Signing below means that you have received and understand this notice. You also receive a copy.

I. Signature:	J. Date:

According to the Paperwork Reduction Act of 1995, no persons are required to respond to a collection of information unless it displays a valid OMB control number. The valid OMB control number for this information collection is 0938-0566. The time required to complete this information collection is estimated to average 7 minutes per response, including the time to review instructions, search existing data resources, gather the data needed, and complete and review the information collection. If you have comments concerning the accuracy of the time estimate or suggestions for improving this form, please write to: CMS, 7500 Security Boulevard, Attn: PRA Reports Clearance Officer, Baltimore, Maryland 21244-1850.

Form CMS-R-131 (03/11) Form Approved OMB No. 0938-0566

Fig. 6.1

7 Medicaid and Other State Programs

Linda M. Smith

KEY TERMS

Your instructor may wish to select some words pertinent to this chapter for a test. For definitions of the terms, further study, and/or reference, the words, phrases, and abbreviations may be found in the glossary at the end of the Textbook. *Key terms for this chapter follow.*

categorically needy
coinsurance
copayment
covered services
Early and Periodic Screening, Diagnosis, and Treatment
federal poverty level
fiscal agent
Medicaid
Medi-Cal
medically needy
Medicare Savings Programs
payer of last resort
prior approval
recipient
share of cost
Children's Health Insurance Program
Supplemental Security Income

KEY ABBREVIATIONS

See how many abbreviations and acronyms you can translate and then use this as a handy reference list. Definitions for the key abbreviations are located near the back of the Textbook *in the glossary.*

CHIP ______________________

DEFRA ______________________

EPSDT ______________________

FPL ______________________

MN ______________________

MSP ______________________

OBRA ______________________

OOY claims ______________________

POS machine ______________________

QI program ______________________

QMB ______________________

RA ______________________

SLMB ______________________

SSI ______________________

TANF ______________________

PERFORMANCE OBJECTIVES

The student will be able to:

- Define and spell the key terms and key abbreviations for this chapter, given the information from the *Textbook* glossary, within a reasonable time period and with enough accuracy to obtain a satisfactory evaluation.
- After reading the chapter, answer the fill in the blank, multiple choice, and true/false review questions with enough accuracy to obtain a satisfactory evaluation.
- Determine if prior authorization is required for a specific scenario.

STUDY OUTLINE

Medicaid
- History

Medicaid Programs
- Children's Health Insurance Program
- Medicare Savings Programs

Medicaid Eligibility
- Verifying Eligibility
- Categorically Needy
- Medically Needy
- Spousal Impoverishment Protection Law
- Accepting Medicaid Patients

Medicaid Benefits
- Covered Services
- Disallowed Services

Medicaid Managed Care

Claim Procedures
- Copayment
- Prior Approval
- Hospital-Acquired Condition
- Time Limit
- Reciprocity
- Claim Form

After Claim Submission
- Remittance Advice
- Appeals

ASSIGNMENT 7.1 REVIEW QUESTIONS

Part I Fill in the Blank

Review the objectives, key terms, glossary definitions of key terms, chapter information, and figures before completing the following review questions.

1. Medicaid is not considered an insurance program. It is a/an _________ program.

2. The Medicaid program is jointly funded by the _______ and _______ governments.

3. Because the federal government sets minimum requirements, states are free to enhance the Medicaid program. Name two ways in which Medicaid programs vary from state to state.

   a. ______________________________

   b. ______________________________

4. Title XIX of the Social Security Act became federal law and created Medicaid in the year ______________.

5. Health care reform legislation passed in 2010, known as ________________affected the Medicaid program by expanding access for childless adults and nonelderly and nonpregnant individuals.

6. To help compensate for budget cuts, many Medicaid programs instituted required specific dollar amounts, known as ______________, to be collected at each office visit from the individual seeking medical services.

7. The measure of income issued every year by HHS and used to determine Medicaid eligibility is known as __________________.

8. In all other states, the program is known as *Medicaid*, but in California the program is called ______________________________.

9. Name the four Medicare Savings Programs for low-income Medicare patients.

   a. ______________________________

   b. ______________________________

   c. ______________________________

   d. ______________________________

10. Medicare beneficiaries who are disabled but have annual incomes below the federal poverty level may be eligible for the __________________ program.

11. _______________ is the portion the patient pays of the Medicare allowed amount.

12. States have the option to cover nonimmigrant and unauthorized aliens who are pregnant or who are children and can meet the definition of __________ in the U.S.

13. When health care services are rendered, the Medicaid identification card or electronic verification must show eligibility for the _________.

14. Name two broad classifications of people eligible for Medicaid assistance.

a. ______________________________

b. ______________________________

15. A __________ is an individual certified by the local welfare department to receive benefits of Medicaid.

16. The name of the program for the prevention, early detection, and treatment of conditions of children receiving welfare is known as ______________________.

It is abbreviated as ______________________.

17. Your Medicaid patient seen today needs long-term hemodialysis services. You telephone for authorization to get verbal approval. Four important items to obtain are:

a. ______________________________

b. ______________________________

c. ______________________________

d. ______________________________

18. The time limit for submitting a Medicaid claim varies from ______________

to ______________________________

from the date the service is rendered.

19. The insurance claim form for submitting Medicaid claims in all states is

______________________________.

20. Your Medicaid patient also has TRICARE. What billing procedure do you follow? Be exact in your steps for a dependant of an active military person.

a. ______________________________

b. ______________________________

21. Five categories of adjudicated claims that may appear on a Medicaid remittance advice document are:

a. ______________________________

b. ______________________________

c. ______________________________

d. ______________________________

e. ______________________________

22. Name three levels of Medicaid appeals.

a. ______________________________

b. ______________________________

c. ______________________________

23. ______________ is the processing of an insurance claim through a series of edits for final determination of coverage (benefits) for possible payment.

Part II Multiple Choice

Choose the best answer.

24. An organization under contract with the state to process claims for a state Medicaid program is a/the:
   a. Medicaid administrative contractor.
   b. Department of Social Services.
   c. Center for Medicare and Medicaid Services.
   d. fiscal agent.

25. A patient's Medicaid eligibility may be verified by:
   a. touch-tone telephone.
   b. modem.
   c. special Medicaid terminal equipment.
   d. all of the above.

26. When a Medicaid patient requires a piece of durable medical equipment, the physician must:
   a. write a prescription.
   b. obtain prior authorization, preferably written.
   c. instruct the patient on how to use the equipment.
   d. give the name and address of where to purchase the equipment.

27. Which of the following services are mandated Medicaid basic benefits?
   a. Ambulance services
   b. Podiatric care
   c. Immunizations
   d. Dental care

28. If a patient is eligible for group health insurance coverage through an employer and they are also eligible for Medicaid benefits, Medicaid is referred to as the:
   a. payer of last resort.
   b. primary payer.
   c. co-insurance.
   d. fiscal agent.

29. If a patient is eligible for Medicare and Medicaid, Medicare is referred to as the:
   a. payer of last resort.
   b. primary payer.
   c. co-insurance.
   d. fiscal agent.

Part III True/False

Write "T" or "F" in the blank to indicate whether you think the statement is true or false.

_______ 30. Hospital-acquired conditions are payable by the Medicaid program.

_______ 31. All states have a Medicaid time limit of 12 months from the date of service for filing claims.

_______ 32. Medicaid spend down eligibility is determined annually to find out the patient's monthly copayment amount.

_______ 33. In some states, the phrase *prior approval* may be referred to as *prior authorization*.

_______ 34. There is only one type of copayment requirement in the Medicaid program.

_______ 35. Providers must enroll for participation in the Medicaid program with the fiscal agent for their region.

_______ 36. A state agency that investigates complaints of mistreatment in long-term care facilities is the Medicaid Fraud Control Unit (MFCU).

_______ 37. If a Medicaid patient requires medical care while out of state, the claim for services should be filed with the patient's home state Medicaid program.

_______ 38. If a Medicaid managed care patient requires medical care, the claim for services should be filed with the state Medicaid's fiscal agent.

ASSIGNMENT 7.2 CRITICAL THINKING

Performance Objective

Task: After reading the scenario, answer the following questions, using critical thinking skills.
Conditions: Use a pen or pencil.

Standards: Time: ________________ minutes

Accuracy: ________________

(Note: The time element and accuracy criteria may be given by your instructor.)

Directions: After reading the scenario, answer the question, using your critical thinking skills. Record your answers on the blank lines.

Scenario: Mrs. Ho suddenly experiences a pain in her right lower abdominal area and rushes to a local hospital for emergency care. Laboratory work verifies that she has a ruptured appendix, and immediate surgery is recommended. Is prior authorization required in a bona fide emergency situation like this?

1. ____

Reason: ____

8 TRICARE and Veterans' Health Care

Linda M. Smith

KEY TERMS

Your instructor may wish to select some words pertinent to this chapter for a test. For definitions of the terms, further study, and/or reference, the words, phrases, and abbreviations may be found in the glossary at the end of the Textbook. *Key terms for this chapter follow.*

active duty service member
allowable charge
authorized provider
beneficiary
catastrophic cap
catchment area
Civilian Health and Medical Program of the Uniformed Services
cooperative care
coordination of benefits
cost share
Defense Enrollment Eligibility Reporting System
Department of Veterans Affairs
emergency
health benefits advisor
health care finder
medically (or psychologically) necessary
Military Treatment Facility
Non-Availability Statement
nonparticipating provider
other health insurance
participating provider
partnership program
point-of-service option
preauthorization
primary care manager
regional contractor
service benefit program
service-connected injury
service retiree (military retiree)
sponsor
summary payment voucher
total, permanent, service-connected disability
TRICARE
TRICARE Extra
TRICARE for Life
TRICARE Prime
TRICARE service center
TRICARE Select
TRICARE Standard
urgent care
veteran
Veterans Health Administration

KEY ABBREVIATIONS

See how many abbreviations and acronyms you can translate and then use this as a handy reference list. Definitions for the key abbreviations are located near the back of the Text-book *in the glossary.*

ADSM ____________________

CHAMPUS ____________________

CHAMPVA ____________________

DEERS ____________________

HBA ____________________

HCF ____________________

MHS ____________________

MTF ____________________

NAS ____________________

nonpar ____________________

OHI ____________________

par ____________________

PCM ____________________

POS ____________________

SHCP ____________________

TFL ____________________

TMA ____________________

TPR ____________________

TSC ____________________

VA ____________________

PERFORMANCE OBJECTIVES

The student will be able to:

- Define and spell the key terms and key abbreviations for this chapter, given the information from the *Textbook* glossary, within a reasonable time period and with enough accuracy to obtain a satisfactory evaluation.
- After reading the chapter, answer the fill in the blank, multiple choice, and true/false review questions with enough accuracy to obtain a satisfactory evaluation.

STUDY OUTLINE

TRICARE
History of TRICARE
- Eligibility
- Nonavailability Statement

Health Plans
- TRICARE Select
- TRICARE Prime
- TRICARE Prime Remote
- TRICARE Prime Overseas
- U.S. Family Health Plan
- TRICARE Reserve Select
- TRICARE Retired Reserve
- TRICARE Young Adult
- TRICARE for Life
- TRICARE Plus
- Supplemental Health Care Program
- TRICARE Hospice Program

Veterans Health Administration Program
- Eligibility
- Enrollment
- Identification Card
- Benefits
- Provider
- Preauthorization

Claims Procedure
- Regional Contractor
- TRICARE Select and Veterans Health Administration (CHAMPVA)
- Access to Health Records
- Computer Matching and Privacy Protection Act of 1988

After Claims Submission
- TRICARE Summary Payment Voucher

ASSIGNMENT 8.1 REVIEW QUESTIONS

Part I Fill in the Blank

Review the objectives, key terms, glossary definitions of key terms, chapter information, and figures before completing the following review questions.

1. CHAMPUS, the acronym for Civilian Health and Medical Program of the Uniformed Services, is now called ______________________ and was organized to control escalating medical costs and to standardize benefits for active duty families and military retirees.

2. The regional contractor for TRICARE East is ____________________________.

3. An active duty service member is known as a/an ______________; once retired, this former member is called a/an ______________________________________.

4. An individual who qualifies for TRICARE is known as a/an __________________.

5. A system for verifying an individual's TRICARE eligibility is called

    ____.

6. Mrs. Hancock, a TRICARE beneficiary, lives 2 miles from a Uniformed Services Medical Treatment Facility but needs to be hospitalized for mental health care services at Orlando Medical Center, a civilian hospital. What type of certification does she require to receive care from a civilian hospital?

    ____

7. Active duty uniformed service personnel are issued a/an _______________ to be used for standard identification.

8. Military family members and retirees are issued a/an _______________to access health care benefits.

9. The maximum dollar amount that a TRICARE member has to pay in any fiscal year for covered medical benefits is referred to as the ______________________, after which TRICARE pays 100% of the allowable charges for the rest of the year.

10. The two primary TRICARE programs are _______________and _______________.

11. Programs that allow TRICARE Standard beneficiaries to receive treatment, services, or supplies from civilian providers are called ____________________________ and

    ____.

12. An individual who is located at TRICARE service centers who can help TRICARE beneficiaries and providers with preauthorization of medical services is a/an ________.

    ____

13. A voluntary TRICARE health maintenance organization type of option is known as

    ____.

14. A physician who is responsible for coordinating and managing all of the TRICARE Prime beneficiary's health care unless there is an emergency is a/an ______________.

15. TRICARE Prime provides the same covered services as TRICARE Select beneficiaries, plus there are additional __________________ and ________________ services.

16. A _______________ is an individual at military hospitals or clinics who is available to assist TRICARE beneficiaries to obtain medical care through the military and through TRICARE.

17. TRICARE Young Adult enrollees must be a dependant of an eligible uniformed service sponsor, unmarried, at least age ________, and not eligible to enroll in an employer-sponsored health plan.

18. TRICARE for Life is a program for TRICARE-eligible beneficiaries who are age _____.

19. The TRICARE ___________ program is designed to provide care and comfort to patients who are terminally ill.

20. CHAMPVA is the acronym for __________________________ now known as the ____.

21. Those individuals who serve in the United States Armed Forces, finish their service, and are honorably discharged are known as ____________.

22. Veterans Health Administration (CHAMPVA) is not an insurance program but is considered as a/an _________________ program.

23. Which individuals are entitled to Veterans Health Administration (CHAMPVA) medical benefits?

    a. ____

    b. ____

    ____

    c. ____

    ____

24. The public law establishing a person's right to review and contest inaccuracies in personal medical records is known as the ______________________________.

25. An organization that contracts with the government to process TRICARE and Veterans Health Administration (CHAMPVA) health insurance claims is known as a/an ____.

26. The time limit for submitting a TRICARE Standard or CHAMPVA claim for out-patient service is ________________________________; for inpatient service, it is ______________________________.

Part II Multiple Choice

Choose the best answer.

27. Effective January 1, 2018, the two TRICARE regions are designated as:
    a. Region West and Region South.
    b. Region North and Region South.
    c. Region East and Region West.
    d. Region South and Region East.

28. The catchment area for a specific geographic region is defined by zip code and is based on an area surrounding each Medical Treatment Facility in the U.S. of approximate radius:
    a. 30 miles.
    b. 40 miles.
    c. 50 miles.
    d. 100 miles.

29. An authorized civilian provider who has not signed a contract with a regional TRICARE contractor to give medical care to TRICARE beneficiaries but agrees to accept assignment on a case-by-case basis is known as a/an:
    a. authorized provider.
    b. network provider.
    c. nonnetwork participating provider.
    d. nonnetwork notparticipating provider.

30. The TRICARE fiscal year:
    a. begins January 1 and ends December 31.
    b. begins April 1 and ends March 30.
    c. begins June 1 and ends May 30.
    d. begins October 1 and ends September 30.

31. A health care professional who helps a patient who is under the TRICARE program obtain preauthorization for care is called a:
    a. primary care physician (PCP).
    b. health care finder (HCF).
    c. health benefits advisor (HBA).
    d. participating provider.

32. TRICARE Prime Remote is a managed plan that can only be used if the distance from both the sponsor's home and work addresses to a military hospital or clinic is more than:
    a. 30 miles.
    b. 40 miles.
    c. 50 miles.
    d. 100 miles.

33. TRICARE Prime Remote Overseas is an HMO-style managed care plan available in the designated remote overseas locations of:
    a. Europe-Australia, and Canada.
    b. Africa, Canada, and the Pacific.
    c. Latin America, Australia, and Canada.
    d. Eurasia-Africa, Latin America, Canada, and the Pacific.

34. Under the U.S. Family Health Plan, the designated provider for Upstate New York is:
    a. Johns Hopkins Medicine.
    b. Martin's Point Health Care.
    c. Brighton Marine Health Center.
    d. St. Vincent Catholic Medical Centers.

35. To qualify for TRICARE for Life (TFL), a beneficiary must be:
    a. a TRICARE beneficiary.
    b. eligible for Medicare Part A.
    c. enrolled in Medicare Part B.
    d. all of the above.

Part III True/False

Write "T" or "F" in the blank to indicate whether you think the statement is true or false.

_______ 36. TRICARE is funded by both the state and federal governments.

_______ 37. A Nonavailability Statement is for individuals who are seeking any type of emergency care service.

_______ 38. TRICARE beneficiaries who use nonauthorized providers and receive medical services may be responsible for their entire bill.

_______ 39. The catastrophic cap does not apply to noncovered TRICARE services.

_______ 40. The TRICARE Select program became effective January 1, 2017.

_______ 41. Referrals are not required for the TRICARE Select program.

_______ 42. TRICARE Prime Remote (TPR) is a program designed for military retirees and their families.

_______ 43. Beneficiaries of the Veterans Health Administration (CHAMPVA) program have complete freedom of choice in selecting their civilian health care providers.

_______ 44. A patient enrolled in the Veterans Health Administration (CHAMPVA) program does not need preauthorization for hospice services.

_______ 45. Service members move often, so it is prudent to ask beneficiaries enrolled in TRICARE to update their information during each office visit.

_______ 46. When transmitting a TRICARE claim, always send it to the TRICARE claims office nearest to the residence of the military sponsor.

_______ 47. TRICARE is considered primary to Medicare for persons younger than age 65 who have Medicare Part A as a result of a disability and who have enrolled in Medicare Part B.

_______ 48. CHAMPVA is considered primary to Medicare for persons younger than age 65 who are enrolled in Medicare Parts A and B.

_______ 49. TRICARE is considered primary to Worker's Compensation if the beneficiary is injured on the job or becomes ill because of his or her work.

_______ 50. If a provider participates with TRICARE, accepts assignment, and receives payment directly from the regional contractor, the patient will receive a copy of the voucher.

ASSIGNMENT 8.2 CRITICAL THINKING

Performance Objective

Task: After reading the scenarios, answer the following questions, using critical thinking skills.

Conditions: Use a pen or pencil.

Standards: Time: _______________ minutes

Accuracy: _______________

(Note: The time element and accuracy criteria may be given by your instructor.)

Directions: After reading the scenarios, answer the following questions, using your critical thinking skills. Record your answers on the blank lines.

1. If Bertha Evans is seen for an office visit and has other insurance besides TRICARE, and she is the dependant of an active military person, whom do you bill first?

   ____

   Reason: ____

2. If Jason Williams, a TRICARE beneficiary who became disabled at age 10 years and who is also receiving Medicare Part A and Medicare Part B benefits, is seen for a consultation, whom do you bill first?

   ____

   Reason: ____

3. If Tanner Vine, a Veterans Health Administration (CHAMPVA) and Medicaid beneficiary, is seen on an emergency basis in the office, whom do you bill first?

   ____

   Reason: ____

9 Workers' Compensation

Linda M. Smith

KEY TERMS

Your instructor may wish to select some words pertinent to this chapter for a test. For definitions of the terms, further study, and/or reference, the words, phrases, and abbreviations may be found in the glossary at the end of the Textbook. *Key terms for this chapter follow.*

accident
adjudication
claims examiner
compromise and release
deposition
ergonomic
extraterritorial
Federal Employees' Compensation Act
injury
insurance adjuster
lien
medical service order
nondisability claim
occupational illness or disease
Occupational Safety and Health Administration
Office of Workers' Compensation Programs
permanent and stationary
permanent disability
petition
reexamination report
second-injury fund
sequelae
state-run program
sub rosa films
subsequent-injury fund
temporary disability
third-party liability
third-party subrogation
waiting period
work hardening
Workers' Compensation Appeals Board
workers' compensation insurance

KEY ABBREVIATIONS

See how many abbreviations and acronyms you can translate and then use this as a handy reference list. Definitions for the key abbreviations are located near the back of the Textbook *in the glossary.*

AME ______________________

C and R ______________________

ERISA ______________________

FECA ______________________

IME ______________________

LHWCA ______________________

OSHA ______________________

OWCP ______________________

P and S ______________________

PD ______________________

QME ______________________

ROM ______________________

SIF ______________________

TD ______________________

WCAB ______________________

WP ______________________

PERFORMANCE OBJECTIVES

The student will be able to:

- Define and spell the key terms and key abbreviations for this chapter, given the information from the *Textbook* glossary, within a reasonable time period and with enough accuracy to obtain a satisfactory evaluation.
- After reading the chapter, answer the fill in the blank, multiple choice, and true/false review questions with enough accuracy to obtain a satisfactory evaluation.
- Given a list of common medical abbreviations and symbols that appear in chart notes, fill in the correct meaning of each abbreviation within a reasonable time period and with enough accuracy to obtain a satisfactory evaluation. Students may use a medical dictionary or internet resource.
- Given the patients' medical chart notes and blank workers' compensation forms, complete each workers' compensation form related to billing within a reasonable time period and with enough accuracy to obtain a satisfactory evaluation.

STUDY OUTLINE

History
- Workers' Compensation Statutes
- Workers' Compensation Reform

Workers' Compensation Laws and Insurance
- Purposes of Workers' Compensation Laws
- Program Funding
- Self-Insurance
- Managed Care

Eligibility
- Work-Related Accident
- Occupational Illness

Coverage
- Federal Laws
- State Laws

Types of State Compensation Benefits

Types of State Workers' Compensation Claims
- Nondisability Claim
- Temporary Disability Claim
- Permanent Disability Claim

Fraud and Abuse

Legal Situations
- Medical Evaluator
- Depositions
- Medical Testimony
- Liens
- Third-Party Subrogation

Medical Reports
- Health Information Record Keeping
- Terminology

Reporting Requirements
- Employer's Report
- Medical Service Order
- Physician's First Report
- Progress or Supplemental Report
- Final Report

Claim Submission
- Financial Responsibility
- Fee Schedules
- Helpful Billing Tips
- Billing Claims
- Out-of-State Claims
- Delinquent or Slow Pay Claims

ASSIGNMENT 9.1 REVIEW QUESTIONS

Part I Fill in the Blank

Review the objectives, key terms, glossary definitions of key terms, chapter information, and figures before completing the following review questions.

1. Individuals who are paid by someone in exchange for labor or services are referred to as

   ______________________________.

2. Name two kinds of statutes under workers' compensation.

   a. ______________________________

   b. ______________________________

3. List five reasons that workers' compensation laws were developed.

   a. ______________________________

   b. ______________________________

   c. ______________________________

   d. ______________________________

   e. ______________________________

4. ____________ pays the workers' compensation insurance premiums.

5. State three methods used for funding workers' compensation.

   a. ______________________________

   b. ______________________________

   c. ______________________________

6. Self-insured employers are governed by ______________, a federal law that sets minimum requirements for group health plans.

7. A form of self-insurance that is owned by its policyholders and serves smaller or mid-size companies is known as __________.

8. When an employee with a preexisting condition is injured at work and the injury produces a disability greater than what would have been caused by the second injury alone, the benefits are drawn from a/an

   ______________________________.

9. An unexpected, unintended event that occurs at a particular time and place, causing injury to an individual not of his or her own making, is called a/an

   ______________________________.

10. Maria Cardoza works in a plastics manufacturing company and inhales some fumes that cause bronchitis. Because this condition is associated with her employment, it is called a/an

    ______________________________.

11. Name the federal workers' compensation acts that cover workers.

a. ______________________________

b. ______________________________

c. ______________________________

d. ______________________________

12. Federal law mandates that states set up laws to meet ______________ requirements.

13. State compensation laws that require each employer to accept its provisions and to provide for specialized benefits for employees who are injured at work are called

______________________________.

14. State compensation laws that may be accepted or rejected by the employer are known as ______________________________

______________________________.

15. When billing for an injury of a patient who lives out-of-state, the insurance billing specialist should follow the rules and fee schedule of the state in which the workers' compensation claim was ___________ filed.

16. The waiting period for income and medical benefits in your state is ______________.

17. List five types of workers' compensation benefits.

a. ______________________________

b. ______________________________

c. ______________________________

d. ______________________________

e. ______________________________

18. Who can treat an industrial injury?

____

____

19. What are three types of workers' compensation claims and the differences among them?

a. ______________________________

b. ______________________________

c. ______________________________

20. Weekly temporary disability payments are based on

______________________________.

21. After suffering an industrial injury, Mr. Fields is in a treatment program in which he is given real work tasks for building strength and endurance. This form of therapy is called ______________________________.

22. When an industrial case reaches the time for rating the disability, this is accomplished by what state agency? ______________________________

23. May an injured person appeal his or her case if he or she is not satisfied with the rating? ______________________ If so, to whom does he or she appeal? ______________________ or ______________________

24. When fraud or abuse is suspected in a workers' compensation case, the physician should report the situation to ______________________.

25. Physicians who conduct medical–legal evaluations of injured workers must pass a complex medical examination to become certified by the ______________ Council.

26. A proceeding that generally takes place in an attorney's office in which an attorney asks a witness questions about a case and the witness answers under oath is referred to as a/an ______________________.

27. In a workers' compensation case, when a claim is made against a separate person or company, but not the employer, it is referred to as a ______________ liability.

28. Explain third-party subrogation.

____

____

29. When an individual suffers a work-related injury or illness, the employer must complete and send a form called a/an ______________________ to the insurance company and workers' compensation state offices, and if the employee is sent to a physician's office for medical care, the employer must complete a form called a/an ______________________, which authorizes the physician to treat the employee.

30. Temporary disability ends when the patient is able to return to work or if the disability lasts longer than __________ months.

Part II Multiple Choice

Choose the best answer.

31. Employers are required to meet health and safety standards for their employees under federal and state statutes known as the:
    a. Occupational Safety and Health Administration (OSHA) Act of 1970.
    b. Health Insurance Portability and Accountability Act (HIPAA).
    c. Clinical Laboratory Improvement Amendment (CLIA).
    d. Employee Retirement Income Security Act (ERISA).

32. The process of carrying on a lawsuit is called:
    a. lien.
    b. litigation.
    c. deposition.
    d. adjudication.

33. A proceeding during which an attorney questions a witness who answers under oath but not in open court is called a:
    a. subpoena.
    b. subrogation.
    c. petition.
    d. deposition.

34. The legal claim on the property of another for payment of a debt is termed a:
    a. medical service order.
    b. subpoena.
    c. lien.
    d. promissory note.

35. The contract for treatment and the financial responsibility in a workers' compensation case is between:
    a. the health care organization and the patient.
    b. the health care organization and the employer.
    c. the health care organization and the workers' compensation insurance carrier.
    d. the employer and the workers' compensation insurance carrier.

36. Workers' compensation fee schedules that consider the time, skills, and extent of the service provided by the physician are:
    a. maximum fee schedules.
    b. relative value scale fee schedules.
    c. Medicare-based fee schedules.
    d. compulsory fee schedules.

Part III True/False

Write "T" or "F" in the blank to indicate whether you think the statement is true or false.

_______ 37. When working for the ABC Machining Company, an employee cuts his finger off while using a lathe. He is covered under workers' compensation.

_______ 38. A roofer takes his girlfriend to a roofing job and she is injured. She is covered under workers' compensation insurance.

_______ 39. A private duty nurse employed by the XYZ homecare service is injured while moving a patient. She is covered under workers' compensation insurance.

_______ 40. A Department of Energy subcontractor diagnosed with a disease resulting from exposure to radiation is covered under workers' compensation.

_______ 41. A postal worker twists his ankle while delivering mail. He is covered under workers' compensation.

_______ 42. An employee who is at an official company retreat suffers from a concussion due to a fall. The injury would be covered under workers' compensation.

_______ 43. An independent contractor is injured while working for a local construction company. The construction company's workers' compensation would cover the related medical bills.

_______ 44. If an individual seeks medical care for a workers' compensation injury from another state, the state's regulations are followed in which the injured person's claim was originally filed.

_______ 45. When a patient arrives at a medical office and says he or she was hurt at work, you should verify insurance information with the benefits coordinator for the employer.

_______ 46. A stamped physician's signature is acceptable on the Doctor's First Report of Occupational Injury or Illness form.

ASSIGNMENT 9.2 COMPLETE A DOCTOR'S FIRST REPORT OF OCCUPATIONAL INJURY OR ILLNESS FORM FOR A WORKERS' COMPENSATION CASE

Performance Objective

Task: Complete a Doctor's First Report of Occupational Injury or Illness form and define patient record abbreviations.

Conditions: Use the patient's record (Fig. 9.1), a Doctor's First Report of Occupational Injury or Illness form (Fig. 9.2), and a computer.

Standards: Claim Productivity Measurement

Time: ________________ minutes

Accuracy: ________________

(Note: The time element and accuracy criteria may be given by your instructor.)

Directions:

1. Complete the Doctor's First Report of Occupational Injury or Illness form (see Fig. 9.2) for this nondisability type of claim.

2. Using a medical dictionary or an internet resource, define abbreviations found in the patient's medical record.

After the instructor has returned your work to you, either make the necessary corrections and place your work in a three-ring notebook for future reference or, if you received a high score, place it in your portfolio for reference when applying for a job.

Abbreviations pertinent to this record:

apt ________________

lt ________________

pt ________________

ED ________________

hosp ________________

ER ________________

C ________________

HX ________________

PX ________________

c/o ________________

L ________________

CT ________________

neg ________________

MC ________________

MDM ________________

DC ________________

PD ________________

FU ________________

wks ________________

approx ________________

RTW ________________

WC ________________

PATIENT RECORD NO. 15-2-3

LAST NAME	FIRST NAME	MIDDLE NAME	BIRTH DATE	SEX	HOME PHONE
Hiranuma	Glen	M.	12-24-55	M	555-467-3383

ADDRESS	CITY	STATE	ZIP CODE
4372 Hanley Avenue	Woodland Hills	XY	12345

CELL PHONE	PAGER NO.	FAX NO.	E-MAIL ADDRESS
555-908-3433		555-467-3383	hiranuma@wb.net

PATIENT'S SOC. SEC. NO.	DRIVER'S LICENSE
558-XX-9960	U3402189

PATIENT'S OCCUPATION	NAME OF COMPANY
house painter	Pittsburgh Paint Company (commercial painting company)

ADDRESS OF EMPLOYER	PHONE
3725 Bonfeld Avenue, Woodland Hills, XY 12345	555-486-9070

SPOUSE OR PARENT	OCCUPATION
Esme M. Hiranuma	homemaker

EMPLOYER	ADDRESS	PHONE

NAME OF INSURANCE: State Compensation Insurance Fund, 14156 Magnolia Boulevard, Torres, XY 12349

POLICY/CERTIFICATE NO.	GROUP NO.
016-2432-211	

REFERRED BY: Pittsburgh Paint Company

DATE	PROGRESS NOTES
5-22-xx	At 9:30 a.m. this ♂ house painter was painting an apt ceiling (apt located at 3540 W. 87th Street, Woodland Hills, XY 12345, County of Woodland Hills) when he slipped and fell from a tall ladder landing on his head and lt side of body; brief unconsciousness for approximately 15 minutes. Employer was notified by coworker and pt was sent to College Hosp ED. I was called to the hosp at request of employer and saw pt in ER at 5 PM (performed a C HX/PX). Pt c/o L shoulder pain and swelling; L leg and hip pain; neck and head pain. X-rays were taken of lt hip (complete), lt femur (2 views), and cervical spine (3 views) as well as CT of brain (without contrast)—all neg. I admitted pt for overnight stay in hosp for concussion. Applied sling for L shoulder sprain. Cleaned and dressed L hip and leg abrasions (MC/MDM). Plan to DC 5/23/xx. No PD expected. Pt to FU in 2 wks. Approx. RTW 6/6 xx. Prepared WC report.
	GP/llf Gerald Practon, MD
5-23-xx	Pt's HA gone. Vital signs normal. Discharged home. RTO 1 wk.
	GP/llf Gerald Practon, MD

Fig. 9.1

STATE OF CALIFORNIA

DOCTOR'S FIRST REPORT OF OCCUPATIONAL INJURY OR ILLNESS

Within 5 days of your initial examination, for every occupational injury or illness, send two copies of this report to the employer's workers' compensation insurance carrier or the insured employer. Failure to file a timely doctor's report may result in assessment of a civil penalty. In the case of diagnosed or suspected pesticide poisoning, send a copy of the report to Division of Labor Statistics and Research, P.O. Box 420603, San Francisco, CA 94142-0603, and notify your local health officer by telephone within 24 hours.

			PLEASE DO NOT USE THIS COLUMN
1. INSURER NAME AND ADDRESS			
2. EMPLOYER NAME			Case No.
3. Address No. and Street City Zip			Industry
4. Nature of business (e.g., food manufacturing, building construction, retailer of women's clothes.)			County
5. **PATIENT NAME** (first name, middle initial, last name)	6. Sex ☐ Male ☐ Female	7. Date of Birth Mo. Day Yr.	Age
8. Address: No. and Street City Zip		9. Telephone number ( )	Hazard
10. Occupation (Specific job title)		11. Social Security Number - -	Disease
12. Injured at: No. and Street City County			Hospitalization
13. Date and hour of injury or onset of illness Mo. Day Yr. Hour ______ a.m. ______ p.m.		14. Date last worked Mo. Day Yr.	Occupation
15. Date and hour of first examination or treatment Mo. Day Yr. Hour ______ a.m. ______ p.m.		16. Have you (or your office) previously treated patient? ☐ Yes ☐ No	Return Date/Code

Patient please complete this portion, if able to do so. Otherwise, doctor please complete immediately, inability or failure of a patient to complete this portion shall not affect his/her rights to workers' compensation under the California Labor Code.

17. **DESCRIBE HOW THE ACCIDENT OR EXPOSURE HAPPENED.** (Give specific object, machinery or chemical. Use reverse side if more space is required.)

18. **SUBJECTIVE COMPLAINTS** (Describe fully. Use reverse side if more space is required.)

19. **OBJECTIVE FINDINGS** (Use reverse side if more space is required.)
A. Physical examination

B. X-ray and laboratory results (State if non or pending.)

20. **DIAGNOSIS** (if occupational illness specify etiologic agent and duration of exposure.) Chemical or toxic compounds involved? ☐ Yes ☐ No
ICD-9 Code ___ ___ ___ - ___ ___

21. Are your findings and diagnosis consistent with patient's account of injury or onset of illness? ☐ Yes ☐ No If "no", please explain.

22. Is there any other current condition that will impede or delay patient's recovery? ☐ Yes ☐ No If "yes", please explain.

23. **TREATMENT RENDERED** (Use reverse side if more space is required.)

24. If further treatment required, specify treatment plan/estimated duration.

25. If hospitalized as inpatient, give hospital name and location Date admitted Mo. Day Yr. Estimated stay

26. WORK STATUS -- Is patient able to perform usual work? ☐ Yes ☐ No
If "no", date when patient can return to: Regular work ___/___/___
Modified work ___/___/___ Specify restrictions ______________________

Doctor's Signature ______________________ CA License Number ______________________

Doctor Name and Degree (please type) ______________________ IRS Number ______________________

Address ______________________ Telephone Number (____)______________________

FORM 5021 (Rev. 4)
1992

Any person who makes or causes to be made any knowingly false or fraudulent material statement or material representation for the purpose of obtaining or denying workers' compensation benefits or payments is guilty of a felony.

Fig. 9.2

ASSIGNMENT 9.3 COMPLETE A DOCTOR'S FIRST REPORT OF OCCUPATIONAL INJURY OR ILLNESS FORM FOR A WORKERS' COMPENSATION CASE

Performance Objective

Task: Complete a Doctor's First Report of Occupational Injury or Illness form and define patient record abbreviations.

Conditions: Use the patient's record (Fig. 9.3a and 9.3b), a Doctor's First Report of Occupational Injury or Illness form (Fig. 9.4), and a computer.

Standards: Claim Productivity Measurement

Time: ______________ minutes

Accuracy: ________________

(Note: The time element and accuracy criteria may be given by your instructor.)

Directions:

1. Complete the Doctor's First Report of Occupational Injury or Illness form for this temporary disability type of claim. Refer to Carlos A. Giovanni's patient record for November 11 through November 15.

2. Using a medical dictionary or an internet resource, define abbreviations found in the patient's medical record.

After the instructor has returned your work to you, either make the necessary corrections and place your work in a three-ring notebook for future reference or, if you received a high score, place it in your portfolio for reference when applying for a job.

Abbreviations pertinent to this record:

pt	______________	H	______________
ER	______________	MDM	______________
C	______________	TD	______________
HX	______________	RTW	______________
PX	______________	approx	______________
CT	______________	HV	______________
R	______________	EPF	______________
tr	______________	M	______________
adm	______________	PO	______________
DC	______________	PF	______________
hosp	______________	SF	______________
OV	______________	X	______________
LC	______________	adv	______________
HA	______________	trt	______________
BP	______________	reg	______________
RTO	______________	W	______________
wks	______________	cons	______________

PATIENT RECORD NO. 15-4-5

LAST NAME	FIRST NAME	MIDDLE NAME	BIRTH DATE	SEX	HOME PHONE
Giovanni	Carlos	A.	10-24-55	M	555-677-3485

ADDRESS	CITY	STATE	ZIP CODE
89 Beaumont Court	Woodland Hills	XY	12345

CELL PHONE	PAGER NO.	FAX NO.	E-MAIL ADDRESS
	555-230-7788	555-677-3485	giovannic@wb.net

PATIENT'S SOC. SEC. NO.	DRIVER'S LICENSE
556-XX-9699	Y0394876

PATIENT'S OCCUPATION	NAME OF COMPANY
TV repairman	Giant Television Co. (TV repair company)

ADDRESS OF EMPLOYER	PHONE
8764 Ocean Avenue, Woodland Hills, XY 12345	555-647-8851

SPOUSE OR PARENT	OCCUPATION
Maria B. Giovanni	homemaker

EMPLOYER	ADDRESS	PHONE

NAME OF INSURANCE
State Compensation Insurance Fund, 600 S. Lafayette Park Place, Ehrlich, XY 12350

POLICY/CERTIFICATE NO.	GROUP NO.
57780	

REFERRED BY: Giant Television Company

Fig. 9.3a

Patient: Giovanni, Carlos A. Patient Record No. 15-04-05

DATE	PROGRESS NOTES
11-11-xx	Pt referred to College Hospital ER by employer for workers' compensation injury. I was called in as on-call neurosurgeon to evaluate the pt. Pt states that today at 2 PM he fell from the roof of a private home while installing an antenna at 2231 Duarte St., Woodland Hills, XY 12345 in Woodland Hills County. He describes the incident as follows: "When I was attaching the base of an antenna, the weight of the antenna shifted and knocked me off the roof." Pt complains of head pain and indicates brief loss of consciousness. I performed a C HX/PX. Complete skull x-rays showed fractured skull. CT of head/brain (without contrast) indicates well-defined R. subdural hematoma. Pt suffering from cerebral concussion; no open wound. Tr plan: Adm pt to College Hospital (5 PM) and schedule R infratentorial craniotomy to evacuate hematoma. (H/MDM). Obtained authorization and prepared Dr.'s First Report.
	AP/llf Astro Parkinson, MD
11-12-xx	Performed R infratentorial craniotomy and evacuated subdural hematoma. Pt stable and returned to room; will be seen daily. TD: Estimated RTW 1-15-xx. Possible cranial defect & head disfigurement resulting. Pt to be hospitalized for approx 2 weeks.
	AP/llf Astro Parkinson, MD
11-13-xx	HV (EPF HX/PX M/MDM). Pt improving; recommend consult with Dr. Graff for cranial defect. Authorization obtained from adjuster (Steve Burroughs) at State Comp.
	AP/llf Astro Parkinson, MD
11-14-xx	Pt seen in cons by Dr. Cosmo Graff who stated he does not recommend correcting PO cranial defect. Both Dr. Graff and I explained how the defect resulted from the injury; there may be some improvement over time. Pt states he is grateful to be alive (EPF HX/PX M/MDM).
	AP/llf Astro Parkinson, MD
11-15-xx	Daily HV (EPF HX/PX M/MDM). Pt progressing appropriately; no complications have occurred.
thru	
11-29-xx	AP/llf Astro Parkinson, MD
11-30-xx	DC from hosp. Permanent cranial defect resulting from fracture and surgery. RTO 1 wk.
	AP/llf Astro Parkinson, MD
12-7-xx	OV (EPF HX/PX LC/MDM) Pt doing very well. No HA or visual disturbances, BP 120/80, alert and oriented. He is anxious to return to work. Pt cautioned about maintaining low activity level until released. RTO 2 wks.
	AP/llf Astro Parkinson, MD
12-21-xx	OV (PF HX/PX SF/MDM). Pt continues to improve. Suggested he start a walking program 3 x wk and monitor symptoms. May do light activity and lifting (10 lbs). Adv to call if any symptoms return. RTO 10 days.
	AP/llf Astro Parkinson, MD
12-29-xx	OV (PF HX/PX SF/MDM). Pt did not experience any symptoms with increased activity. No further trt necessary. Pt will increase activity and call if any problems occur. Pt scheduled to resume reg W on 1-15-xx. Final report submitted to workers' compensation carrier.
	AP/llf Astro Parkinson, MD

Fig. 9.3b, cont'd

STATE OF CALIFORNIA

DOCTOR'S FIRST REPORT OF OCCUPATIONAL INJURY OR ILLNESS

Within 5 days of your initial examination, for every occupational injury or illness, send two copies of this report to the employer's workers' compensation insurance carrier or the insured employer. Failure to file a timely doctor's report may result in assessment of a civil penalty. In the case of diagnosed or suspected pesticide poisoning, send a copy of the report to Division of Labor Statistics and Research, P.O. Box 420603, San Francisco, CA 94142-0603, and notify your local health officer by telephone within 24 hours.

	PLEASE DO NOT USE THIS COLUMN
1. **INSURER NAME AND ADDRESS**	
2. **EMPLOYER NAME**	Case No.
3. Address No. and Street City Zip	Industry
4. Nature of business (e.g., food manufacturing, building construction, retailer of women's clothes.)	County
5. **PATIENT NAME** (first name, middle initial, last name) / 6. Sex ☐ Male ☐ Female / 7. Date of Birth Mo. Day Yr.	Age
8. Address: No. and Street City Zip / 9. Telephone number ( )	Hazard
10. Occupation (Specific job title) / 11. Social Security Number - -	Disease
12. Injured at: No. and Street City County	Hospitalization
13. Date and hour of injury or onset of illness Mo. Day Yr. Hour ______ a.m. ______ p.m. / 14. Date last worked Mo. Day Yr.	Occupation
15. Date and hour of first examination or treatment Mo. Day Yr. Hour ______ a.m. ______ p.m. / 16. Have you (or your office) previously treated patient? ☐ Yes ☐ No	Return Date/Code

Patient please complete this portion, if able to do so. Otherwise, doctor please complete immediately, inability or failure of a patient to complete this portion shall not affect his/her rights to workers' compensation under the California Labor Code.

17. **DESCRIBE HOW THE ACCIDENT OR EXPOSURE HAPPENED.** (Give specific object, machinery or chemical. Use reverse side if more space is required.)

18. **SUBJECTIVE COMPLAINTS** (Describe fully. Use reverse side if more space is required.)

19. **OBJECTIVE FINDINGS** (Use reverse side if more space is required.)
 A. Physical examination

 B. X-ray and laboratory results (State if non or pending.)

20. **DIAGNOSIS** (if occupational illness specify etiologic agent and duration of exposure.) Chemical or toxic compounds involved? ☐ Yes ☐ No
ICD-9 Code ___ ___ ___ - ___ ___

21. Are your findings and diagnosis consistent with patient's account of injury or onset of illness? ☐ Yes ☐ No If "no", please explain.

22. Is there any other current condition that will impede or delay patient's recovery? ☐ Yes ☐ No If "yes", please explain.

23. **TREATMENT RENDERED** (Use reverse side if more space is required.)

24. If further treatment required, specify treatment plan/estimated duration.

25. If hospitalized as inpatient, give hospital name and location Date admitted Mo. Day Yr. Estimated stay

26. WORK STATUS -- Is patient able to perform usual work? ☐ Yes ☐ No
 If "no", date when patient can return to: Regular work ___/___/___
 Modified work ___/___/___ Specify restrictions ______________________

Doctor's Signature ______________________ CA License Number ______________________

Doctor Name and Degree (please type) ______________________ IRS Number ______________________

Address ______________________ Telephone Number (____)______________________

FORM 5021 (Rev. 4)
1992

Any person who makes or causes to be made any knowingly false or fraudulent material statement or material representation for the purpose of obtaining or denying workers' compensation benefits or payments is guilty of a felony.

Fig. 9.4

10 Disability Income Insurance and Disability Benefits Programs

Linda M. Smith

KEY TERMS

Your instructor may wish to select some words pertinent to this chapter for a test. For definitions of the terms, further study, and/or reference, the words, phrases, and abbreviations may be found in the glossary at the end of the Textbook.

Some of the insurance terms presented in this chapter are shown marked with an asterisk (*) and may seem familiar from previous chapters. However, their meanings may or may not have a slightly different connotation when referring to disability income insurance. Key terms for this chapter follow.

accidental death and dismemberment
Armed Services Disability
benefit period*
Civil Service Retirement System
consultative examiner
cost-of-living adjustment
Disability Determination Services
disability income insurance
double indemnity
exclusions*
Federal Employees Retirement System
future purchase option
guaranteed renewable*
hearing
long-term disability insurance
noncancelable clause*
Non-VA Medical Care Program
partial disability*
reconsideration
residual benefits*
residual disability
short-term disability insurance
Social Security Administration
Social Security Disability Insurance program
State Disability Insurance
supplemental benefits
Supplemental Security Income
temporary disability*
temporary disability insurance
total disability*
unemployment compensation disability
Veterans Affairs disability program
Veterans Affairs outpatient clinic card
voluntary disability insurance
waiting period*
waiver of premium*

KEY ABBREVIATIONS

See how many abbreviations and acronyms you can translate and then use this as a handy reference list. Definitions for the key abbreviations are located near the back of the Textbook *in the glossary.*

AIDS ______________________

CE ______________________

COLA ______________________

CSRS ______________________

DDS ______________________

FERS ______________________

HIV ______________________

OASDI ______________________

SDI ______________________

SSA ______________________

SSDI program ______________________

SSI ______________________

TDI ______________________

UCD ______________________

VA ______________________

PERFORMANCE OBJECTIVES

The student will be able to:

- Define and spell the key terms and key abbreviations for this chapter, given the information from the *Textbook* glossary, within a reasonable time period, and with enough accuracy to obtain a satisfactory evaluation.
- After reading the chapter, answer the fill in the blank, multiple choice, and true/false review questions with enough accuracy to obtain a satisfactory evaluation.
- Fill in the correct meaning of each abbreviation, given a list of common medical abbreviations and symbols that appear in chart notes, within a reasonable time period and with enough accuracy to obtain a satisfactory evaluation.
- Complete each state disability form, given the patients' medical chart notes and blank state disability forms, within a reasonable time period and with enough accuracy to obtain a satisfactory evaluation.

STUDY OUTLINE

Disability Claims
History
Disability Income Insurance
  Individual
  Group
Federal Disability Programs
  Workers' Compensation
  Disability Benefit Programs
State Disability Insurance
  Background
  Funding
  Eligibility
  Benefits
  Time Limits
  Medical Examinations
  Restrictions
Voluntary Disability Insurance
Claims Submission Guidelines
  Disability Income Claims
Conclusion

ASSIGNMENT 10.1 REVIEW QUESTIONS

Part I Fill in the Blank

Review the objectives, key terms, glossary definitions of key terms, chapter information, and figures before completing the following review questions.

1. Insurance that provides monthly or weekly income when an individual is unable to work because of a nonindustrial illness or injury is called

   ____.

2. A ______________ is the maximum amount of time that benefits will be paid to the injured or ill person for the disability.

3. When an individual who is insured under a disability income insurance policy cannot perform one or more of his or her regular job duties, this is known as

   ______________ or ______________________________
   disability.

4. Ezra Jackson has disability income insurance under a group policy paid for by his employer. Ezra makes no contribution toward the policy premiums. One evening he goes inline skating and suffers a complex fracture of the patella, which necessitates several months off from work. Are his monthly disability benefits taxable?

   ______________________ Why or why not? ______________________

   ____

5. Some insurance contracts that pay twice the face amount of the policy if accidental death occurs may have a provision titled ______________________.

6. When an individual becomes permanently disabled and cannot pay the insurance premium, a desirable provision in an insurance contract is ______________________.

7. Give three examples of preexisting conditions that may be written into a disability contract as exclusions:

   a. ____

   b. ____

   c. ____

8. Two federal programs for individuals younger than 65 years of age who have a severe disability are:

   a. ____

   b. ____

9. The strict definition of *Disability* given by Social Security is ______________

   ____.

10. When applying for SSDI benefits, there is a ______________ waiting period during which time the individual will not receive SSA benefits.

11. The __________ program pays monthly income benefits to adults and children with limited income and resources who are disabled, blind, or age 65 or older.

12. The Social Security Administration may hire a physician to evaluate an applicant's disability. A physician's role may be any one of the following:

a. ____________________

b. ____________________

c. ____________________

13. If Disability Determination Services determines that the claimant is not eligible for disability benefits, the first level of the appeals process is referred to as ____________________.

14. The two types of federal retirement which have provisions for those who become disabled are ____________________ and ____________________.

15. Jamie Woods, a Navy petty officer, suffered an accident aboard the USS *Denebola* three weeks after his honorable discharge. To receive veteran's benefits for this injury, the time limit in which a claim must be filed is ____________________.

16. Name the states and the territory that have nonindustrial state disability programs.

a. ____________________

b. ____________________

c. ____________________

d. ____________________

e. ____________________

f. ____________________

17. In your state, temporary disability insurance claims must be filed within __________ days.

18. How long can a person continue to draw state disability insurance benefits?

____

19. After a claim begins, when do basic state disability benefits become payable if the patient is confined to his or her home? ____________________ If the patient is hospitalized? ____________________

20. Nick Tyson has recovered since a previous illness ended and becomes ill again with the same ailment. Is he entitled to state disability benefits? ____________________

21. John S. Thatcher stubbed his toe as he was leaving work and going to his car parked on the street. Because the injury was only slightly uncomfortable, he thought no more about it. The next morning he found that his foot was too swollen to fit in his shoe, so he stayed home. When the swelling did not subside after three days, John went to the doctor. Radiographs showed a broken toe, which kept John home for two weeks. After one week he applied for temporary state disability benefits.

    Will he be paid? ____________________

    Why or why not? ____________________

22. Peggy Jonson has an ectopic pregnancy and is unable to work because of complications of this condition. Can she receive state temporary disability benefits?

    ____

23. Four states that allow for maternity benefits in normal pregnancy are:

    a. ____________________

    b. ____________________

    c. ____________________

    d. ____________________

24. Betty T. Kraft had to stay home from her job because her 10-year-old daughter had measles. She applied for temporary state disability benefits.

    Will she be paid? ____________________

    Why or why not? ____________________

25. Vincent P. Michael was ill with a bad cold for one week. Will he receive temporary state disability benefits? ____________________

    Why or why not? ____________________

26. Betsy C. Palm works in Hawaii and had an emergency appendectomy. She was hospitalized for three days. Will she receive state disability benefits?

    ____

    Why or why not? ____________________

27. Frank E. Thompson is a box boy at a supermarket on Saturdays and Sundays while a full-time student at college. He broke his leg while skiing and cannot work at the market, but he is able to attend classes with his leg in a cast. Can he collect state disability benefits for his part-time job? ____________________

    Why or why not? ____________________

28. Jerry L. Slate is out of a job and is receiving unemployment insurance benefits. He is now suffering from severe intestinal flu. The employment office calls him to interview for a job, but he is too ill to go. Can he collect temporary state disability benefits for this illness when he might have been given a job?

____

Why or why not? ______________________________

29. While walking the picket line with other employees on strike, Gene J. Berry came down with pneumonia and was ill for two weeks. Can he collect temporary state disability benefits?

Why or why not? ______________________________

Gene went back to work for three weeks and then developed a slight cold and cough, which again was diagnosed as pneumonia. The doctor told him to stay home from work. Would he be able to collect temporary disability benefits?

____

Why or why not? ______________________________

30. A month after he retired, Roger Reagan had a gallbladder operation. Can he receive temporary state disability benefits?

Why or why not? ______________________________

31. Jane M. Lambert fell in the back yard of her home and fractured her left ankle. She had a nonunion fracture and could not work for 28 weeks. For how long will she collect temporary state disability benefits? ______________________________

32. Dr. Kay examines Ben Yates and completes a disability income claim form because of a prolonged illness. On receiving the information, the insurance adjuster notices some conflicting data. Name other documents that may be requested to justify payment of benefits.

a. ______________________________

b. ______________________________

c. ______________________________

33. Trent Walters, a permanently disabled individual, applies for federal disability benefits. To establish eligibility for benefits under this program, data allowed must be __________ year/years old.

34. A Veterans Affairs patient is seen on an emergency basis by Dr. Onion. Name the two methods or options for billing this case.

a. ______________________________

b. ______________________________

Part II Multiple Choice

Choose the best answer.

35. Another disability income insurance term for benefits is:
    a. indemnity.
    b. supplemental benefits.
    c. guarantee.
    d. compensation.

36. When the purchase of insurance is investigated, the words to look for in the insurance contract that mean the premium cannot be increased at renewal time are:
    a. guaranteed renewable.
    b. conditional provision.
    c. noncancelable clause.
    d. optional provision.

37. Provisions that limit the scope of insurance coverage are known as:
    a. clauses.
    b. deductibles.
    c. conditions.
    d. exclusions.

38. A Social Security Administration division that determines an individual's eligibility to be placed under the federal disability program is called:
    a. Disability Determination Services.
    b. Social Security Disability.
    c. Supplemental Security Income.
    d. none of the above.

39. The time period from the beginning of disability to receiving the first payment of benefits is called a/an:
    a. exclusion period.
    b. waiting period.
    c. insurance period.
    d. elimination phase.

40. The entity responsible for notifying the insurance company of a disability income claim is:
    a. the insured.
    b. the claimant.
    c. the physician.
    d. both a and b.

Part III True/False

Write "T" or "F" in the blank to indicate whether you think the statement is true or false.

________ 41. When a person insured under a disability income insurance policy cannot, for a limited period of time, perform all functions of his or her regular job duties, it is known as *permanent disability*.

________ 42. Disability income policies provide medical expense benefits.

________ 43. There is no standard definition for total disability.

________ 44. Eligibility for the SSI program is based strictly on financial need.

________ 45. To be eligible to apply for disability benefits under Social Security, an individual must be unable to perform any type of work for a period of not less than 12 months.

________ 46. Hospital benefits may be paid for nonoccupational illness or injury under state temporary disability benefits.

________ 47. If a woman has an abnormal condition that arises from her pregnancy (e.g., diabetes or varicose veins) and is unable to work because of the condition, she may not receive state disability benefits.

________ 48. When a claim form is submitted for a patient applying for state disability benefits, the most important item required on the form is the claimant's Social Security number.

________ 49. To justify payment of disability benefits, an insurance company may request an employee's wage statements.

________ 50. A person receiving state disability benefits must report any income received to the state disability insurance office because it can affect benefits.

ASSIGNMENT 10.2 COMPLETE TWO STATE DISABILITY INSURANCE FORMS

Performance Objective

Task: Complete two state disability insurance forms and define patient record abbreviations.

Conditions: Use the patient's record (Fig. 10.1), a New York State Notice and Proof of Claim for Disability Benefits (Fig. 10.2), and a computer.

Standards: Time: ____________ minutes

Accuracy: ____________

(Note: The time element and accuracy criteria may be given by your instructor.)

Directions:

1. To familiarize you with what information the employee must furnish, this assignment will encompass completing the New York State Notice and Proof of Claim for Disability Benefits.

2. Mr. Broussard (see Fig. 10.1) is applying for state disability benefits, and he does not receive sick leave pay from his employer. The language he prefers is English. He does not want any disclosure of benefit payment information to his employer. During his disability, he was not in the custody of law enforcement authorities for any violation and he has no alcoholic tendencies.

3. Date the Claimant's Information November 5 of the current year, and date the Health Care Provider's Statement November 10 of the current year.

4. Refer to Chapter 10 and Fig. 10.2 of the *Textbook* to assist you in completing this form.

After the instructor has returned your work to you, either make the necessary corrections and place your work in a three-ring notebook for future reference or, if you received a high score, place it in your portfolio for reference when applying for a job.

Abbreviations pertinent to this record:

NP	____________	c/o	____________
LBP	____________	pt	____________
lt	____________	wk	____________
reg	____________	exam	____________
SLR	____________	rt	____________
WNL	____________	STAT	____________
MRI	____________	RTO	____________
imp	____________	retn	____________

PATIENT RECORD

Broussard	Jeff	L.	03-09-52	M	555-466-2490
LAST NAME	FIRST NAME	MIDDLE NAME	BIRTH DATE	SEX	HOME PHONE

3577 Plain Street	Woodland Hills	XY	12345
ADDRESS	CITY	STATE	ZIP CODE

555-667-7654	555-399-5903	555-466-2490	broussard@wb.net
CELL PHONE	PAGER NO.	FAX NO.	E-MAIL ADDRESS

566-XX-0090	F0394588
PATIENT'S SOC. SEC. NO.	DRIVER'S LICENSE

carpenter Payroll #2156	Ace Construction Company
PATIENT'S OCCUPATION	NAME OF COMPANY

4556 West Eighth Street, Dorland, XY 12347	555-447-8900
ADDRESS OF EMPLOYER	PHONE

Harriet M. Broussard	secretary
SPOUSE OR PARENT	OCCUPATION

Merit Accounting Company, 6743 Main Street, Woodland Hills, XY 12345	555-478-0980
EMPLOYER ADDRESS	PHONE

Blue Cross	Jeff L. Broussard
NAME OF INSURANCE	INSURED OR SUBSCRIBER

466-XX-9979	6131
POLICY/CERTIFICATE NO.	GROUP NO.

REFERRED BY: Harold B. Hartburn (friend)

DATE	PROGRESS NOTES
10-21-xx	8:30 a.m. NP seen c/o ongoing LBP. On 9-12-xx after swinging a golf club, pt had sudden onset of severe pain in low back with radiation to lt side. Pt unable to work 9-13 but resumed wk on 8-17 and has been working full time but doing no lifting while working. Pain is exacerbating affecting his work and reg duties. Exam showed SLR strongly positive on lt, on rt causes pain into lt side. Neurological exam WNL. Ordered STAT MRI. Off work. RTO.
	RS/mtf Raymond Skeleton, MD
10-23-xx	Pt returns for test results. MRI showed huge defect of L4-5. Imp: acute herniated disc L4-5 with spinal stenosis. Recommended laminotomy, foraminotomy, and diskectomy L4-5.
	RS/mtf Raymond Skeleton, MD
11-1-xx	Admit to College Hospital. Operation: Lumbar laminotomy with exploration and decompression of spinal cord with diskectomy L4-5; lumbar anterior arthrodesis.
	RS/mtf Raymond Skeleton, MD
11-5-xx	Pt seen daily in hosp. At 3 p.m. pt discharged to home. Will retn to wk 12-15-XX.
	RS/mtf Raymond Skeleton, MD

Fig. 10.1

DB-450 9-17

New York State

NOTICE AND PROOF OF CLAIM FOR DISABILITY BENEFITS

Use this form if you became disabled **while employed** or if you became disabled **within four (4) weeks after termination of employment** OR if you became **disabled after having been unemployed for more than four (4) weeks**. Please answer all questions in Part A and questions 1 through 3 in Part B. Read all instructions on this form carefully. Health care providers must complete Part B on page 2.

PART A - CLAIMANT'S INFORMATION (Please Print or Type)

1. Last Name: ______ First Name: ______ MI: ___

2. Mailing Address (Street & Apt. #): ______

City: ______ State: ___ Zip: ______ Country: ______

3. Daytime Phone #: ______ 4. Email Address: ______

5. Social Security #: ___ - ___ - ___ 6. Date of Birth: ___ - ___ - ___ 7. Gender: ☐ Male ☐ Female

8. My disability is (if injury, also state how, when and where it occurred): ______

9. I became disabled or became ineligible for Unemployment Insurance because of this disability on: ___ / ___ / ___

I worked on that day: ☐ Yes ☐ No

Have you recovered from this disability? ☐ Yes ☐ No If Yes, what was the date you were able to work: ___ / ___ / ___

Have you since worked for wages or profit? ☐ Yes ☐ No If Yes, list dates: ______

10. Give name of last employer. If more than one employer during last eight (8) weeks, name all employers. Average Weekly Wage is based on all wages earned in last eight (8) weeks worked.

LAST EMPLOYER			PERIOD OF EMPLOYMENT		Average Weekly Wage (Include Bonuses, Tips, Commissions, Reasonable Value of Board, Rent, etc.)
Firm or Trade Name	Address	Phone Number	First Day	Last Day Worked	
			Mo. Day Yr.	Mo. Day Yr.	
OTHER EMPLOYER (during last eight (8) weeks)			**PERIOD OF EMPLOYMENT**		**Average Weekly Wage** (Include Bonuses, Tips, Commissions, Reasonable Value of Board, Rent, etc.)
Firm or Trade Name	Address	Phone Number	First Day	Last Day Worked	
			Mo. Day Yr.	Mo. Day Yr.	
			Mo. Day Yr.	Mo. Day Yr.	

11. My job is or was: ______ (Occupation) 12. Union Member: ☐ Yes ☐ No If "Yes": ______ (Name of Union or Local Number)

13. Were you claiming or receiving unemployment prior to this disability? ☐ Yes ☐ No

If you did **not** claim or if you claimed but did **not** receive unemployment insurance benefits after LAST DAY WORKED, explain reasons fully: ______

14. For the period of disability covered by this claim:

A. Are you **receiving** wages, salary or separation pay: ☐ Yes ☐ No

B. Are you **receiving** or **claiming**:

1. Workers' compensation for work-connected disability: ☐ Yes ☐ No
2. Paid Family Leave: ☐ Yes ☐ No
3. No-Fault motor vehicle accident (check box): ☐ Yes ☐ No or personal injury involving third party (check box): ☐ Yes ☐ No
4. Long-term disability benefits under the Federal Social Security Act for this disability: ☐ Yes ☐ No

IF "YES" IS CHECKED IN ANY OF THE ITEMS IN 14, COMPLETE THE FOLLOWING:

I have: ☐ received ☐ claimed from: ______ for the period: ___ / ___ / ___ to: ___ / ___ / ___

15. In the year (52 weeks) **before** your disability began, have you received disability benefits for other periods of disability? ☐ Yes ☐ No

If "Yes", fill in the following: Paid by: ______ from: ___ / ___ / ___ to: ___ / ___ / ___

16. In the year (52 weeks) **before** your disability began, have you received Paid Family Leave? ☐ Yes ☐ No

If "Yes", fill in the following: Paid by: ______ from: ___ / ___ / ___ to: ___ / ___ / ___

I hereby claim Disability Benefits and certify that for the period covered by this claim I was disabled. If my disability began while I was unemployed, I certify that I had been unemployed for more than four (4) weeks. I have read the instructions on page 2 of this form and that the foregoing statements, including any accompanying statements are, to the best of my knowledge, true and complete.

______ Claimant's Signature ______ Date

An individual may sign on behalf of the claimant only if he or she is legally authorized to do so and the claimant is a minor, mentally incompetent or incapacitated. If signed by other than claimant, print information below and complete and submit Form OC-110A, Claimant's Authorization to Disclose Workers' Compensation Records.

______ On behalf of Claimant ______ Address ______ Relationship to Claimant

DB-450 (9-17) Page 1 of 2

Fig. 10.2 (From New York State Workers' Compensation Board.)

Continued

PART B - HEALTH CARE PROVIDER'S STATEMENT (Please Print or Type)

THE HEALTH CARE PROVIDER'S STATEMENT MUST BE FILLED IN COMPLETELY. THE ATTENDING HEALTH CARE PROVIDER SHALL COMPLETE AND RETURN TO THE CLAIMANT WITHIN SEVEN (7) DAYS OF RECEIPT OF THIS FORM. For item 7-d, you must give estimated date. If disability is caused by or arising in connection with pregnancy, enter estimated delivery date in item 9. **INCOMPLETE ANSWERS MAY DELAY PAYMENT OF BENEFITS.**

1. Last Name: ____________________ First Name: ____________________ MI: ___

2.Gender: ☐ Male ☐ Female 3. Date of Birth: ___ / ___ / ___

4. Diagnosis/Analysis: ____________________ Diagnosis Code: ____________

a. Claimant's symptoms: ____________________

b. Objective findings: ____________________

5. Claimant hospitalized?: ☐ Yes ☐ No From: ___ / ___ / ___ To: ___ / ___ / ___

6. Operation indicated?: ☐ Yes ☐ No a. Type ____________ b. Date ___ / ___ / ___

7. ENTER DATES FOR THE FOLLOWING	MONTH	DAY	YEAR
a Date of your first treatment for this disability			
b. Date of your most recent treatment for this disability			
c. Date Claimant was unable to work because of this disability			
d. Date Claimant will again be able to perform work (Even if considerable question exists, estimate date. Avoid use of terms such as unknown or undetermined.)			
e. If pregnancy related, please check box and enter the date ☐ estimated delivery date OR ☐ actual delivery date			

8. In your opinion, is this disability the result of injury arising out of and in the course of employment or occupational disease?: ☐ Yes ☐ No If "Yes", has Form C-4 been filed with the Board? ☐ Yes ☐ No

I certify that I am a:

(Physician, Chiropractor, Dentist, Podiatrist, Psychologist, Nurse-Midwife) **Licensed or Certified in the State of** **License Number**

Health Care Provider's Printed Name **Health Care Provider's Signature** **Date**

Health Care Provider's Address **Phone #**

CLAIMANT: READ THESE INSTRUCTIONS CAREFULLY

PLEASE NOTE: Do not date and file this form prior to your first date of disability. In order for your claim to be processed, Parts A and B must be completed.

1. If you are using this form because you became disabled **while employed** or you became disabled **within four (4) weeks after termination of employment**, your completed claim should be mailed **within thirty (30) days to your employer or your last employer's insurance carrier**. You may find your employer's disability insurance carrier on the Workers' Compensation Board's website using Employer Coverage Search.

2. If you are using this form because you became **disabled after having been unemployed for more than four (4) weeks**, your completed claim should be mailed to: **Workers' Compensation Board, Disability Benefits Bureau, 328 State Street, Schenectady, NY 12305.** If you answered "Yes" to question 14.B.3, please complete and attach Form DB-450.1.

If you have any questions about claiming disability benefits, you may contact the Board's Disability Benefits Bureau at (800) 353-3092. Additional information may be obtained at the Board's website: www.wcb.ny.gov, or you may write to the Disability Benefits Bureau at the address listed above.

Notification Pursuant to the New York Personal Privacy Protection Law (Public Officers Law Article 6-A) and the Federal Privacy Act of 1974 (5 U.S.C. § 552a). The Workers' Compensation Board's (Board's) authority to request that claimants provide personal information, including their social security number, is derived from the Board's investigatory authority under Workers' Compensation Law (WCL) § 20, and its administrative authority under WCL § 142. This information is collected to assist the Board in investigating and administering claims in the most expedient manner possible and to help it maintain accurate claim records. Providing your social security number to the Board is voluntary. There is no penalty for failure to provide your social security number on this form; it will not result in a denial of your claim or a reduction in benefits. The Board will protect the confidentiality of all personal information in its possession, disclosing it only in furtherance of its official duties and in accordance with applicable state and federal law

HIPAA NOTICE - In order to adjudicate a workers' compensation claim or disability benefits claim, WCL 13-a(4)(a) and 12 NYCRR 325-1.3 require health care providers to regularly file medical reports of treatment with the Board and the insurance carrier or employer. Pursuant to 45 CFR 164.512 these legally required medical reports are exempt from HIPAA's restrictions on disclosure of health information.

Disclosure of Information: The Board will not disclose any information about your case to any unauthorized party without your consent. If you choose to have such information disclosed to an unauthorized party, you must file with the Board an original signed Form OC-110A, Claimant's Authorization to Disclose Workers' Compensation Records, or an original signed, notarized authorization letter. You may telephone your local WCB office to have Form OC-110A sent to you, or you may download it from our website, www.wcb.ny.gov. It can be found under Forms on the 'List of All Common Workers' Compensation Board Forms' web page. Mail the completed authorization form to the address listed above.

An employer or insurer, or any employee, agent, or person acting on behalf of an employer or insurer, who KNOWINGLY MAKES A FALSE STATEMENT OR REPRESENTATION as to a material fact in the course of reporting, investigation of, or adjusting a claim for any benefit or payment under this chapter for the purpose of avoiding provision of such payment or benefit SHALL BE GUILTY OF A CRIME AND SUBJECT TO SUBSTANTIAL FINES AND IMPRISONMENT.

DB-450 (9-17) Page 2 of 2

Fig. 10.2, cont'd

ASSIGNMENT 10.3 COMPLETE TWO STATE DISABILITY INSURANCE FORMS

Performance Objective

Task: Complete two state disability insurance forms and define patient record abbreviations.

Conditions: Use the patient's record (Fig. 10.3), a New York State Notice and Proof of Claim for Disability Benefits (Fig. 10.4), and a computer.

Standards: Time: ____________ minutes

Accuracy: ____________

(Note: The time element and accuracy criteria may be given by your instructor.)

Directions:

1. Assume that the Claim Statement of Employee has been completed satisfactorily by Mr. Fred E. Thorndike (see Fig. 10.3). Complete the New York State Notice and Proof of Claim for Disability Benefits (Fig. 10.4) and date it December 2. In completing this portion of the assignment, look at the first entry made by Dr. Practon on November 25 only.

2. Mr. Thorndike returns to see Dr. Practon on December 7, at which time his disability leave needs to be extended. Complete the Health Care Provider's Statement (Fig. 10.4) by referring to the entry made during the second visit, and date the certificate December 7. Remember that this is not a claim for payment to the physician, so no ledger card has been furnished for this patient.

3. Refer to Chapter 10 and Fig. 10.2 of the *Textbook* to assist you in completing these forms.

After the instructor has returned your work to you, either make the necessary corrections and place your work in a three-ring notebook for future reference or, if you received a high score, place it in your portfolio for reference when applying for a job.

Abbreviations pertinent to this record:

pt ____________________

PE ____________________

dx ____________________

RTO ____________________

est ____________________

$\overline{c}$ ____________________

reg ____________________

SDI ____________________

wks ____________________

Cont ____________________

wk ____________________

FU ____________________

CXR ____________________

PATIENT RECORD

Thorndike	Fred	E.	02-17-54	M	555-465-7820
LAST NAME	FIRST NAME	MIDDLE NAME	BIRTH DATE	SEX	HOME PHONE

5784 Helen Street	Woodland Hills	XY	12345
ADDRESS	CITY	STATE	ZIP CODE

555-432-7744	555-320-5500	555-466-7820	thorndike@wb.net
CELL PHONE	PAGER NO.	FAX NO.	E-MAIL ADDRESS

549-XX-8721	M00430548
PATIENT'S SOC. SEC. NO.	DRIVER'S LICENSE

salesman Payoll No. 6852	Easy on Paint Company
PATIENT'S OCCUPATION	NAME OF COMPANY

4586 West 20th Street, Woodland Hills, XY 12345	555-467-8898
ADDRESS OF EMPLOYER	PHONE

Jennifer B. Thorndike	homemaker
SPOUSE OR PARENT	OCCUPATION

EMPLOYER	ADDRESS	PHONE

Pacific Mutual Insurance Company, 120 South Main Street, Merck, XY 12346
NAME OF INSURANCE

	6709	Fred E. Thorndike
POLICY/CERTIFICATE NO.	GROUP NO.	INSURED OR SUBSCRIBER

REFERRED BY: John Diehl (Friend)

DATE	PROGRESS NOTES
11-25-xx	On or about 11-3-xx, pt began to have chest pain and much coughing. On 11-24-xx, pt too ill to work and decided to file for SDI benefits. Pt states illness is not work connected and he does not receive sick pay. PE: Pt examined and complained of productive cough of 3 wks duration and chest pain. Chest x-rays confirmed dx-mucopurulent chronic bronchitis. Cont home rest and prescribed antibiotic medication. RTO 12-7-xx. Pt will be capable of returning to wk 12-8-xx.
	GP/mtf Gerald Practon, MD
12-07-xx	Est pt returns for F/U c bronchitis. Chest pain improved. Still running low grade temp c̄ productive cough. F/U CXR shows clearing. Recommended bed rest x 7d. Will extend disability to 12-15-xx at which time pt can resume reg work. No complications anticipated.
	GP/mtf Gerald Practon, MD

Fig. 10.3

DB-450 9-17

New York State

NOTICE AND PROOF OF CLAIM FOR DISABILITY BENEFITS

Use this form if you became disabled **while employed** or if you became disabled **within four (4) weeks after termination of employment** OR if you became **disabled after having been unemployed for more than four (4) weeks**. Please answer all questions in Part A and questions 1 through 3 in Part B. Read all instructions on this form carefully. Health care providers must complete Part B on page 2.

PART A - CLAIMANT'S INFORMATION (Please Print or Type)

1. Last Name: ____ First Name: ____ MI: __
2. Mailing Address (Street & Apt. #): ____
   City: ____ State: ____ Zip: ____ Country: ____
3. Daytime Phone #: ____ 4. Email Address: ____
5. Social Security #: ___ - ___ - ___ 6. Date of Birth: ___ - ___ - ___ 7. Gender: ☐ Male ☐ Female
8. My disability is (if injury, also state <u>how</u>, <u>when</u> and <u>where</u> it occurred): ____
9. I became disabled or became ineligible for Unemployment Insurance because of this disability on: ___ / ___ / ___
   I worked on that day: ☐ Yes ☐ No
   Have you recovered from this disability? ☐ Yes ☐ No If Yes, what was the date you were able to work: ___ / ___ / ___
   Have you since worked for wages or profit? ☐ Yes ☐ No If Yes, list dates: ____
10. Give name of last employer. If more than one employer during last eight (8) weeks, name all employers. Average Weekly Wage is based on all wages earned in last eight (8) weeks worked.

LAST EMPLOYER			PERIOD OF EMPLOYMENT		Average Weekly Wage (Include Bonuses, Tips, Commissions, Reasonable Value of Board, Rent, etc.)
Firm or Trade Name	Address	Phone Number	First Day	Last Day Worked	
			Mo. Day Yr.	Mo. Day Yr.	
OTHER EMPLOYER (during last eight (8) weeks)			**PERIOD OF EMPLOYMENT**		**Average Weekly Wage** (Include Bonuses, Tips, Commissions, Reasonable Value of Board, Rent, etc.)
Firm or Trade Name	Address	Phone Number	First Day	Last Day Worked	
			Mo. Day Yr.	Mo. Day Yr.	
			Mo. Day Yr.	Mo. Day Yr.	

11. My job is or was: ____ (Occupation) 12. Union Member: ☐ Yes ☐ No If "Yes": ____ (Name of Union or Local Number)
13. Were you claiming or receiving unemployment prior to this disability? ☐ Yes ☐ No
    If you did **not** claim or if you claimed but did **not** receive unemployment insurance benefits after LAST DAY WORKED, explain reasons fully: ____
14. For the period of disability covered by this claim:
    A. Are you <u>**receiving**</u> wages, salary or separation pay: ☐ Yes ☐ No
    B. Are you <u>**receiving**</u> or <u>**claiming**</u>:
       1. Workers' compensation for work-connected disability: ☐ Yes ☐ No
       2. Paid Family Leave: ☐ Yes ☐ No
       3. No-Fault motor vehicle accident **(check box)**: ☐ Yes ☐ No or personal injury involving third party **(check box)**: ☐ Yes ☐ No
       4. Long-term disability benefits under the Federal Social Security Act for this disability: ☐ Yes ☐ No

IF "YES" IS CHECKED IN ANY OF THE ITEMS IN 14, COMPLETE THE FOLLOWING:

I have: ☐ received ☐ claimed from: ____ for the period: ___ / ___ / ___ to: ___ / ___ / ___

15. In the year (52 weeks) **before** your disability began, have you received disability benefits for other periods of disability? ☐ Yes ☐ No
    If "Yes", fill in the following: Paid by: ____ from: ___ / ___ / ___ to: ___ / ___ / ___
16. In the year (52 weeks) **before** your disability began, have you received Paid Family Leave? ☐ Yes ☐ No
    If "Yes", fill in the following: Paid by: ____ from: ___ / ___ / ___ to: ___ / ___ / ___

I hereby claim Disability Benefits and certify that for the period covered by this claim I was disabled. If my disability began while I was unemployed, I certify that I had been unemployed for more than four (4) weeks. I have read the instructions on page 2 of this form and that the foregoing statements, including any accompanying statements are, to the best of my knowledge, true and complete.

____ **Claimant's Signature** ____ **Date**

An individual may sign on behalf of the claimant only if he or she is legally authorized to do so and the claimant is a minor, mentally incompetent or incapacitated. If signed by other than claimant, print information below and complete and submit Form OC-110A, Claimant's Authorization to Disclose Workers' Compensation Records.

____ **On behalf of Claimant** ____ **Address** ____ **Relationship to Claimant**

DB-450 (9-17) Page 1 of 2

Fig. 10.4 (From Employment Development Department, State of California.)

Continued

PART B - HEALTH CARE PROVIDER'S STATEMENT (Please Print or Type)

THE HEALTH CARE PROVIDER'S STATEMENT MUST BE FILLED IN COMPLETELY. THE ATTENDING HEALTH CARE PROVIDER SHALL COMPLETE AND RETURN TO THE CLAIMANT WITHIN SEVEN (7) DAYS OF RECEIPT OF THIS FORM. For item 7-d, you must give estimated date. If disability is caused by or arising in connection with pregnancy, enter estimated delivery date in item 9. **INCOMPLETE ANSWERS MAY DELAY PAYMENT OF BENEFITS.**

1. Last Name: ______________________ First Name: ______________________ MI: ___

2.Gender: ☐ Male ☐ Female 3. Date of Birth: ___ / ___ / _____

4. Diagnosis/Analysis: ______________________ Diagnosis Code: ____________

a. Claimant's symptoms: ______________________

b. Objective findings: ______________________

5. Claimant hospitalized?: ☐ Yes ☐ No From: ___ / ___ / _____ To: ___ / ___ / _____

6. Operation indicated?: ☐ Yes ☐ No a. Type ____________ b. Date ___ / ___ / _____

7. ENTER DATES FOR THE FOLLOWING	MONTH	DAY	YEAR
a Date of your first treatment for this disability			
b. Date of your most recent treatment for this disability			
c. Date Claimant was unable to work because of this disability			
d. Date Claimant will again be able to perform work (Even if considerable question exists, estimate date. Avoid use of terms such as unknown or undetermined.)			
e. If pregnancy related, please check box and enter the date ☐ estimated delivery date OR ☐ actual delivery date			

8. In your opinion, is this disability the result of injury arising out of and in the course of employment or occupational disease?:
☐ Yes ☐ No If "Yes", has Form C-4 been filed with the Board? ☐ Yes ☐ No

I certify that I am a:

(Physician, Chiropractor, Dentist, Podiatrist, Psychologist, Nurse-Midwife) | **Licensed or Certified in the State of** | **License Number**

Health Care Provider's Printed Name | **Health Care Provider's Signature** | **Date**

Health Care Provider's Address | **Phone #**

CLAIMANT: READ THESE INSTRUCTIONS CAREFULLY

PLEASE NOTE: Do not date and file this form prior to your first date of disability. In order for your claim to be processed, Parts A and B must be completed.

1. If you are using this form because you became disabled **while employed** or you became disabled **within four (4) weeks after termination of employment**, your completed claim should be mailed **within thirty (30) days to your employer or your last employer's insurance carrier**. You may find your employer's disability insurance carrier on the Workers' Compensation Board's website using Employer Coverage Search.

2. If you are using this form because you became **disabled after having been unemployed for more than four (4) weeks**, your completed claim should be mailed to: **Workers' Compensation Board, Disability Benefits Bureau, 328 State Street, Schenectady, NY 12305.** If you answered "Yes" to question 14.B.3, please complete and attach Form DB-450.1.

If you have any questions about claiming disability benefits, you may contact the Board's Disability Benefits Bureau at (800) 353-3092. Additional information may be obtained at the Board's website: www.wcb.ny.gov, or you may write to the Disability Benefits Bureau at the address listed above.

Notification Pursuant to the New York Personal Privacy Protection Law (Public Officers Law Article 6-A) and the Federal Privacy Act of 1974 (5 U.S.C. § 552a). The Workers' Compensation Board's (Board's) authority to request that claimants provide personal information, including their social security number, is derived from the Board's investigatory authority under Workers' Compensation Law (WCL) § 20, and its administrative authority under WCL § 142. This information is collected to assist the Board in investigating and administering claims in the most expedient manner possible and to help it maintain accurate claim records. Providing your social security number to the Board is voluntary. There is no penalty for failure to provide your social security number on this form; it will not result in a denial of your claim or a reduction in benefits. The Board will protect the confidentiality of all personal information in its possession, disclosing it only in furtherance of its official duties and in accordance with applicable state and federal law

HIPAA NOTICE - In order to adjudicate a workers' compensation claim or disability benefits claim, WCL 13-a(4)(a) and 12 NYCRR 325-1.3 require health care providers to regularly file medical reports of treatment with the Board and the insurance carrier or employer. Pursuant to 45 CFR 164.512 these legally required medical reports are exempt from HIPAA's restrictions on disclosure of health information.

Disclosure of Information: The Board will not disclose any information about your case to any unauthorized party without your consent. If you choose to have such information disclosed to an unauthorized party, you must file with the Board an original signed Form OC-110A, Claimant's Authorization to Disclose Workers' Compensation Records, or an original signed, notarized authorization letter. You may telephone your local WCB office to have Form OC-110A sent to you, or you may download it from our website, www.wcb.ny.gov. It can be found under Forms on the 'List of All Common Workers' Compensation Board Forms' web page. Mail the completed authorization form to the address listed above.

An employer or insurer, or any employee, agent, or person acting on behalf of an employer or insurer, who KNOWINGLY MAKES A FALSE STATEMENT OR REPRESENTATION as to a material fact in the course of reporting, investigation of, or adjusting a claim for any benefit or payment under this chapter for the purpose of avoiding provision of such payment or benefit SHALL BE GUILTY OF A CRIME AND SUBJECT TO SUBSTANTIAL FINES AND IMPRISONMENT.

DB-450 (9-17) Page 2 of 2

Fig. 10.4, cont'd

ASSIGNMENT 10.4 COMPLETE A STATE DISABILITY INSURANCE FORM

Performance Objective

Task: Complete a state disability insurance form and define patient record abbreviations.

Conditions: Use the patient's record (Fig. 10.5), a New York State Notice and Proof of Claim for Disability Benefits (Fig. 10.6), and a computer.

Standards: Time: __________ minutes

Accuracy: __________

(Note: The time element and accuracy criteria may be given by your instructor.)

Directions:

1. Assume that the Claimant's Information has been completed satisfactorily by Mr. James T. Fujita (see Fig. 10.5). Complete the Health Care Provider's Statement (see Fig. 10.6) and date it December 15.

2. Refer to Chapter 10 of the *Textbook* to assist you in completing this form.

After the instructor has returned your work to you, either make the necessary corrections and place your work in a three-ring notebook for future reference or, if you received a high score, place it in your portfolio for reference when applying for a job.

Abbreviations pertinent to this record:

pt ______________________ exam ______________________

hx ______________________ neg ______________________

WBC ______________________ imp ______________________

wk ______________________ SDI ______________________

PATIENT RECORD

Fujita	James	T.	03-27-54	M	555-677-2881
LAST NAME	FIRST NAME	MIDDLE NAME	BIRTH DATE	SEX	HOME PHONE

3538 South A Street	Woodland Hills	XY	12345
ADDRESS	CITY	STATE	ZIP CODE

555-499-6556	555-988-4100	555-677-2881	fujita@wb.net
CELL PHONE	PAGER NO.	FAX NO.	E-MAIL ADDRESS

567-XX-8898	M4387931
PATIENT'S SOC. SEC. NO.	DRIVER'S LICENSE

electrician Payoll No. 8834	Macy Electric Company
PATIENT'S OCCUPATION	NAME OF COMPANY

2671 North C Street, Woodland Hills, XY 12345	555-677-2346
ADDRESS OF EMPLOYER	PHONE

Mary J. Fujita	homemaker
SPOUSE OR PARENT	OCCUPATION

EMPLOYER	ADDRESS	PHONE

Atlantic Mutual Insurance Company, 111 South Main Street, Woodland Hills, XY 12345
NAME OF INSURANCE

F20015		James T. Fujita
POLICY/CERTIFICATE NO.	GROUP NO.	INSURED OR SUBSCRIBER

REFERRED BY: Cherry Hotta (aunt)

DATE	PROGRESS NOTES
12-07-XX	Today pt could not go to work and came for exam complaining of pain in abdomen, nausea, and no vomiting. Pt has hx of mesentery adenopathy. Exam neg except abdomen showed tenderness all over with voluntary guarding. WBC 10,000. Imp: Mesenteric adenitis. Advised strict bed rest at home and bland diet. To return in 1 wk. Will file for SDI benefits. Pt states illness is not work connected and he receives sick leave pay of $150/wk.
	GI/mtf Gaston Input, MD
12-15-xx	Exam showed normal nontender abdomen. No nausea. Pt tolerating food well. WBC 7,500. Pt will be capable of returning to work 12-22-xx.
	GI/mtf Gaston Input, MD

Fig. 10.5

DB-450 9-17

New York State
NOTICE AND PROOF OF CLAIM FOR DISABILITY BENEFITS

Use this form if you became disabled **while employed** or if you became disabled **within four (4) weeks after termination of employment** OR if you became **disabled after having been unemployed for more than four (4) weeks**. Please answer all questions in Part A and questions 1 through 3 in Part B. Read all instructions on this form carefully. Health care providers must complete Part B on page 2.

PART A - CLAIMANT'S INFORMATION (Please Print or Type)

1. Last Name: ________________ First Name: ________________ MI: ___
2. Mailing Address (Street & Apt. #): ________________

   City: ________ State: ____ Zip: ______ Country: ______
3. Daytime Phone #: ________ 4. Email Address: ________________
5. Social Security #: ____ - ___ - ____ 6. Date of Birth: ___ - ___ - ____ 7. Gender: ☐ Male ☐ Female
8. My disability is (if injury, also state <u>how</u>, <u>when</u> and <u>where</u> it occurred): ________________
9. I became disabled or became ineligible for Unemployment Insurance because of this disability on: ___ / ___ / ______

   I worked on that day: ☐ Yes ☐ No

   Have you recovered from this disability? ☐ Yes ☐ No If Yes, what was the date you were able to work: ___ / ___ / ______

   Have you since worked for wages or profit? ☐ Yes ☐ No If Yes, list dates: ________________
10. Give name of last employer. If more than one employer during last eight (8) weeks, name all employers. Average Weekly Wage is based on all wages earned in last eight (8) weeks worked.

LAST EMPLOYER			PERIOD OF EMPLOYMENT		Average Weekly Wage (Include Bonuses, Tips, Commissions, Reasonable Value of Board, Rent, etc.)
Firm or Trade Name	Address	Phone Number	First Day	Last Day Worked	
			Mo. Day Yr.	Mo. Day Yr.	

OTHER EMPLOYER (during last eight (8) weeks)			PERIOD OF EMPLOYMENT		Average Weekly Wage (Include Bonuses, Tips, Commissions, Reasonable Value of Board, Rent, etc.)
Firm or Trade Name	Address	Phone Number	First Day	Last Day Worked	
			Mo. Day Yr.	Mo. Day Yr.	
			Mo. Day Yr.	Mo. Day Yr.	

11. My job is or was: ________________ (Occupation) 12. Union Member: ☐ Yes ☐ No If "Yes": ________________ (Name of Union or Local Number)
13. Were you claiming or receiving unemployment prior to this disability? ☐ Yes ☐ No

    If you did **not** claim or if you claimed but did **not** receive unemployment insurance benefits after LAST DAY WORKED, explain reasons fully: ________________
14. For the period of disability covered by this claim:

    A. Are you <u>**receiving**</u> wages, salary or separation pay: ☐ Yes ☐ No

    B. Are you <u>**receiving**</u> or <u>**claiming**</u>:

    1. Workers' compensation for work-connected disability: ☐ Yes ☐ No
    2. Paid Family Leave: ☐ Yes ☐ No
    3. No-Fault motor vehicle accident (**check box**): ☐ Yes ☐ No or personal injury involving third party (**check box**): ☐ Yes ☐ No
    4. Long-term disability benefits under the Federal Social Security Act for this disability: ☐ Yes ☐ No

IF "YES" IS CHECKED IN ANY OF THE ITEMS IN 14, COMPLETE THE FOLLOWING:

I have: ☐ received ☐ claimed from: ________________ for the period: ___ / ___ / ______ to: ___ / ___ / ______

15. In the year (52 weeks) **before** your disability began, have you received disability benefits for other periods of disability? ☐ Yes ☐ No

    If "Yes", fill in the following: Paid by: ________________ from: ___ / ___ / ______ to: ___ / ___ / ______
16. In the year (52 weeks) **before** your disability began, have you received Paid Family Leave? ☐ Yes ☐ No

    If "Yes", fill in the following: Paid by: ________________ from: ___ / ___ / ______ to: ___ / ___ / ______

I hereby claim Disability Benefits and certify that for the period covered by this claim I was disabled. If my disability began while I was unemployed, I certify that I had been unemployed for more than four (4) weeks. I have read the instructions on page 2 of this form and that the foregoing statements, including any accompanying statements are, to the best of my knowledge, true and complete.

________________ Claimant's Signature ________ Date

An individual may sign on behalf of the claimant only if he or she is legally authorized to do so and the claimant is a minor, mentally incompetent or incapacitated. If signed by other than claimant, print information below and complete and submit Form OC-110A, Claimant's Authorization to Disclose Workers' Compensation Records.

________________ On behalf of Claimant ________________ Address ________________ Relationship to Claimant

DB-450 (9-17) Page 1 of 2

Fig. 10.6 (From Employment Development Department, State of California.)

Continued

PART B - HEALTH CARE PROVIDER'S STATEMENT (Please Print or Type)

THE HEALTH CARE PROVIDER'S STATEMENT MUST BE FILLED IN COMPLETELY. THE ATTENDING HEALTH CARE PROVIDER SHALL COMPLETE AND RETURN TO THE CLAIMANT WITHIN SEVEN (7) DAYS OF RECEIPT OF THIS FORM. For item 7-d, you must give estimated date. If disability is caused by or arising in connection with pregnancy, enter estimated delivery date in item 9. **INCOMPLETE ANSWERS MAY DELAY PAYMENT OF BENEFITS.**

1. Last Name: ____________________ First Name: ____________________ MI: ___

2.Gender: ☐ Male ☐ Female 3. Date of Birth: ___/___/_____

4. Diagnosis/Analysis: ____________________ Diagnosis Code: __________

a. Claimant's symptoms: ____________________

b. Objective findings: ____________________

5. Claimant hospitalized?: ☐ Yes ☐ No From: ___/___/_____ To: ___/___/_____

6. Operation indicated?: ☐ Yes ☐ No a. Type __________ b. Date ___/___/_____

7. ENTER DATES FOR THE FOLLOWING	MONTH	DAY	YEAR
a Date of your first treatment for this disability			
b. Date of your most recent treatment for this disability			
c. Date Claimant was unable to work because of this disability			
d. Date Claimant will again be able to perform work (Even if considerable question exists, estimate date. Avoid use of terms such as unknown or undetermined.)			
e. If pregnancy related, please check box and enter the date ☐ estimated delivery date OR ☐ actual delivery date			

8. In your opinion, is this disability the result of injury arising out of and in the course of employment or occupational disease?: ☐ Yes ☐ No If "Yes", has Form C-4 been filed with the Board? ☐ Yes ☐ No

I certify that I am a:

(Physician, Chiropractor, Dentist, Podiatrist, Psychologist, Nurse-Midwife)	Licensed or Certified in the State of	License Number

Health Care Provider's Printed Name	Health Care Provider's Signature	Date

Health Care Provider's Address	Phone #

CLAIMANT: READ THESE INSTRUCTIONS CAREFULLY

PLEASE NOTE: Do not date and file this form prior to your first date of disability. In order for your claim to be processed, Parts A and B must be completed.

1. If you are using this form because you became disabled **while employed** or you became disabled **within four (4) weeks after termination of employment**, your completed claim should be mailed **within thirty (30) days to your employer or your last employer's insurance carrier**. You may find your employer's disability insurance carrier on the Workers' Compensation Board's website using Employer Coverage Search.

2. If you are using this form because you became **disabled after having been unemployed for more than four (4) weeks**, your completed claim should be mailed to: **Workers' Compensation Board, Disability Benefits Bureau, 328 State Street, Schenectady, NY 12305.** If you answered "Yes" to question 14.B.3, please complete and attach Form DB-450.1.

If you have any questions about claiming disability benefits, you may contact the Board's Disability Benefits Bureau at (800) 353-3092. Additional information may be obtained at the Board's website: www.wcb.ny.gov, or you may write to the Disability Benefits Bureau at the address listed above.

Notification Pursuant to the New York Personal Privacy Protection Law (Public Officers Law Article 6-A) and the Federal Privacy Act of 1974 (5 U.S.C. § 552a). The Workers' Compensation Board's (Board's) authority to request that claimants provide personal information, including their social security number, is derived from the Board's investigatory authority under Workers' Compensation Law (WCL) § 20, and its administrative authority under WCL § 142. This information is collected to assist the Board in investigating and administering claims in the most expedient manner possible and to help it maintain accurate claim records. Providing your social security number to the Board is voluntary. There is no penalty for failure to provide your social security number on this form; it will not result in a denial of your claim or a reduction in benefits. The Board will protect the confidentiality of all personal information in its possession, disclosing it only in furtherance of its official duties and in accordance with applicable state and federal law

HIPAA NOTICE - In order to adjudicate a workers' compensation claim or disability benefits claim, WCL 13-a(4)(a) and 12 NYCRR 325-1.3 require health care providers to regularly file medical reports of treatment with the Board and the insurance carrier or employer. Pursuant to 45 CFR 164.512 these legally required medical reports are exempt from HIPAA's restrictions on disclosure of health information.

Disclosure of Information: The Board will not disclose any information about your case to any unauthorized party without your consent. If you choose to have such information disclosed to an unauthorized party, you must file with the Board an original signed Form OC-110A, Claimant's Authorization to Disclose Workers' Compensation Records, or an original signed, notarized authorization letter. You may telephone your local WCB office to have Form OC-110A sent to you, or you may download it from our website, www.wcb.ny.gov. It can be found under Forms on the 'List of All Common Workers' Compensation Board Forms' web page. Mail the completed authorization form to the address listed above.

An employer or insurer, or any employee, agent, or person acting on behalf of an employer or insurer, who KNOWINGLY MAKES A FALSE STATEMENT OR REPRESENTATION as to a material fact in the course of reporting, investigation of, or adjusting a claim for any benefit or payment under this chapter for the purpose of avoiding provision of such payment or benefit SHALL BE GUILTY OF A CRIME AND SUBJECT TO SUBSTANTIAL FINES AND IMPRISONMENT.

DB-450 (9-17) Page 2 of 2

Fig. 10.6, cont'd

ASSIGNMENT 10.5 COMPLETE A STATE DISABILITY INSURANCE FORM

Performance Objective

Task:	Complete a state disability insurance form and define patient record abbreviations.
Conditions:	Use the patient's record (Fig. 10.7), a New York State Notice and Proof of Claim for Disability Benefits (Fig. 10.8), and a computer.
Standards:	Time: ___________ minutes
	Accuracy: ___________
	(Note: The time element and accuracy criteria may be given by your instructor.)

Directions:

1. Mr. Vincent P. Michael (see Fig. 10.7) is applying for state disability benefits. Complete the New York State Notice and Proof of Claim for Disability Benefits (Fig. 10.8) and date it September 22. Assume that the Claimant's Information has been completed satisfactorily by Mr. Michael. Remember that this is not a claim for payment to the physician, so no ledger card has been furnished for this patient.

2. Refer to Chapter 10 of the *Textbook* to assist you in completing this form.

After the instructor has returned your work to you, either make the necessary corrections and place your work in a three-ring notebook for future reference or, if you received a high score, place it in your portfolio for reference when applying for a job.

Abbreviations pertinent to this record:

Pt	______________________	exam	______________________
ESR	______________________	mm	______________________
hr	______________________	imp	______________________
CVA	______________________	adv	______________________
retn	______________________	wk	______________________
approx	______________________	L	______________________

PATIENT RECORD

Michael	Vincent	P.	05-17-55	M	555-567-9001
LAST NAME	FIRST NAME	MIDDLE NAME	BIRTH DATE	SEX	HOME PHONE

1529 1/2 Thompson Boulevard	Woodland Hills	XY	12345
ADDRESS	CITY	STATE	ZIP CODE

555-398-5677	555-311-0098	555-567-9001	michael@wb.net
CELL PHONE	PAGER NO.	FAX NO.	E-MAIL ADDRESS

562-XX-8888	E0034578
PATIENT'S SOC. SEC. NO.	DRIVER'S LICENSE

assembler "A"	Burroughs Corporation
PATIENT'S OCCUPATION	NAME OF COMPANY

5411 North Lindero Canyon Road, Woodland Hills, XY 12345	555-560-9008
ADDRESS OF EMPLOYER	PHONE

Helen J. Michael	homemaker
SPOUSE OR PARENT	OCCUPATION

EMPLOYER	ADDRESS	PHONE

Blue Shield	Vincent P. Michael
NAME OF INSURANCE	INSURED OR SUBSCRIBER

T8411981A	677899AT
POLICY/CERTIFICATE NO.	GROUP NO.

REFERRED BY: Robert T. Smith (friend)

DATE	PROGRESS NOTES
9-20-xx	Patient calls the office complaining of having had the flu, headache, dizziness, and of being tired. Pt unable to
	go to work today. Exam shows weakness of L hand. Pt exhibits light dysphasia and confusion. Pt is referred to
	XYZ Radiology for chest x-ray, frontal and lateral, and to the lab at College Hospital for ESR. Pt to return tomorrow
	at 11 AM for results.
	BC/mtf *Brady Coccidioides, MD*
9-21-xx	Chest x-rays show cardiomegaly and slight pulmonary congestion. ESR 46 mm/hr. Imp.
	Post flu syndrome, transient ischemic attack, possible CVA. Prescribed medication for the congestion and adv. pt.
	to take aspirin 1/day. Pt to stay off work and retn in 1 week. Approx. date of retn to work 10-16-xx.
	BC/mtf *Brady Coccidioides, MD*

Fig. 10.7

DB-450 9-17

New York State
NOTICE AND PROOF OF CLAIM FOR DISABILITY BENEFITS

Use this form if you became disabled **while employed** or if you became disabled **within four (4) weeks after termination of employment** OR if you became **disabled after having been unemployed for more than four (4) weeks**. Please answer all questions in Part A and questions 1 through 3 in Part B. Read all instructions on this form carefully. Health care providers must complete Part B on page 2.

PART A - CLAIMANT'S INFORMATION (Please Print or Type)

1. Last Name: ______ First Name: ______ MI: ___
2. Mailing Address (Street & Apt. #): ______
   City: ______ State: ___ Zip: ______ Country: ______
3. Daytime Phone #: ______ 4. Email Address: ______
5. Social Security #: ___ - ___ - ___ 6. Date of Birth: ___ - ___ - ___ 7. Gender: ☐ Male ☐ Female
8. My disability is (if injury, also state how, when and where it occurred): ______
9. I became disabled or became ineligible for Unemployment Insurance because of this disability on: ___ / ___ / ___
   I worked on that day: ☐ Yes ☐ No
   Have you recovered from this disability? ☐ Yes ☐ No If Yes, what was the date you were able to work: ___ / ___ / ___
   Have you since worked for wages or profit? ☐ Yes ☐ No If Yes, list dates: ______
10. Give name of last employer. If more than one employer during last eight (8) weeks, name all employers. Average Weekly Wage is based on all wages earned in last eight (8) weeks worked.

LAST EMPLOYER			PERIOD OF EMPLOYMENT		Average Weekly Wage (Include Bonuses, Tips, Commissions, Reasonable Value of Board, Rent, etc.)
Firm or Trade Name	Address	Phone Number	First Day	Last Day Worked	
			Mo. Day Yr.	Mo. Day Yr.	
OTHER EMPLOYER (during last eight (8) weeks)			**PERIOD OF EMPLOYMENT**		**Average Weekly Wage** (Include Bonuses, Tips, Commissions, Reasonable Value of Board, Rent, etc.)
Firm or Trade Name	Address	Phone Number	First Day	Last Day Worked	
			Mo. Day Yr.	Mo. Day Yr.	
			Mo. Day Yr.	Mo. Day Yr.	

11. My job is or was: ______ (Occupation) 12. Union Member: ☐ Yes ☐ No If "Yes": ______ (Name of Union or Local Number)
13. Were you claiming or receiving unemployment prior to this disability? ☐ Yes ☐ No
    If you did **not** claim or if you claimed but did **not** receive unemployment insurance benefits after LAST DAY WORKED, explain reasons fully: ______
14. For the period of disability covered by this claim:
    A. Are you **receiving** wages, salary or separation pay: ☐ Yes ☐ No
    B. Are you **receiving** or **claiming**:
       1. Workers' compensation for work-connected disability: ☐ Yes ☐ No
       2. Paid Family Leave: ☐ Yes ☐ No
       3. No-Fault motor vehicle accident (check box): ☐ Yes ☐ No or personal injury involving third party (check box): ☐ Yes ☐ No
       4. Long-term disability benefits under the Federal Social Security Act for this disability: ☐ Yes ☐ No

IF "YES" IS CHECKED IN ANY OF THE ITEMS IN 14, COMPLETE THE FOLLOWING:
I have: ☐ received ☐ claimed from: ______ for the period: ___ / ___ / ___ to: ___ / ___ / ___

15. In the year (52 weeks) **before** your disability began, have you received disability benefits for other periods of disability? ☐ Yes ☐ No
    If "Yes", fill in the following: Paid by: ______ from: ___ / ___ / ___ to: ___ / ___ / ___
16. In the year (52 weeks) **before** your disability began, have you received Paid Family Leave? ☐ Yes ☐ No
    If "Yes", fill in the following: Paid by: ______ from: ___ / ___ / ___ to: ___ / ___ / ___

I hereby claim Disability Benefits and certify that for the period covered by this claim I was disabled. If my disability began while I was unemployed, I certify that I had been unemployed for more than four (4) weeks. I have read the instructions on page 2 of this form and that the foregoing statements, including any accompanying statements are, to the best of my knowledge, true and complete.

______ **Claimant's Signature** ______ **Date**

An individual may sign on behalf of the claimant only if he or she is legally authorized to do so and the claimant is a minor, mentally incompetent or incapacitated. If signed by other than claimant, print information below and complete and submit Form OC-110A, Claimant's Authorization to Disclose Workers' Compensation Records.

______ **On behalf of Claimant** ______ **Address** ______ **Relationship to Claimant**

DB-450 (9-17) Page 1 of 2

Fig. 10.8 (From Employment Development Department, State of California.)

Continued

PART B - HEALTH CARE PROVIDER'S STATEMENT (Please Print or Type)

THE HEALTH CARE PROVIDER'S STATEMENT MUST BE FILLED IN COMPLETELY. THE ATTENDING HEALTH CARE PROVIDER SHALL COMPLETE AND RETURN TO THE CLAIMANT WITHIN SEVEN (7) DAYS OF RECEIPT OF THIS FORM. For item 7-d, you must give estimated date. If disability is caused by or arising in connection with pregnancy, enter estimated delivery date in item 9. **INCOMPLETE ANSWERS MAY DELAY PAYMENT OF BENEFITS.**

1. Last Name: ______________ First Name: ______________ MI: ___

2.Gender: ☐ Male ☐ Female 3. Date of Birth: ___ / ___ / ___

4. Diagnosis/Analysis: ______________ Diagnosis Code: ______________

a. Claimant's symptoms: ______________

b. Objective findings: ______________

5. Claimant hospitalized?: ☐ Yes ☐ No From: ___ / ___ / ___ To: ___ / ___ / ___

6. Operation indicated?: ☐ Yes ☐ No a. Type ______________ b. Date ___ / ___ / ___

7. ENTER DATES FOR THE FOLLOWING	MONTH	DAY	YEAR
a Date of your first treatment for this disability			
b. Date of your most recent treatment for this disability			
c. Date Claimant was unable to work because of this disability			
d. Date Claimant will again be able to perform work (Even if considerable question exists, estimate date. Avoid use of terms such as unknown or undetermined.)			
e. If pregnancy related, please check box and enter the date ☐ estimated delivery date OR ☐ actual delivery date			

8. In your opinion, is this disability the result of injury arising out of and in the course of employment or occupational disease?: ☐ Yes ☐ No If "Yes", has Form C-4 been filed with the Board? ☐ Yes ☐ No

I certify that I am a:

(Physician, Chiropractor, Dentist, Podiatrist, Psychologist, Nurse-Midwife) ______ **Licensed or Certified in the State of** ______ **License Number** ______

Health Care Provider's Printed Name ______ **Health Care Provider's Signature** ______ **Date** ______

Health Care Provider's Address ______ **Phone #** ______

CLAIMANT: READ THESE INSTRUCTIONS CAREFULLY

PLEASE NOTE: Do not date and file this form prior to your first date of disability. In order for your claim to be processed, Parts A and B must be completed.

1. If you are using this form because you became disabled **while employed** or you became disabled **within four (4) weeks after termination of employment**, your completed claim should be mailed **within thirty (30) days to your employer or your last employer's insurance carrier**. You may find your employer's disability insurance carrier on the Workers' Compensation Board's website using Employer Coverage Search.

2. If you are using this form because you became **disabled after having been unemployed for more than four (4) weeks**, your completed claim should be mailed to: **Workers' Compensation Board, Disability Benefits Bureau, 328 State Street, Schenectady, NY 12305.** If you answered "Yes" to question 14.B.3, please complete and attach Form DB-450.1.

If you have any questions about claiming disability benefits, you may contact the Board's Disability Benefits Bureau at (800) 353-3092. Additional information may be obtained at the Board's website: www.wcb.ny.gov, or you may write to the Disability Benefits Bureau at the address listed above.

Notification Pursuant to the New York Personal Privacy Protection Law (Public Officers Law Article 6-A) and the Federal Privacy Act of 1974 (5 U.S.C. § 552a). The Workers' Compensation Board's (Board's) authority to request that claimants provide personal information, including their social security number, is derived from the Board's investigatory authority under Workers' Compensation Law (WCL) § 20, and its administrative authority under WCL § 142. This information is collected to assist the Board in investigating and administering claims in the most expedient manner possible and to help it maintain accurate claim records. Providing your social security number to the Board is voluntary. There is no penalty for failure to provide your social security number on this form; it will not result in a denial of your claim or a reduction in benefits. The Board will protect the confidentiality of all personal information in its possession, disclosing it only in furtherance of its official duties and in accordance with applicable state and federal law

HIPAA NOTICE - In order to adjudicate a workers' compensation claim or disability benefits claim, WCL 13-a(4)(a) and 12 NYCRR 325-1.3 require health care providers to regularly file medical reports of treatment with the Board and the insurance carrier or employer. Pursuant to 45 CFR 164.512 these legally required medical reports are exempt from HIPAA's restrictions on disclosure of health information.

Disclosure of Information: The Board will not disclose any information about your case to any unauthorized party without your consent. If you choose to have such information disclosed to an unauthorized party, you must file with the Board an original signed Form OC-110A, Claimant's Authorization to Disclose Workers' Compensation Records, or an original signed, notarized authorization letter. You may telephone your local WCB office to have Form OC-110A sent to you, or you may download it from our website, www.wcb.ny.gov. It can be found under Forms on the 'List of All Common Workers' Compensation Board Forms' web page. Mail the completed authorization form to the address listed above.

An employer or insurer, or any employee, agent, or person acting on behalf of an employer or insurer, who KNOWINGLY MAKES A FALSE STATEMENT OR REPRESENTATION as to a material fact in the course of reporting, investigation of, or adjusting a claim for any benefit or payment under this chapter for the purpose of avoiding provision of such payment or benefit SHALL BE GUILTY OF A CRIME AND SUBJECT TO SUBSTANTIAL FINES AND IMPRISONMENT.

DB-450 (9-17) Page 2 of 2

Fig. 10.8, cont'd

11 Medical Documentation and the Electronic Health Record

Cheryl Fassett

KEY TERMS

Your instructor may wish to select some words pertinent to this chapter for a test. For definitions of the terms, further study, and/or reference, the words, phrases, and abbreviations may be found in the glossary at the end of the Textbook. *Key terms for this chapter follow.*

acute
attending physician
chief complaint
chronic
clinical documentation improvement
cloned note
comorbidity
comprehensive
concurrent care
consultation
consulting physician
continuity of care
counseling
critical care
degaussing
detailed
documentation
electronic health record
emergency care
eponym
established patient
expanded problem focused
external audit
family history
health record
high complexity
history of present illness
internal review
legible
low complexity
medical decision making
medical necessity
moderate complexity
morbidity
mortality
new patient
non-physician practitioner
ordering physician
past history
physical examination
prepayment audit
primary care physician
problem focused
prospective review
query
referral
referring physician
resident physician
retrospective review
review of systems
social history
straightforward
subacute
subpoena
subpoena duces tecum
teaching physician
treating or performing physician
zeroization

KEY ABBREVIATIONS

See how many abbreviations and acronyms you can translate and then use this as a handy reference list. Definitions for the key abbreviations are located near the back of the Textbook *in the glossary.*

ARRA ______________________

C level of history or examination ______________________

CC ______________________

CDI ______________________

CCU ______________________

D level of history or examination ______________________

dx or Dx ________________

ED or ER ________________

EHR ________________

E/M service ________________

EMR ________________

EPF level of history or examination ________________

ESI ________________

FH ________________

HC medical decision making ________________

HIM ________________

HIV ________________

HPI ________________

ICU ________________

LC medical decision making ________________

LLQ ________________

LUQ ________________

MC medical decision making ________________

MDM ________________

NPP ________________

PCP ________________

PE or PX ________________

PF level of history or examination ________________

PFSH ________________

PH ________________

POMR system ________________

RCU ________________

RLQ ________________

R/O ________________

ROS ________________

RUQ ________________

SF medical decision making ________________

SH ________________

SOAP style ________________

SOR system ________________

WNL ________________

PERFORMANCE OBJECTIVES

The student will be able to:

- Define and spell the key terms and key abbreviations for this chapter, given the information from the *Textbook* glossary, within a reasonable time period and with enough accuracy to obtain a satisfactory evaluation.
- Answer the fill in the blank, mix and match, multiple choice, and true/false review questions after reading the chapter, with enough accuracy to obtain a satisfactory evaluation.
- Use critical thinking to solve an office problem about patients' medical records.
- Abstract subjective and objective data from patient records, within a reasonable time period and with enough accuracy to obtain a satisfactory evaluation.
- Review a patient record and obtain answers to questions about the documentation presented, within a reasonable time period and with enough accuracy to obtain a satisfactory evaluation.
- Select the correct medicolegal form, create a letter with appropriate content, prepare an envelope, and properly complete US Postal Service documents for the physician's signature, given the patients' chart notes and ledger cards, within a reasonable time period and with enough accuracy to obtain a satisfactory evaluation.

STUDY OUTLINE

The Documentation Process
- Health Record
- Electronic Health Records

Incentive Programs for Adoption of Electronic Health Records

General Principles of Health Record Documentation
- Documenters
- Clinical Documentation Improvement
- Legible Documentation
- Common Documentation Errors
- Medical Necessity
- Legalities of Health Record Billing Patterns
- Termination of a Case

Documentation Terminology
- Terminology for Evaluation and Management Services
- Diagnostic Terminology and Abbreviations
- Directional Terms
- Surgical Terminology

Abstracting From Medical Records
- Life or Health Insurance Applications

Review and Audit of Health Records
- Internal Reviews
- External Reviews
- Software Edit Checks

Release and Retention of Health Records
- Subpoena
- Retention of Records
- Data Storage
- Data Disposal
- Electronic Power Protection
- Prevention of Legal Problems

Documentation Guidelines for Evaluation and Management Services
- Audit Point System
- Documentation of History
- Documentation of Examination
- Documentation of Medical Decision Making

ASSIGNMENT 11.1 REVIEW QUESTIONS

Part I Fill in the Blank

Review the objectives, key terms, glossary definitions to key terms, chapter information, and figures before completing the following review questions.

1. Written or graphic information about patient care is termed a/an ________________.

2. List the two types of health record systems that can be used in a medical practice.

   a. ________________________________

   b. ________________________________

3. The difference between an EMR and an EHR is that the __________ is an individual physician's record of the patient's care, whereas the __________ is all of the patient's health records, from many different information systems and providers.

4. The greatest advantage of an EHR system is the improvement of quality of care and patient safety through the __________ of medical records between providers and other health care organizations.

5. What is the Centers for Medicare and Medicaid Services (CMS) definition of *legible documentation?*

   ____

   ____

6. ____________________ is the performance of services or procedures consistent with the diagnosis, done with standards of good medical practice and a proper level of care given in the appropriate setting.

7. Medicare administrative contractors have __________ to access a medical practice without an appointment or search warrant to conduct a review of documentation, audits, and evaluations.

8. If a medical practice is audited by Medicare officials and intentional miscoding is discovered, __________ may be levied and providers may be ________________.

9. Define the following terms in relationship to billing.

   a. New patient ________________________________

   ____

   b. Established patient ________________________________

   ____

10. Explain the difference between a consultation and the referral of a patient.

    a. Consultation:

    ____

    ____

    b. Referral:

    ____

    ____

11. Medical care for a patient who has received treatment for an illness and is referred to a second physician for treatment of the same condition is a situation called ______________.

12. An emergency medical condition, as defined by Medicare, is a medical condition manifesting itself by ____________________ of ____________________ such that the absence of immediate medical attention could reasonably be expected to result in placing the patient's health in serious jeopardy, serious impairment to body functions, or serious dysfunction of any body organ or part.

13. For EHRs, how should an insurance billing specialist correct an error on a patient's record?

____

14. For paper-based records, how should an error be corrected on a patient's record?

____

15. Name the six documentation components of a patient's history.

 a. ____
 b. ____
 c. ____
 d. ____
 e. ____
 f. ____

16. List the eight descriptive elements that can be documented in the HPI.

 a. ____
 b. ____
 c. ____
 d. ____
 e. ____
 f. ____
 g. ____
 h. ____

17. List four of the body systems that are recognized for the reporting of the review of systems (ROS).

 a. ____
 b. ____
 c. ____
 d. ____

18. A problem-focused examination is a/an __________ examination of the affected body area or organ system.

19. Medical decision making (MDM) is the process performed after taking the patient's history and performing the examination, which results in a/an ________________________.

20. Any charts that are amended with additional notes must be labeled "________________" or "late entry," dated on the day of the amendment, and signed by the physician.

Part II Mix and Match

21. Match the following terms in the right column with their descriptions, and fill in the blank with the appropriate letter.

_______ Renders a service to a patient

_______ Directs selection, preparation, and administration of tests, medication, or treatment

_______ Legally responsible for the care and treatment given to a patient

_______ Gives an opinion regarding a specific problem that is requested by another doctor

_______ Sends the patient for tests or treatment or to another doctor for consultation

_______ Oversees care of patients in managed care plans and refers patients to see specialists when needed

_______ Responsible for training and supervising medical students

_______ Clinical nurse specialist or licensed social worker who treats a patient for a specific medical problem and uses the results of a diagnostic test in managing a patient's medical problem

_______ Performs one or more years of training in a specialty area while working at a hospital (medical center)

a. Attending physician
b. Consulting physician
c. Non-physician practitioner
d. Ordering physician
e. Primary care physician
f. Referring physician
g. Resident physician
h. Teaching physician
i. Treating or performing physician

Part III Multiple Choice

Choose the best answer.

22. Chart chasing is eliminated when using which type of record system?
   a. Paper-based
   b. EHR
   c. Problem-oriented
   d. Integrated record

23. Regarding the SOAP style of documentation that a physician uses to chart a patient's progress in the health record, SOAP stands for:
   a. signature, observation, assessment, and progress.
   b. subjective, objective, assessment, and plan.
   c. symptoms, objective findings, and professional services.
   d. subjective, opinions, assistance, and present illness.

24. During the performance of an external audit to review a medical practice's health records, the system used to show deficiencies in documentation is called a/an:
   a. SOAP system.
   b. electronic recording system.
   c. information record system.
   d. point system.

25. Which of these elements is a requirement for all levels of history?
   a. Chief complaint (CC)
   b. History of present illness (HPI)
   c. Review of systems (ROS)
   d. Past, family, or social history (PFSH)

26. When there is an underlying disease or other conditions are present at the time of the patient's office visit, this is termed:
    a. mortality.
    b. continuity.
    c. comorbidity.
    d. complexity.

27. Critical care is rendered in:
    a. the coronary care unit.
    b. the intensive care unit.
    c. the emergency room.
    d. all of the above.

28. Verification of successful backups by comparing original records with copied records should be performed:
    a. once a day.
    b. once a week.
    c. once a month.
    d. once a year.

29. An acceptable method for ensuring that electronic PHI (ePHI) cannot be recovered from a hard drive that is being disposed of is by:
    a. deletion of files.
    b. formatting drives.
    c. incineration.
    d. all of the above.

Part IV True/False

Write "T" or "F" in the blank line to indicate whether you think the statement is true or false.

_______ 30. A patient's hospital discharge summary contains the discharge diagnosis but not the admitting diagnosis.

_______ 31. An eponym should not be used when a comparable anatomic term can be used in its place.

_______ 32. If the phrase "rule out" appears in a patient's health record in connection with a disease, then code the condition as if it existed.

_______ 33. During a prospective review or prebilling audit, all procedures or services and diagnoses listed on the encounter form must match the data on the insurance claim form.

_______ 34. Willful disregard of a subpoena is punishable as contempt of court.

_______ 35. Based on Medicare Conditions of Participation, hospitals must retain medical records for a period of at least 4 years.

_______ 36. Assigned insurance claims for Medicaid and Medicare cases must be kept for a period of 7 years.

_______ 37. If a patient fails to make payment on an overdue account, the physician has the right to formally withdraw from providing care to the patient.

_______ 38. There are very few circumstances that insurance billers may be faced with when executing their job duties that may lead to a case of lawsuit.

_______ 39. Deleting files or formatting the hard drive is sufficient to keep electronic protected health information from being accessed.

ASSIGNMENT 11.2 REVIEW DIAGNOSTIC TERMINOLOGY AND ABBREVIATIONS

In the Textbook, review Fig. 11.6, and use a medical dictionary to complete the assignment.

1. Place the appropriate letter on a blank line before the phrase.

_______ Taking or letting out fluids from a body part	a. alteration
_______ Act of cutting out	b. bypass
_______ Modifying a body part without affecting function	c. control
_______ Taking out or off a device from a body part	d. drainage
_______ Stop or attempt to stop bleeding	e. excision
_______ Altering the route of passage with anastomoses	f. removal

2. Write in the meaning of these abbreviations and/or symbols commonly encountered in a patient's medical record:

   RLQ ____

   DC ____

   WNL ____

   R/O ____

   URI ____

3. When documenting incisions, the unit of measure for length should be listed in __________.

Multiple Choice Questions

4. If a physician called and asked for a patient's medical record STAT, what does he or she mean?
   a. The physician wants a statistic from a patient's record.
   b. The physician wants the record delivered on Tuesday.
   c. The physician wants the record delivered immediately.

5. If a physician asks you to locate the results of the last UA, what would you be searching for?
   a. A urinalysis report
   b. An x-ray report of the ulna
   c. Uric acid test results

6. If a physician telephoned and asked for a copy of the last H&P to be emailed, what is being requested?
   a. Heart and pulmonary findings
   b. H2 antagonist test results
   c. A history and physical

7. If a hospital nurse telephoned and asked you to read the results of the patient's last CBC, what would you be searching for?
   a. Carcinoma basal cell report
   b. Complete blood count
   c. Congenital blindness, complete report

8. If you were asked to make a photocopy of the patient's last CT, what would you be searching for?
   a. Chemotherapy record
   b. Connective tissue report
   c. Computed tomography scan

ASSIGNMENT 11.3 CRITICAL THINKING: SOLVE AN OFFICE PROBLEM

Performance Objective

Task: Answer questions after reviewing the case study using critical thinking skills.

Conditions: Use a case study and a pen or pencil.

Standards: Time: _________ minutes

Accuracy: _____________

Directions: Answer questions after reviewing the case study using your critical thinking skills. Record your answer on the blank lines.

1. A patient comes into the office for treatment. He does not return, because he is dissatisfied with Dr. Practon's treatment. Is it necessary to keep his records when he obviously will not return? ______________________________

   Why? ______________________________

   ____

ASSIGNMENT 11.4 ABSTRACT SUBJECTIVE OBSERVATIONS AND OBJECTIVE FINDINGS FROM PATIENT RECORDS

Performance Objective

Task: List subjective observations and objective findings after reading each of the case studies.

Conditions: Use a pencil and four case studies.

Standards: Time: __________ minutes

Accuracy: ___________

(Note: The time element and accuracy criteria may be given by your instructor.)

Case Study 1 Mrs. Smith is 25 years old and was brought into the emergency department of College Hospital with complaints of difficulty breathing and chest pain. Her vital signs show an elevated temperature of 101°F and pulse rate of 90. Respirations are labored at 30 per minute. Blood pressure is 140/80. Her skin is warm and diaphoretic (perspiring). She states, "This condition has been going on for the past three days."

Subjective observations: ____

Objective findings: ____

Case Study 2 Mr. Jones is 56 years old and was admitted to the hospital with chest pain and elevated pulse and blood pressure. His skin is cold and clammy.

Subjective observations: ____

Objective findings: ____

Case Study 3 You are assisting the radiology technician with Sally Salazar, a 6-year-old Hispanic girl who was brought into the pediatrician's office with a suspected fracture of the right arm. Sally states she was "running at school, tripped on my shoelace, and fell." She tells you her "arm hurts," points out how "funny my arm looks," and starts to cry. You notice her arm looks disfigured and is covered with dirt. Sally is cradling her arm against her body and is unwilling to let go because "it's going to fall off."

Subjective observations: ____

Objective findings: ____

Case Study 4 You are working in the business office of College Hospital. A former patient in your hospital comes in complaining of his billing. He states he was never catheterized, never had any of the medications listed on his itemized bill, and has "never been in this hospital for that length of time." His face is red, his voice is gradually getting louder, and you notice he is standing with the aid of crutches because his left leg is in a full cast.

Subjective observations: ____

Objective findings: ____

ASSIGNMENT 11.5 REVIEW OF A PATIENT RECORD

Performance Objective

Task: Answer questions after reviewing a patient's record.

Conditions: Use a pencil, internal record review sheet, medical dictionary, abbreviation reference list, drug reference book (e.g., *Mosby's MD Consult*), and laboratory reference book.

Standards: Time: __________ minutes

Accuracy: ____________

(Note: The time element and accuracy criteria may be given by your instructor.)

Directions: In many instances, when developing the skill of reviewing a patient record, you may need critical thinking in addition to efficient use of reference books. Answer only those questions you think can be justified by the documentation presented in the patient's record. Because the content of each record is variable, you may or may not have answers to all eight questions.

Answer the questions by recording on the blank lines the documentation found identifying the components from the patient's record.

If your answers vary, perhaps you have a reason for them that may or may not be valid. List your reasons in the response section. Differences may be reviewed with your instructor privately or via class discussion.

Patient Record

10-21-20xx

HPI

This new pt is an 80-year-old white male who has had problems with voiding since 9-5-20xx.

During the night, the pt had only 50 mL output and was catheterized this morning because of his poor urinary output (200 mL). He was thought to have a distended bladder; he complains of pressure in the suprapubic region. He has not had any gross hematuria. He has difficulty voiding, especially lying down. His voiding pattern is improved while standing and sitting.

Gene Ulibarri, MD

1. Location: In what body system is the sign or symptom occurring?

   Response: ____

2. Quality: Is the symptom or pain burning, gnawing, stabbing, pressure-like, squeezing, fullness?

   Response: ____

3. Severity: In this case, how would you rank the symptom (how was distress relieved) or pain (slight, mild, severe, persistent)?

   Response: ____

4. Duration: How long has the symptom been present, or how long does it last?

   Response: ____

5. Timing: When does(do) a sign(s) or symptom(s) occur (AM, PM, after or before meals)?

   Response: ____

6. Context: Is the pain/symptom associated with big meals, dairy products, etc.?

   Response: ____

7. Modifying factors: What actions make symptoms worse or better?

   Response: ____

8. Associated signs and symptoms: What other system or body area produces complaints when the presenting problem occurs? (Example: Chest pain leads to shortness of breath.)

   Response: ____

12 Diagnostic Coding

Cheryl Fassett

KEY TERMS

Your instructor may wish to select some words pertinent to this chapter for a test. For definitions of the terms, further study, and/or reference, the words, phrases, and abbreviations may be found in the glossary at the end of the Textbook. *Key terms for this chapter follow.*

adverse effect
benign tumor
carcinoma in situ
chief complaint
combination code
complication
computer-assisted coding
conventions
eponym
essential modifiers
etiology
Excludes 1
Excludes 2
external causes of morbidity
International Classification of Diseases, Tenth Revision, Clinical Modification
International Classification of Diseases, Tenth Revision, Procedure Coding System
intoxication
late effect
laterality
malignant tumor
manifestation
medical necessity
metastasis
morbidity
mortality
neoplasm
nonessential modifiers
not elsewhere classifiable
not otherwise specified
Official Guidelines for Coding and Reporting
ordinality of encounter
placeholder
poisoning
primary diagnosis
principal diagnosis
prophylaxis
residual subcategories
rule out
secondary diagnosis
sequela
sequencing
syndrome
Uncertain Behavior
Z codes

KEY ABBREVIATIONS

AHA ______________________

AHIMA ______________________

CAC ______________________

CC ______________________

CM ______________________

CPT ______________________

DM ______________________

GEMS ______________________

HIV ______________________

ICD-10-CM ______________________

ICD-10-PCS ______________________

ICD-11 ______________________

MRI ______________________

NCHS ______________________

NEC ______________________

NOS ______________________

WHO ______________________

PERFORMANCE OBJECTIVES

The student will be able to:

- Define and spell the key terms and key abbreviations for this chapter, given the information from the textbook glossary, within a reasonable time period and with enough accuracy to obtain a satisfactory evaluation.
- Answer the fill-in-the-blank, multiple choice, and true/false review questions after reading the chapter, with enough accuracy to obtain a satisfactory evaluation.
- Indicate main terms, subterms, subterms to subterms, and carryover lines, given a section of a page from the ICD-10-CM code book, with enough accuracy to obtain a satisfactory evaluation.
- Answer questions, given a section of a page from the ICD-10-CM code book, with enough accuracy to obtain a satisfactory evaluation.
- Select the correct diagnostic code numbers and given diagnoses, and locate the conditions using Volumes 1 and 2 of the ICD-10-CM code book, with enough accuracy to obtain a satisfactory evaluation.
- Select the correct diagnostic code numbers, given a series of scenarios and diagnoses, using Volumes 1 and 2 of the ICD-10-CM code book, with enough accuracy to obtain a satisfactory evaluation.

STUDY OUTLINE

Diagnosis Coding Overview
- Assigning a Diagnosis Code
- Sequencing of Diagnostic Codes
- Admitting Diagnoses
- Medical Necessity

International Classification of Diseases
- History
- Transition From ICD-9-CM to ICD-10-CM
- ICD-10 Diagnosis and Procedure Codes
- ICD-10-CM
- ICD-10-PCS
- ICD-10-CM and Its Compliance With HIPAA
- Organization and Format of ICD-10-CM
- Alphabetic Index to Diseases and Injuries
- Special Points to Remember in the Alphabetic Index
- Tabular List of Diseases and Injuries
- Special Points to Remember in the Tabular List

Official Coding Guidelines for ICD-10-CM
- Selection of a Coding Manual
- Diagnostic Code Book Conventions
- General Coding Guidelines
- Chapter-Specific Coding Guidelines
- Diagnostic Coding and Reporting Guidelines for Outpatient Services
- Handy Hints for Diagnostic Coding
- Computer-Assisted Coding

The Future of Diagnosis Coding

Basic Steps in Selecting Diagnostic Codes from ICD-10-CM

ASSIGNMENT 12.1 REVIEW QUESTIONS

Part I Fill in the Blank on ICD-10-CM

Review the objectives, key terms, and chapter information before completing the following review questions.

1. When submitting insurance claims for patients seen by a healthcare organization office or in an outpatient hospital setting, the _________ diagnosis is listed first, but in the inpatient hospital setting, the _________ diagnosis is used.

2. Claims to insurance carriers often are denied because of lack of ________________, which indicates that the procedure provided was not payable for the diagnosis submitted.

3. Diagnosis coding for services provided by a healthcare organization are reported using ICD-10-CM effective with dates of service ______________________________.

4. The abbreviation ICD-10-CM means ______________________________.

5. The official version of the International Classification of Disease (ICD) was developed by the ____.

6. ICD-10-CM requires ________________ documentation in the medical record than the previous coding system, ICD-9-CM.

7. ICD-10-PCS is the coding system for reporting inpatient services by hospitals and replaces ________________ of the ICD-9-CM coding system.

8. ICD-10-CM is the standard code set required under ________________ legislation and must be used by covered entities when assigning diagnostic codes.

9. Volume 2, Diseases, is a/an ______________ index or listing of code numbers.

10. Volume 1, Diseases, is a/an ______________ listing of code numbers.

11. When using the ICD-10-CM coding system, the ________________ is used as a placeholder to save space for future code expansion.

12. Conventions are ____________________ used in the diagnostic code books to assist in the selection of correct codes for the diagnosis encountered.

13. The abbreviation NEC appearing in the ICD-10-CM code book means ____.

14. ________________________ are used to enclose synonyms in the Tabular List.

15. If a condition is documented in the medical record, but it is not specified as to whether the condition is acute or chronic, then the ______________ code should be assigned.

16. When selecting a code that corresponds with the condition stated in the medical record, the coder should first locate the term in the ____________________ and then confirm the code in the ____________________.

17. The instructional note ________________ listed in the Tabular List assists the coder as to when it is appropriate to report a secondary code.

18. A condition that is produced after the acute phase of an illness is listed as the main term ________________________ in the Alphabetic Index.

19. When reporting a condition that affects the left side of the patient, the character ________________________ is reported to indicate laterality.

20. The Neoplasm Table has column headings for ______________, ______________, ________________________, and ________________________.

21. In juvenile diabetes, the patient's _________ does not function and produce enough insulin.

22. When coding for diabetes in pregnancy, a code from category _________ is assigned as the primary diagnosis.

23. _________ hypertension is indicative of a life-threatening condition.

24. Full-term uncomplicated _________ deliveries are always reported with the code O80.

25. When reporting accidents and injuries, a seventh character of "A" identifies that the encounter is ________________.

26. Additional external cause codes are _________ when reporting poisonings using combination codes from T36 through T65.

27. If documentation states that the incident related to a poisoning was a suspected suicide attempt, the code would be reported from the column titled __________________.

28. If a patient falls and fractures his or her wrist, the fracture code is the primary code, followed by a/an ________________ code to explain how the accident occurred.

29. When a person encounters health services to receive a vaccination, the diagnosis is reported with a/an __________________.

Part II Multiple Choice on ICD-10-CM

Choose the best answer.

30. The consequences of inaccurate assignment of diagnostic codes include:
    a. delay in payment of claim.
    b. denial of claim.
    c. change in level of reimbursement.
    d. all of the above.

31. Diagnosis codes should be reported to the highest level of:
    a. specificity.
    b. medical necessity.
    c. etiology.
    d. sequel.

32. When a provider makes a hospital visit, the encounter should be reported with a diagnosis code that represents:
    a. the reason the patient was admitted to the hospital.
    b. the condition the provider evaluated and treated during the encounter.
    c. the condition that was requested by the admitting physician.
    d. the final discharge diagnosis.

33. To determine the diagnosis codes that would support medical necessity of a specific procedure, such as magnetic resonance imaging (MRI), under Medicare guidelines, the coder should consult:
    a. *Current Procedural Terminology* (CPT) guidelines.
    b. local coverage determinations (LCDs) and national coverage determinations (NCDs).
    c. all of the above.
    d. none of the above.

34. Passage of which legislation, in 1988, placed requirements on physicians to report appropriate diagnosis codes on all claims to Medicare?
    a. Affordable Care Act
    b. Health Insurance Portability and Accountability Act (HIPAA)
    c. American Recovery and Reinvestment Act
    d. Medicare Catastrophic Coverage Act

35. ICD-10-PCS (Procedure Coding System) was developed by 3M Health Information Systems under contract with the:
    a. National Center for Health Statistics.
    b. World Health Organization.
    c. Centers for Disease Control.
    d. Centers for Medicare and Medicaid Services.

36. Annual updates to ICD-10-CM are published:
    a. by the AMA and AHA.
    b. by the AHA and AHIMA.
    c. by the AHA, AHIMA, and US Printing Office.
    d. by the AMA, AHA, AHIMA, and US Printing Office.

37. The Alphabetic Index to Diseases and Injuries is placed:
    a. after Volume 1, the Tabular Index.
    b. first in the coding manual.
    c. after the Table of Drugs and Chemicals.
    d. after the Index to External Causes.

38. How many chapters does the Tabular List contain?
    a. 17
    b. 17 with two supplementary classifications
    c. 19
    d. 21

39. When two diagnoses are classified with a single code, it is referred to as:
    a. a combination code.
    b. a manifestation.
    c. an external cause code.
    d. a Z code.

40. An essential modifier is also referred to as a:
    a. main term.
    b. nonessential modifier.
    c. subterm.
    d. convention.

41. The equivalent of unspecified is:
    a. NEC.
    b. NOS.
    c. nonessential.
    d. secondary.

42. When reporting outpatients' services, signs and symptoms are acceptable for reporting purposes:
    a. in all situations.
    b. in addition to the definitive diagnosis.
    c. when a definitive diagnosis has not been determined.
    d. under no circumstances.

43. When conditions documented as "threatened" are referenced in the Alphabetic Index and there is no entry for the threatened condition, report:
    a. with signs and symptoms.
    b. as if the patient has the condition.
    c. the existing underlying condition.
    d. all of the above.

44. When reporting laterality, the final character "3" is reported to indicate:
    a. right side.
    b. left side.
    c. bilateral.
    d. unspecified.

45. When reporting an encounter for testing of human immunodeficiency virus (HIV), the code should be assigned as:
    a. B20.
    b. R75.
    c. Z11.4.
    d. Z21.

46. When fractures are documented, but there is no indication of whether the fracture is open or closed,
    a. report as closed.
    b. report as open.
    c. it does not matter if it is reported as open or closed.
    d. report as unspecified.

47. When identifying the total body surface area of a burn, the front torso is considered as:
   a. 1%.
   b. 9%.
   c. 18%.
   d. 36%.

48. Why are external cause codes used?
   a. To generate additional revenue
   b. To establish injury prevention programs
   c. All of the above
   d. None of the above

Part III True/False

Write "T" or "F" in the blank to indicate whether you think the statement is true or false.

_______ 49. Diagnoses that relate to the patient's previous medical problem must always be reported.

_______ 50. The concept of "principal diagnosis" is applicable to outpatient and inpatient cases.

_______ 51. The diagnosis coding system is designed to provide statistical mortality rate data that include information about causes of diseases.

_______ 52. The process for looking up a diagnosis code in the ICD-9-CM coding system is the same as in the ICD-10-CM coding system.

_______ 53. ICD-10 was published by the World Health Organization (WHO) and clinically modified by the Centers for Medicare and Medicaid Services (CMS).

_______ 54. The Alphabetic Index contains the Table of Drugs and Chemicals.

_______ 55. ICD-10-CM codes can contain up to seven characters.

_______ 56. Signs and symptoms that are not typically associated with a disease process should be reported when documented.

_______ 57. When a person who is not currently sick encounters health services for some specific purpose, such as to receive a vaccination, a Z code is used.

_______ 58. *Code conventions* are rules or principles for determining a diagnostic code when using a diagnostic code book.

_______ 59. Because there are annual ICD-10-CM code revisions, there is a three-month grace period to implement these changes and revisions.

_______ 60. An external cause code may never be sequenced as the primary diagnosis in the first position.

ASSIGNMENT 12.2 LOCATING INFORMATION IN ICD-10-CM, VOLUME 2

Performance Objective

Task:	Answer questions pertaining to categories G00-G09 of ICD-10-CM, Volume 2.
Conditions:	Use the abstracted section from ICD-10-CM, Volume 2, and pen or pencil.
Standards:	Time: __________ minutes
	Accuracy: ___________
	(Note: The time element and accuracy criteria may be given by your instructor.)

Directions: Refer to a section from a page of ICD-10-CM, Volume 2 (Fig. 12.1), and answer questions pertaining to categories G00 through G09.

1. Locate the section title. ____

2. Place an X in front of each of the following diagnostic statements included in category code G00 and its subcategories.

   __________ bacterial leptomeningitis

   __________ bacterial meningitis

   __________ bacterial meningomyelitis

   __________ leptospirosis

   __________ tuberculous meningitis

   __________ meningoencephalitis

   __________ bacterial arachnoiditis

3. Refer to the *Exclusion* 1 note located under category code G01, titled "Meningitis in bacterial diseases classified elsewhere." Place an X in front of the following code number(s) that are excluded.

   __________ gonococcal meningitis A54.81

   __________ meningitis as a result of measles (B05.1)

   __________ meningitis in neurosyphilis (A52.13)

   __________ *Hemophilus* meningitis (G00.0)

   __________ meningitis as a result of candidal meningitis (B37.5)

   __________ Lyme disease (A69.21)

4. Place an X in front of each of the following diagnostic statements included in category code G04 and its subcategories.

   __________ meningomyelitis

   __________ meningoencephalitis

   __________ pyogenic meningitis

   __________ epidemic meningitis

   __________ tuberculous meningitis

   __________ acute ascending myelitis

5. Write the code numbers for category G04.0 that require a fifth digit.

____

INFLAMMATORY DISEASES OF THE CENTRAL NERVOUS SYSTEM (G00-G09)

● **G00 Bacterial meningitis, not elsewhere classified**
An infection of the cerebrospinal fluid surrounding the spinal cord and brain.

Includes bacterial arachnoiditis
bacterial leptomeningitis
bacterial meningitis
bacterial pachymeningitis

Excludes1 bacterial:
meningoencephalitis (G04.2)
meningomyelitis (G04.2)

G00.0 Hemophilus meningitis
Meningitis due to Hemophilus influenzae

G00.1 Pneumococcal meningitis

G00.2 Streptococcal meningitis
Use additional code to further identify organism (B95.0-B95.5)

G00.3 Staphylococcal meningitis
Use additional code to further identify organism (B95.61-B95.8)

G00.8 Other bacterial meningitis
Meningitis due to Escherichia coli
Meningitis due to Friedländer bacillus
Meningitis due to Klebsiella
Use additional code to further identify organism (B96.-)

■ **G00.9 Bacterial meningitis, unspecified**
Meningitis due to gram-negative bacteria, unspecified
Purulent meningitis NOS
Pyogenic meningitis NOS
Suppurative meningitis NOS

●◗ ***G01 Meningitis in bacterial diseases classified elsewhere***
Code first underlying disease

Excludes1 meningitis (in):
gonococcal (A54.81)
leptospirosis (A27.81)
listeriosis (A32.11)
Lyme disease (A69.21)
meningococcal (A39.0)
neurosyphilis (A52.13)
tuberculosis (A17.0)
meningoencephalitis and meningomyelitis in bacterial diseases classified elsewhere (G05)

Fig. 12.1

●◗ *G02 Meningitis in other infectious and parasitic diseases classified elsewhere*

Code first underlying disease, such as:
African trypanosomiasis (B56.-)
poliovirus infection (A80.-)

Excludes1 candidal meningitis (B37.5)
coccidioidomycosis meningitis (B38.4)
cryptococcal meningitis (B45.1)
herpesviral [herpes simplex] meningitis (B00.3)
infectious mononucleosis complicated by meningitis (B27.- with fourth character 2)
measles complicated by meningitis (B05.1)
meningoencephalitis and meningomyelitis in other infectious and parasitic diseases classified elsewhere (G05)
mumps meningitis (B26.1)
rubella meningitis (B06.02)
varicella [chickenpox] meningitis (B01.0)
zoster meningitis (B02.1)

● **G03 Meningitis due to other and unspecified causes**

Includes arachnoiditis NOS
leptomeningitis NOS
meningitis NOS
pachymeningitis NOS

Excludes1 meningoencephalitis (G04.-)
meningomyelitis (G04.-)

G03.0 Nonpyogenic meningitis
Aseptic meningitis
Nonbacterial meningitis

G03.1 Chronic meningitis

G03.2 Benign recurrent meningitis [Mollaret]

G03.8 Meningitis due to other specified causes

■ **G03.9 Meningitis, unspecified**
Arachnoiditis (spinal) NOS

● **G04 Encephalitis, myelitis and encephalomyelitis**

Includes acute ascending myelitis
meningoencephalitis
meningomyelitis

Excludes1 encephalopathy NOS (G93.40)
other noninfectious acute disseminated encephalomyelitis (noninfectious ADEM) (G04.81)

Excludes2 acute transverse myelitis (G37.3-)
alcoholic encephalopathy (G31.2)
benign myalgic encephalomyelitis (G93.3)
multiple sclerosis (G35)
subacute necrotizing myelitis (G37.4)
toxic encephalitis (G92)
toxic encephalopathy (G92)

● **G04.0 Acute disseminated encephalitis and encephalomyelitis (ADEM)**

Excludes1 acute necrotizing hemorrhagic encephalopathy (G04.3-)

G04.00 Acute disseminated encephalitis and encephalomyelitis, unspecified

G04.01 Postinfectious acute disseminated encephalitis and encephalomyelitis (postinfectious ADEM)

Excludes1 post chickenpox encephalitis (B01.1)
post measles encephalitis (B05.0)
post measles myelitis (B05.1)

G04.02 Postimmunization acute disseminated encephalitis, myelitis and encephalomyelitis
Encephalitis, post immunization
Encephalomyelitis, post immunization
Use additional code to identify the vaccine (T50.A-, T50.B-, T50.Z-)

G04.1 Tropical spastic paraplegia

G04.2 Bacterial meningoencephalitis and meningomyelitis, not elsewhere classified

● **G04.3 Acute necrotizing hemorrhagic encephalopathy**
Sudden and severe CNS disease with pathology of hemorrhages and necrosis of white matter

Excludes1 acute disseminated encephalitis and encephalomyelitis (G04.0-)

G04.30 Acute necrotizing hemorrhagic encephalopathy, unspecified

G04.31 Postinfectious acute necrotizing hemorrhagic encephalopathy

G04.32 Postimmunization acute necrotizing hemorrhagic encephalopathy
Use additional code to identify vaccine (T50.A-, T50.B-, T50.Z-)

G04.39 Other acute necrotizing hemorrhagic encephalopathy
Code also underlying etiology, if applicable

● **G04.8 Other encephalitis, myelitis and encephalomyelitis**
Code also any associated seizure (G40.-, R56.9)

G04.81 Other encephalitis and encephalomyelitis
Noninfectious acute disseminated encephalomyelitis (noninfectious ADEM)

G04.89 Other myelitis

● **G04.9 Encephalitis, myelitis and encephalomyelitis, unspecified**

■ **G04.90 Encephalitis and encephalomyelitis, unspecified**
Ventriculitis (cerebral) NOS

■ **G04.91 Myelitis, unspecified**

Fig. 12.1, cont'd

DIAGNOSTIC CODING ASSIGNMENTS

In this chapter, the points awarded for assignments that require diagnostic codes are 1 point for each correct digit.

ASSIGNMENT 12.3 OBTAIN GENERAL DIAGNOSTIC CODES FOR CONDITIONS

Performance Objective

Task: Locate the correct diagnostic code for each diagnosis listed.

Conditions: Use pen or pencil and ICD-10-CM diagnostic code book.

Standards: Time: ____________ minutes

Accuracy: ______________

(Note: The time element and accuracy criteria may be given by your instructor.)

Directions: Using the ICD-10-CM code book, read each diagnosis and locate the condition in Volume 2, the Alphabetic Index. Then go to Volume 1, to the Tabular List of Diseases. Match the definition as closely as possible to the written description and assign the correct code, entering it on the blank line.

Problems	ICD-10-CM Codes
1. Breast mass	______________
2. *Klebsiella* pneumonia	______________
3. Acute lateral wall myocardial infarction; initial episode	______________
4. Acute cerebrovascular accident	______________
5. Atherosclerotic cardiovascular disease	______________
6. Dyspnea, rule out (R/O) cystic fibrosis	______________
7. Ileitis	______________
8. Osteoarthritis of elbow	______________
9. Tinnitus	______________
10. Acute exacerbation of chronic asthmatic bronchitis	______________

ASSIGNMENT 12.4 CODE DIAGNOSES FROM MEDICAL RECORDS

Performance Objective

Task: Locate the correct diagnostic code for each case scenario.

Conditions: Use pen or pencil and ICD-10-CM diagnostic code book.

Standards: Time: ______________ minutes

Accuracy: ______________

(Note: The time element and accuracy criteria may be given by your instructor.)

Directions: This exercise will give you experience in basic diagnostic coding for physicians' insurance claims. First list the ICD-10-CM code for the diagnosis, condition, problem, or other reason for the admission and/or encounter (visit) shown in the medical record to be chiefly responsible for the services provided. Then list additional diagnostic codes that describe any coexisting conditions that affect patient care. Always assign codes to their highest level of specificity—the more digits, the more specific. Do not code probable, R/O, suspected, or questionable conditions. Assign the correct code(s), entering it (them) on the blank line.

Problems	ICD-10-CM Codes
Problem 1. A patient, Mrs. Jennifer Hanson, calls Dr. Input's office stating she has blood in her stool. Dr. Input suspects a gastrointestinal bleed and tells Mrs. Hanson to come in immediately. It is discovered that the reason for the blood in the stool is a bleeding duodenal ulcer. Code the diagnosis to be listed on the insurance claim for the office visit.	______________
Problem 2. a. Jason Belmen comes in with a fractured humerus. He also has chronic obstructive pulmonary disease (COPD), which is not treated. Code the diagnosis.	______________
b. Assume Mr. Belmen needs general anesthesia for open reduction of the fractured humerus. The COPD could now be considered a risk factor. List the diagnostic code in the second part of this scenario.	______________
Problem 3. Margarita Sanchez came into the office for removal of sutures. Code the diagnosis.	______________
Problem 4. A patient, George Martin, has benign prostatic hypertrophy (BPH). He is seen for catheterization because of urinary retention. Code the primary and secondary diagnoses for the office visit. (Note: BPH is an enlargement of the prostate gland, caused by overgrowth of androgen-sensitive glandular elements, which occurs naturally with aging.)	______________
Problem 5. Mia Bartholomew is seen in the office complaining of a sore throat. A throat culture is done, and the specimen is sent to an outside laboratory for a culture and sensitivity study to determine the presence of *Streptococcus.* List the diagnostic code the physician would use if the insurance claim is submitted before the results are known. List the diagnostic code used if the physician submits the insurance claim after the laboratory report is received indicating *Streptococcus* is present.	______________

ASSIGNMENT 12.5 CODE DIAGNOSES USING Z CODES

Performance Objective

Task: Locate the correct diagnostic code for each case scenario.

Conditions: Use pen or pencil and ICD-10-CM diagnostic code book.

Standards: Time: ______________ minutes

Accuracy: ________________

(Note: The time element and accuracy criteria may be given by your instructor.)

Directions: In this exercise, you will be reviewing Z codes in the ICD-10-CM code book. Assign the correct code, entering it on the blank line. These are some keywords under which Z codes may be located in Volume 2:

admission	checking/checkup	donor	insertion of	status post
aftercare	conflict	evaluation	maintenance	vaccination
attention to	contact	examination	observation	
border	contraception	fitting of	person with	
care of	counseling	follow-up	problem with	
carrier	dialysis	history of	screening	

Problems

ICD-10-CM Codes

1. Kathy Osborn, a patient, is seen in the office for an annual checkup. ________________
2. Daniel Matsui is seen in the office for adjustment of a lumbosacral corset. ________________
3. Philip O'Brien comes into the office to receive a prophylactic flu shot. ________________
4. Bernadette Murphy is seen in the office for a pregnancy test; the result is positive. ________________
5. Michiko Fujita is seen in the office for a fractured rib. No x-rays are taken because Mrs. Fujita thinks she is pregnant. ________________
6. Dr. Perry Cardi sees Kenneth Pickford in the office for a cardiac pacemaker adjustment. The pacemaker was implanted because of sick sinus syndrome. ________________
7. Frank Meadows returns for follow-up, postoperative transurethral prostatic resection (TURP) for prostate cancer after treatment has been completed. ________________

ASSIGNMENT 12.6 CODE NEOPLASTIC DIAGNOSES

Performance Objective

Task: Locate the correct diagnostic code for each diagnosis listed.

Conditions: Use pen or pencil and ICD-10-CM diagnostic code book.

Standards: Time: ______________ minutes

Accuracy: ________________

(Note: The time element and accuracy criteria may be given by your instructor.)

Directions: In this exercise, you will be reviewing diagnostic codes in the ICD-10-CM code book involving neoplasms. Assign the correct code, entering it on the blank line.

Problems	ICD-10-CM Codes
1. Leiomyoma, uterus	________________
2. Ewing's sarcoma, forearm	________________
3. Adenocarcinoma, right breast, central portion, female	________________
4. Dyspnea resulting from carcinoma of the breast, female with metastasis to the upper lobe, right lung	________________
5. Patient is seen for a yearly examination 1 year after a mastectomy for breast cancer; she is disease-free at this time.	________________

ASSIGNMENT 12.7 CODE DIAGNOSES FOR PATIENTS WITH DIABETES

Performance Objective

Task: Locate the correct diagnostic code for each diagnosis listed.

Conditions: Use pen or pencil and ICD-10-CM diagnostic code book.

Standards: Time: ______________ minutes

Accuracy: ______________

(Note: The time element and accuracy criteria may be given by your instructor.)

Directions: In this exercise, you will review diagnostic codes in the ICD-10-CM code book involving cases of patients with diabetes. The diabetes codes are combination codes that include the type of diabetes, the body system affected, and the complications affecting that body system. Use as many codes as are necessary to describe all of the complications of the disease. Assign as many codes from categories E08 through E13 as needed to identify all of the associated conditions that the patient has.

Example: If a patient with type 2 uncontrolled diabetes is treated for a skin ulcer on the lower extremity, look up "diabetes" in Volume 2 and find the subterm "with skin ulcer." The diabetes code listed is E11.622. Go to Volume 1 and verify. Volume 1 instructs you to "*use additional code to identify site of ulcer*" (L97.-, L98.-). The additional code L97.809 is selected, as it describes "Nonpressure chronic ulcer of other part of unspecified lower leg with unspecified severity."

Always verify all codes in Volume 1 before assigning them. Assign the correct code(s) for each case involving diabetes, entering it (them) on the blank line.

Problems	ICD-10-CM Codes
1. Diabetes mellitus	______________
2. Type 2, non–insulin-dependent diabetes mellitus with neuropathy.	______________
3. Diabetic gangrene (type 1 diabetes)	______________
4. Type 2 diabetes with cataract	______________
5. Type 1 diabetes with diabetic polyneuropathy and retinopathy	______________

ASSIGNMENT 12.8 CODE DIAGNOSES FOR PATIENTS WITH HYPERTENSION

Performance Objective

Task: Locate the correct diagnostic code for each diagnosis listed.

Conditions: Use pen or pencil and ICD-10-CM diagnostic code book.

Standards: Time: ______________ minutes

Accuracy: ______________

(Note: The time element and accuracy criteria may be given by your instructor.)

Directions: In this exercise, you will review diagnostic codes in the ICD-10-CM code book involving patients who have hypertension. To begin coding, look in Volume 2 under "hypertension."

Assign the correct code(s) for each case, entering it (them) on the blank line.

Problems	ICD-10-CM Codes
1. High blood pressure reading	______________
2. Malignant hypertension	______________
3. Hypertension complicating pregnancy	______________
4. Hypertension with kidney disease	______________
5. Hypertension as a result of arteriosclerotic cardiovascular disease (ASCVD) and systolic congestive heart failure (CHF)	______________
6. Myocarditis and CHF as a result of malignant hypertension	______________

ASSIGNMENT 12.9 CODE DIAGNOSES FOR INJURIES, FRACTURES, BURNS, LATE EFFECTS, AND COMPLICATIONS

Performance Objective

Task: Locate the correct diagnostic code for each diagnosis listed.

Conditions: Use pen or pencil and ICD-10-CM diagnostic code book.

Standards: Time: ____________ minutes

Accuracy: ____________

(Note: The time element and accuracy criteria may be given by your instructor.)

Directions: In this exercise, you will review diagnostic codes from the ICD-10-CM code book involving patients who have suffered injuries, burns, fractures, and late effects. Here are some guidelines for coding injuries, fractures, burns, late effects, and complications.

Injuries

When coding injuries, assign separate codes for each injury unless a combination code is provided, in which case the combination code is assigned. The code for the most serious injury, as determined by the provider and the focus of treatment, is sequenced first.

Fractures

Fractures are presumed to be closed unless otherwise specified. Fracture not indicated, whether displaced or not displaced, should be coded as displaced.

Burns

Multiple burns at the same site, but of different degrees, are coded to the most severe degree.

Code the extent of body surface involved (percentage of body surface), when specified, as an additional code.

Late Effects

A residual, late effect is defined as the current condition resulting from a previous acute illness or injury that is no longer the current problem. Late effects are coded using the residual or late effect as the primary diagnosis. The cause of the residual or late effect is coded second.

Complications

For conditions resulting from the malfunction of internal devices, use the subterm "mechanical" found under the main term "complication."

Postoperative complications are sometimes found under the subterm "postoperative," which appears under the main term identifying the condition. If not found there, look for a subterm identifying the type of procedure, type of complication, or surgical procedure under the main term "complication."

Problems	ICD-10-CM Codes
1. Supracondylar fracture of right femur with intracondylar extension of lower end; initial encounter	____________
2. Fracture of left humerus and left foot; subsequent encounter	____________
3. Comminuted fracture of left radius and ulna, not displaced; initial encounter	____________
4. Pathologic fracture of right hip caused by drug-induced osteoporosis; initial encounter for fracture	____________
5. Lacerations of the upper arm with embedded glass; initial encounter	____________
6. Burns on the face and neck; sequela	____________
7. Second- and third-degree burns on chest wall; 20% of body involved, 10% third-degree; initial encounter	____________
8. Bursitis of the knee resulting from crushing injury to the knee 1 year ago	____________

ASSIGNMENT 12.10 CODE DIAGNOSES FOR PREGNANCY, DELIVERY, AND NEWBORN CARE

Performance Objective

Task: Locate the correct diagnostic code for each case scenario.

Conditions: Use pen or pencil and ICD-10-CM diagnostic code book.

Standards: Time: ______________ minutes

Accuracy: ______________

(Note: The time element and accuracy criteria may be given by your instructor.)

Directions: In this exercise, you will review diagnostic codes from the ICD-10-CM code book involving patients who have conditions involving pregnancy and delivery, and newborn infants.

For the supervision of a normal pregnancy, turn to Volume 2 and look up "pregnancy." This is a long category. Look up the subterm "supervision" and find the sub-subterm "normal" (NEC Z34.8-) and "first" (Z34.0-). Check Volume 1 to verify these codes. Also see code Z33.1, "pregnancy state, incidental." This code is used in the second position to tell the insurance carrier that the patient is pregnant in addition to any other diagnosis.

If a patient has complications, turn to Volume 2 and look under the main term "pregnancy." Find the subterm "complicated by" and find the sub-subterm stating the complication. These are codes from ICD-10-CM Chapter 15: "Pregnancy, Childbirth, and Puerperium" (O00-O9a).

Delivery in a completely normal case is coded O80 and is listed under the main term "delivery, uncomplicated." *Normal* is described as "delivery requiring minimal or no assistance, with or without episiotomy, without fetal manipulation (e.g., rotation version) or instrumentation (forceps) of a spontaneous, cephalic, vaginal, full-term, single, live-born infant." This code is for use as a single diagnosis code and is not to be used with any other code from Chapter 15.

When coding deliveries, always include a code for the status of the infant. Look up "outcome of delivery" in Volume 2, and you will find various Z37 codes listing possible outcomes. These codes would be listed as secondary codes on the insurance claim form for the delivery.

On the insurance claim form for the newborn, turn to "newborn" in Volume 2. You will find codes from Z38.0 to Z38.8 describing the birth of the newborn. Use these codes in the first position when billing for services for the newborn infant.

Assign the correct code(s) for each case, entering it (them) on the blank line.

Problems	ICD-10-CM Codes
1. A pregnant patient who is due to deliver in 6 weeks presents in the office with preeclampsia.	______________
2. A patient presents with a chief complaint of severe episodes of pain and vaginal hemorrhage. The physician determines that the patient has an incomplete spontaneous abortion complicated by excessive hemorrhage; she was 6 weeks pregnant.	______________
3. A patient comes in who is diagnosed with a kidney stone; the patient is pregnant.	______________
4. A patient is delivered of twins, both live born by cesarean section because of cephalopelvic disproportion, which caused an obstruction. Code the mother's chart.	______________

ASSIGNMENT 12.11 CODE DIAGNOSES USING TABLE OF DRUGS AND CHEMICALS

Performance Objective

Task: Locate the correct diagnostic code for each diagnosis listed.

Conditions: Use pen or pencil and the ICD-10-CM diagnostic code book.

Standards: Time: ____________ minutes

Accuracy: ____________

(Note: The time element and accuracy criteria may be given by your instructor.)

Directions: In this exercise, you will be reviewing diagnostic codes from the ICD-10-CM code book involving patients who may have had an adverse effect from ingesting a toxic substance. Read the definitions for poisoning and drug intoxication in the *Textbook.*

Injury codes T36 through T65 are combination codes that include the substances related to adverse effects, poisonings, toxic effects, and underdosing, as well as the external cause. No additional external cause code is required to report poisonings, toxic effects, adverse effects, or underdosing codes.

A code from categories T36 through T65 is sequenced first, followed by the code or codes that specify the nature of the adverse effect, poisoning, or toxic effect.

Assign the correct code(s) for each case and enter it (them) on the blank line.

Problems	ICD-10-CM Codes
1. Light-headedness caused by digitalis intoxication; initial encounter	____________
2. Treatment of a rash after an initial dose of penicillin is given	____________
3. Initial encounter for accidental overdose of meperidine (Demerol)	____________
4. A 20-month-old baby accidentally ingests approximately 15 aspirin and is severely nauseated.	____________
5. A patient presents in the physician's office with a vague complaint of not feeling well. The physician notices that the patient has ataxia (a staggering gait). After reviewing the patient's history, the physician determines the ataxia is caused by the meprobamate the patient is taking.	____________
6. Initial visit for internal bleeding: abnormal reaction to a combination of chloramphenicol and warfarin (Coumadin)	____________

13 Procedural Coding

Cheryl Fassett

KEY TERMS

Your instructor may wish to select some words pertinent to this chapter for a test. For definitions of the terms, further study, and/or reference, the words, phrases, and abbreviations may be found in the glossary at the end of the textbook. *Key terms for this chapter follow.*

bilateral
bundled codes
comprehensive code
conversion factor
Current Procedural Terminology
customary fee
downcoding
durable medical equipment
emergency department
fee schedule
global surgery policy
Healthcare Common Procedure Coding System
modifiers
National Correct Coding Initiative
never event
physical status modifiers
procedure code numbers
professional component
qualifying circumstance modifiers
reasonable fee
relative value studies
relative value unit
resource-based relative value scale
surgical package
technical component
unbundling
upcoding
usual, customary, and reasonable

KEY ABBREVIATIONS

See how many abbreviations and acronyms you can translate and then use this as a handy reference list. Definitions for the key abbreviations are located near the back of the textbook in the glossary.

CF ____________________

CPT ____________________

DME ____________________

ECG ____________________

ED ____________________

E/M ____________________

EOB ____________________

FTC ____________________

GAF ____________________

GPCIs ____________________

HCPCS ____________________

NCCI edits ____________________

PC ____________________

PS ____________________

QC ____________________

RBRVS ____________________

RVS ____________________

RVU ____________________

TC ____________________

UCR ____________________

PERFORMANCE OBJECTIVES

The student will be able to:

- Define and spell the key terms and key abbreviations for this chapter, given the information from the textbook glossary, within a reasonable time period and with enough accuracy to obtain a satisfactory evaluation.
- Answer the fill-in-the-blank, mix and match, multiple choice, and true/false review questions after reading the chapter, with enough accuracy to obtain a satisfactory evaluation.
- Select the five-digit procedure code numbers, modifiers, and/or descriptors of each service, given a series of problems relating to various medical procedures and services and using the *Current Procedural Terminology* (CPT) code book, with enough accuracy to obtain a satisfactory evaluation.
- Fill in the correct meaning of each abbreviation given in a list of common medical abbreviations and symbols that appear in chart notes, with enough accuracy to obtain a satisfactory evaluation.

STUDY OUTLINE

Understanding the Importance of Procedural Coding Skills
A Coding Specialist's Tools
Health Care Procedure Coding System
- Level I: CPT Codes
- Level II: HCPCS Codes

CPT Content and Format
- Category I: Codes
- Category II: Performance Measurement Codes
- Category III: New and Emerging Technology Codes
- Code Book Symbols
- Unlisted Procedures
- Evaluation and Management Services
- Anesthesia Services
- Surgery Guidelines
- Integumentary System
- Musculoskeletal System
- Respiratory System
- Cardiovascular System
- Urinary System
- Male Genital System
- Female Reproductive System
- Endocrine System
- Nervous System
- Eye and Auditory System
- Radiology
- Pathology and Laboratory
- Medicine Section

Code Modifiers
- Common CPT Modifiers
- HCPCS Modifiers

Correct Coding Edits and Practices
- National Correct Coding Initiative (NCCI)
- Bundling
- Unbundling
- Downcoding
- Upcoding
- Code Monitoring

Methods of Payment
- Fee Schedule
- Usual, Customary, and Reasonable
- Relative Value Studies
- Resource-Based Relative Value Scale
- Medicare Fee Schedule
- Developing a Fee Schedule Using RBRVS

Procedure 13.1: Choose Correct Procedural Codes for Professional Services
Procedure 13.2: Locate Correct Level II HCPCS Codes for Professional Services

ASSIGNMENT 13.1 REVIEW QUESTIONS

Part I Fill in the Blank

Review the objectives, key terms, and chapter information before completing the following review questions.

1. The coding system used for billing professional medical services and procedures is found in a book titled ______________________________.

2. The Medicare program uses a system of coding composed of two levels, and this is called ______________________________.

3. A medical service or procedure performed that differs in some way from the code description may be shown by using a CPT code with a/an ______________.

4. A *relative value scale* or *schedule* is a listing of procedure codes indicating the relative value of services performed, which is shown by ______________.

5. Name three methods for basing payments adopted by insurance companies and by state and federal programs.

   a. ______________________________

   b. ______________________________

   c. ______________________________

6. List four of the situations that can occur in a medical practice when referring to charges and payments from a fee schedule.

   a. ______________________________

   b. ______________________________

   c. ______________________________

   d. ______________________________

7. Name the six sections of Category I in the CPT code book published by the American Medical Association.

   a. ______________________________

   b. ______________________________

   c. ______________________________

   d. ______________________________

   e. ______________________________

   f. ______________________________

8. Name five criteria for Medicare's definition of DME.

   a. ______________________________

   b. ______________________________

   c. ______________________________

   d. ______________________________

   e. ______________________________

9. A surgical package includes:

   ____

   ____

   ____

   ____

10. A function of computer software that performs online checking of codes on an insurance claim to detect improper code submission is called a/an ____________________.

11. A single code that describes two or more component codes bundled together as one unit is known as a/an ____________________.

12. Grouping related codes together is commonly referred to as ____________________.

13. Use of many procedural codes to identify procedures that may be described by one code is termed ____________________.

14. A code used on a claim that does not match the code system used by the third-party payer and is converted to the closest code rendering less payment is termed

    ____________________.

15. Intentional manipulation of procedural codes to generate increased reimbursement is called ____________________.

16. Give eight reasons for using modifiers on insurance claims.

    a. ______________________________

    b. ______________________________

    c. ______________________________

    d. ______________________________

    e. ______________________________

    f. ______________________________

    g. ______________________________

    h. ______________________________

17. What modifier is usually used when billing for an assistant surgeon who is not in a teaching hospital?

____

18. Explain when to use the -99 modifier code.

____

____

Part II Mix and Match

19. Match the symbols in the first column with the definitions in the second column. Write the correct letters on the blanks.

_______	▶◀	a. New code
_______	●	b. Modifier -51 exempt
_______	↗	c. Add-on code
_______	⊘	d. New or revised text
_______	+	e. Revised code
_______	▲	f. Reference material

20. Match the two-digit modifiers in the first column with the definitions in the second column. Write the correct letters on the blanks.

_______ -23	a. Increased procedural service
_______ -22	b. Multiple procedures
_______ -25	c. Staged or related procedure
_______ -26	d. Decision for surgery
_______ -51	e. Significant, separately identifiable evaluation and management (E/M) service by the same physician on the same day of the procedure or other service
_______ -52	f. Unusual anesthesia
_______ -57	g. Reduced services
_______ -58	h. Professional component

Part III Multiple Choice Questions

Choose the best answer.

21. The codes used to bill ambulance services, surgical supplies, and durable medical equipment are:
    a. CPT codes.
    b. CPT modifiers
    c. Level I HCPCS CPT codes.
    d. Level II HCPCS national codes.

22. A complex reimbursement system in which three fees are considered in calculating payment is known as:
    a. usual, customary, and reasonable (UCR).
    b. relative value studies (RVS).
    c. resource-based relative value scale (RBRVS).
    d. relative value unit (RVU).

23. Medicare defines the postoperative global periods as:
    a. 0, 25, 50, or 100 days.
    b. 0, 10, or 90 days.
    c. 0, 10, 20, or 50 days.
    d. 0, 20, 50, or 90 days.

24. To code numerous CPT codes to identify a procedure that can be described in a single comprehensive code is referred to as:
    a. unbundling.
    b. downcoding.
    c. bundling.
    d. upcoding.

25. When two surgeons work together as primary surgeons performing distinct parts of a procedure, and each doctor bills for performing his or her distinct part of the procedure, the CPT surgical code is listed with modifier:
    a. -62.
    b. -66.
    c. -80.
    d. -82.

Part IV True/False

Write "T" or "F" in the blank to indicate whether you think the statement is true or false.

________26. Procedure coding is the transformation of written descriptions of procedures and professional services into numeric designations (code numbers).

________27. Category II codes describe clinical components that may be typically included in evaluation and management services or clinical services and do not have a relative value associated with them.

________28. When multiple lacerations have been repaired using the same technique and are in the same anatomic category, each repair should be assigned a separate code when billing an insurance claim.

________29. When listing a sterile tray for an in-office surgical procedure, the tray is bundled with the procedure, unless other supplies are needed in addition to those usually used.

________30. HCPCS Level II modifiers consist of only two numeric characters.

PROCEDURE CODING ASSIGNMENTS

In this chapter, the points awarded for assignments that require procedure codes are 1 point for each correct digit.

ASSIGNMENT 13.2 INTRODUCTION TO CPT AND CODING EVALUATION AND MANAGEMENT SERVICES

Performance Objective

Task: Locate the correct information and/or procedure code for each question and/or case scenario.

Conditions: Use pen or pencil and the CPT code book.

Standards: Time: ______________ minutes

Accuracy: ______________

(Note: The time element and accuracy criteria may be given by your instructor.)

1. To become acquainted with the sections of the CPT code book, match the code number in the left column with the appropriate description in the right column by writing the letters in the blanks. Locate each code number in the CPT code book. As you progress through the assignment, the problems get more difficult and complex.

99231	______	a.	Chest x-ray
59400	______	b.	Anesthesia for procedures on cervical spine and cord
71045	______	c.	Subsequent hospital care
00600	______	d.	Supplies and materials
85025	______	e.	Routine OB care, antepartum and postpartum
99070	______	f.	CBC

2. Name the section of the CPT where each of the following codes is located.

a. 65091 ________________________________

b. 86038 ________________________________

c. 92596 ________________________________

d. 75984 ________________________________

e. 0042T ________________________________

f. 01320 ________________________________

g. 99324 ________________________________

h. 0503F ________________________________

3. Evaluation and Management (E/M) codes are used by physicians to report a significant portion of their services. Remember, it is the physician's responsibility to assign E/M codes, and the exercises presented here are only for familiarization. The problems will acquaint you with terminology for this section of the CPT code book. Select the appropriate **new patient** office visit codes using the key components:

   a. This is a Level 3 case: Detailed history

      Detailed examination

      Low-complexity decision making ______________

   b. This is a Level 1 case: Problem-focused history

      Problem-focused examination

      Straightforward decision making ______________

   c. This is a Level 5 case: Comprehensive history

      Comprehensive examination

      High-complexity decision making ______________

4. Select the appropriate **established patient** office visit codes using the key components. Coding these cases illustrates consideration of two of three components.

   a. This is a Level 4 case: Detailed history

      Detailed examination

      Low-complexity decision making ______________

   b. This is a Level 5 case: Comprehensive history

      Comprehensive examination

      Moderate-complexity decision making ______________

   c. This is a Level 5 case: Detailed history

      Comprehensive examination

      High-complexity decision making ______________

5. Evaluation and Management (E/M) codes **99201** to **99239** are used for services provided in the physician's office or in a hospital facility. Read the brief statement and then locate the code number in the *Current Procedural Terminology* code book.

   a. Office visit of a 20-year-old patient seen within the past 3 years for instruction in diabetes injection sites by RN (minimal problem). Patient not seen by physician at this brief visit. ______________

   b. Office visit of a 30-year-old new patient with allergic rhinitis. This case had an expanded problem-focused history & examination and straightforward decision making. ______________

   c. Discussion of medication with the son of an 80-year-old patient with dementia on discharge from the observation unit. ______________

   d. Admission to hospital of 60-year-old established patient in acute respiratory distress with bronchitis. Comprehensive history & examination and medical decision making of moderate complexity. ______________

   e. Hospital visit of a 4-year-old boy, now stable, who will be discharged the next day. This is a problem-focused interval history & examination and medical decision making of low complexity. ______________

   f. New patient seen in the office for chest pain, congestive heart failure, and hypertension. Comprehensive history & examination and highly complex decision making. ______________

6. Evaluation and Management codes **99241** to **99255** are used for consultations provided in the physician's office or in an outpatient or inpatient hospital facility. A *consultation* is a service provided by a physician whose opinion about a case is requested by another physician. Read the brief statement and then locate the code number in the *Current Procedural Terminology* code book.

   a. Office consultation for a 30-year-old woman complaining of palpitations and chest pains. Her family physician described a mild systolic click. This is an expanded problem-focused history & examination and straightforward decision making. ______________

   b. Subsequent inpatient consultation for a 54-year-old woman, who is now stable, admitted 2 days ago for a bleeding ulcer. This case requires a detailed history & examination and low-complexity decision making. ______________

   c. Office consultation for a 14-year-old boy with poor grades in school and suspected alcohol abuse. This is a comprehensive history & examination and medical decision making of moderate complexity. ______________

   d. Subsequent inpatient consultation for a 50-year-old man who is diabetic and is suffering with fever, chills, gangrenous heel ulcer, rhonchi, and dyspnea (difficulty breathing), an unstable condition. The patient appears lethargic and tachypneic (rapid breathing). This case is a comprehensive history & examination with highly complex medical decision making. ______________

   e. Initial emergency department (ED) consultation for a senior who presents with thyrotoxicosis, exophthalmos, cardiac arrhythmia, and congestive heart failure. This case is a comprehensive history & examination with highly complex medical decision making. ______________

   f. Initial hospital consultation for a 30-year-old woman, post-abdominal surgery, who is exhibiting a fever. This case is an expanded problem-focused history & examination and straightforward medical decision making. ______________

7. Evaluation and Management codes **99281** to **99499** are used for emergency department, critical care, nursing facility, rest home, custodial care, home, prolonged, physician standby, and preventive medicine services. Read the brief statement and then locate the code number in the *Current Procedural Terminology* code book.

   a. First hour of critical care of a senior who, after major surgery, suffers a cardiac arrest from a pulmonary embolus. ____________

   b. A 40-year-old woman is admitted to the Obstetrical unit, and the primary care physician has requested the neonatologist to stand by for possible cesarean section and neonatal resuscitation. Code for a 1-hour standby. ____________

   c. A child is seen in the ED with a fever, diarrhea, abdominal cramps, and vomiting. This case had an expanded problem-focused history & examination, and a moderately complex medical decision was made. ____________

   d. A patient is seen for an annual visit at a nursing facility for detailed history & comprehensive examination and low-complexity medical decision making. ____________

   e. An initial visit is made to a domiciliary care facility for a developmentally disabled individual with a mild rash on hands and face. This case had an expanded problem-focused history & examination and low-complexity medical decision making. ____________

   f. A 50-year-old man with a history of asthma comes into the office with acute bronchospasm and moderate respiratory distress. Office treatment is initiated. The case requires intermittent physician face-to-face time with the patient for 2 hours and prolonged services. Assume the appropriate E/M code has been assigned for this case. ____________

ASSIGNMENT 13.3 CODE ANESTHESIA PROBLEMS

Performance Objective

Task: Locate the correct procedure and modifier, if necessary, for each question and/or case scenario.

Conditions: Use pen or pencil and CPT code book.

Standards: Time: ______________ minutes

Accuracy: ______________

(Note: The time element and accuracy criteria may be given by your instructor.)

Directions: Anesthesia codes **00100** to **01999** may be used by anesthesiologists and physicians. Some plastic surgeons, other medical specialists, and large clinics may have a room set aside to perform surgical procedures that might be performed in a hospital outpatient surgical department. Read the brief statement and then locate the Anesthesia Code in the *Current Procedural Terminology* code book. Special modifiers **P1** through **P6** may be needed when coding for this section, as well as code numbers for cases that have difficult circumstances. Definitions for abbreviations may be found in Appendix A of this *Workbook.*

a. Cesarean delivery after neuraxial labor anesthesia, normal healthy patient ______________ ______________

b. Reduction mammoplasty of a woman with mild systemic disease ______________

c. Total right hip replacement, 71-year-old patient, normal healthy patient ______________ ______________

d. Repair of cleft palate, newborn infant, normal healthy patient ______________ ______________

e. TURP, normal healthy male ______________

ASSIGNMENT 13.4 CODE SURGICAL PROBLEMS

Performance Objective

Task: Locate the correct procedure code and modifier, if necessary, for each question and/or case scenario.

Conditions: Use pen or pencil and *Current Procedural Terminology* code book.

Standards: Time: ______________ minutes

Accuracy: ______________

(Note: The time element and accuracy criteria may be given by your instructor.)

Directions: Surgery codes **10040** to **69979** are used for each anatomic part of the body. Read over each case carefully. Use the *Current Procedural Terminology* code book to obtain the correct code number for each descriptor given. Full descriptors for services rendered have been omitted in some instances to give you practice in abstracting the correct descriptor from the available information. Indicate the correct two-digit modifier if necessary. The skill of critical thinking enters this section of the assignment, in that you may have to use your own judgment to code because the cases do not contain full details. Remember to use the index at the back of the CPT code book.

a. Suppose you work in an office that has an encounter form listing code 43228. Check your edition of CPT and see whether you can locate this code number. If the code does not appear, what code number are you directed to use? ______________

Integumentary System 10040-19499

b. Removal of benign lesion from the back (1.0 cm) and left foot (0.5 cm) ______________

c. Drainage of deep breast abscess ______________

d. Laser destruction of two benign facial lesions ______________

Musculoskeletal System 20000-29909

Reminder: Be sure to read the "Application of casts and strapping" guidelines in your CPT code book that appear before the 29000 codes.

e. Aspiration of fluid (arthrocentesis) from right knee joint; not infectious ______________

f. Deep tissue biopsy of left upper arm ______________

g. Fracture of the left tibia, closed treatment ______________

Does the procedural code include application and removal of the first cast? ______________

If done as an office procedure, may supplies be coded? ______________

Does the procedural code include subsequent replacement of a cast for follow-up care? ______________

If not, list the code number for application of a walking short leg cast. ______________

Respiratory System 30000-32999

h. Parietal pleurectomy ______________

i. Removal of two nasal polyps, simple ______________

j. Diagnostic bronchoscopy with bronchial biopsy ______________

Cardiovascular System 33010-37799

k. Pacemaker insertion with transvenous electrode, atrial ______________

l. Thromboendarterectomy with patch graft ______________

m. Introduction of intracatheter and injection procedure for contrast venography ______________

Hemic/Lymphatic/Diaphragm 38100-39599

n. Repair, esophageal/diaphragmatic hernia, transthoracic ______________

o. Partial splenectomy ______________

p. Excision, two deep cervical nodes ______________

Digestive System 40490-49999

q. T & A, 12-year-old boy ______________

r. Endoscopic balloon dilation of esophagus ______________

Urinary System/Male and Female Genital 50010-55980

s. Removal of urethral diverticulum from female patient ______________

t. Anastomosis of single ureter to bladder ______________

Laparoscopy/Peritoneoscopy/Hysteroscopy/Female Genital/ Maternity 56300-59899

u. Routine OB care, antepartum and postpartum care ______________

v. Therapeutic D & C, nonobstetric ______________

w. Enucleation of eye, with implant, muscles attached to implant ______________

x. Strabismus surgery, superior oblique muscle ______________

y. Cochlear device implantation ______________

z. Bilateral, myringotomy including aspiration, requiring general anesthesia ______________

ASSIGNMENT 13.5 CODE PROBLEMS FOR RADIOLOGY AND PATHOLOGY

Performance Objective

Task: Locate the correct procedure code and modifier, if necessary, for each question and/or case scenario.

Conditions: Use pen or pencil and *Current Procedural Terminology* code book.

Standards: Time: ______________ minutes

Accuracy: ______________

(Note: The time element and accuracy criteria may be given by your instructor.)

Radiologists, as well as other physicians in many specialties, perform these studies. A physician who interprets, dictates, and signs a report may not bill for the report separately because it is considered part of the radiology procedure.

Some medical practices perform basic laboratory tests under a waived test certificate that complies with the rules of the Clinical Laboratory Improvement Amendments (CLIA) of 1988, implemented in September 1992.

a. Upper GI x-ray study with films and KUB ______________

b. Ultrasound, pregnant uterus after first trimester, two gestations ______________ and ______________

c. Routine urinalysis with microscopy, nonautomated ______________

d. Hemoglobin (Hgb), electrophoretic method ______________

ASSIGNMENT 13.6 PROCEDURE CODE AND MODIFIER PROBLEMS

Performance Objective

Task: Locate the correct procedure code and modifiers, if necessary, for each case scenario.

Conditions: Use pen or pencil and *Current Procedural Terminology* code book.

Standards: Time: ______________ minutes

Accuracy: ______________

(Note: The time element and accuracy criteria may be given by your instructor.)

Directions: Find the correct procedure codes and modifiers, if necessary. This assignment will reinforce what you have already learned about procedural coding because code numbers for the case scenarios presented are located in all the sections of the CPT code book. Also search for codes in the Medicine section, if necessary.

1. A new patient had five benign skin lesions on the right arm destroyed with surgical curettement. Complete the coding for the surgery.

Code Number	*Description*
a. ______________	Level 3, detailed history and examination with low-complexity decision making, initial new patient office visit
b. ______________	Destruction of five benign skin lesions rt arm

2. Mrs. Stayman had four moles on her back. Dr. Davis excised the multiple nevi in one new-patient office visit after an expanded problem-focused history & examination and straightforward medical decision making. The information on the pathology report stated nonmalignant lesions measuring 2.2 cm, 1.5 cm, 1 cm, and 0.75 cm.

Code Number		*Description*
a. ______________	________	Initial OV
b. ______________		Excision, benign lesion 2.2 cm
c. ______________	________	Excision, benign lesion 1.5 cm
d. ______________	________	Excision, benign lesion 1 cm
e. ______________	________	Excision, benign lesion 0.75 cm

In another case, if a patient required removal of a 1-cm lesion on the back and a 0.5-cm lesion on the neck, the procedural codes would be ______________ for the back lesion and ______________ for the neck lesion.

3. Dr. Davis stated on his operative report that Mr. Allen was suffering from a complex, complicated nasal fracture. Dr. Davis debrided the wound because it was contaminated and performed an open reduction with internal fixation in a complex and complicated procedure.

Code Number		*Description*
a. ______________	______	Initial OV, complex history & examination, moderate-complexity decision making
b. ______________		Open tx nasal fracture, complicated
c. ______________	______	Debridement, skin, subcutaneous tissue, muscle, and bone

4. A registered nurse (RN), an established patient, age 40 years, sees the doctor for an annual physical. A Pap (Papanicolaou) smear is obtained and sent to an outside laboratory. The patient also has a furuncle on the right axilla at the time of the visit, which the doctor incises and drains (I & D).

Code Number		*Description*
a. ______________	______	Periodic physical examination
b. ______________		Handling of specimen
c. ______________		I & D, furuncle, right axilla
d. ______________		5-mL penicillin IM injection

5. While making his rounds in the hospital during the noon hour, Dr. James sees a new patient in the ED for a laceration of the forehead, 5-cm long. The doctor does a workup for a possible concussion.

Code Number		*Description*
a. ______________	______	ED care, expanded problem-focused history, expanded problem-focused examination, low-complexity decision making
b. ______________		Repair of laceration, simple, face

6. The physician sees a new patient in the office with the same condition as the patient in Problem 5; however, an infection has developed, and the patient is seen for daily dressing changes. On day 11, the sutures are removed, and on day 12, a final dressing change is made, and the patient is discharged.

Code Number		*Description*
a. ______________	______	Level 3, detailed history & examination with low-complexity decision making, initial new patient office visit
b. ______________		Repair of laceration
c. ______________		Tet tox (tetanus toxoid) 0.5 mL
d. ______________		Administration intramuscular injection
e. ______________		Minimal service, OV (suture removal)
f. ______________		Minimal service, OV (dressing change)

Note: Some fee schedules allow no follow-up days; Medicare fee schedule allows 10 follow-up days for the procedural code number for repair of laceration.

7. The physician sees 13-year-old Bobby Jones (established patient) for a Boy Scout physical. Bobby is in good health and well groomed. His troop is going for a 1-week camping trip in 12 days. The physician reviewed safety issues with Bobby, talked to him about school, and counseled him about not getting into drugs or alcohol. Bobby denied any problems with that or of being sexually active. He said that he plays baseball. He has no allergies. The physician performed a detailed examination. The physician completed information for scouting papers and cleared him for camping activity.

Code Number	*Description*
a. ________________	Periodic preventive evaluation and management

8. A new patient, David Ramsey, age 15 years, was seen by Dr. Menter for lapses of memory and frequent headaches. The doctor performed an electroencephalogram (EEG) and some psychological tests (including a psychodiagnostic assessment using personality and psychopathology tests [Rorschach and MMPI]). Dr. Astro Parkinson was called in as a consultant. All the test results were negative, and the patient was advised to come in for weekly psychotherapy.

Code Number	*Description*
Dr. Menter's bill:	
a. ________________	OV, comprehensive history & examination, moderate-complexity decision making
b. ________________	EEG, extended monitoring (1 hour)
c. ________________	Psychological tests (Rorschach and MMPI)
d. ________________	Psychotherapy (60 minutes—done on a different day)
Dr. Parkinson's bill:	
e. ________________	Consultation, expanded problem-focused history & examination, straightforward decision making

9. An established patient, age 70 years, requires repair of a bilateral initial inguinal hernia (reducible). The code for this initial procedure is

a. ________________ ________________

ASSIGNMENT 13.7 HCPCS/MODIFIER CODE MATCH

Performance Objective

Task: Locate the correct HCPCS code and modifier, if necessary, for each medical drug, supply item, or service presented.

Conditions: Use pen or pencil and HCPCS code reference list in Appendix B of this *Workbook*.

Standards: Time: ______________ minutes

Accuracy: ______________

(Note: The time element and accuracy criteria may be given by your instructor.)

Directions: Match the HCPCS code in the first or second column with the description of the drug, supply item, or service presented in the third or fourth column. Write the correct letters on the blanks.

E1280	______	J0760	______	a. Vitamin B_{12}, 1000 mg	k. Blood (whole) for transfusion/unit
E0141	______	A9150	______	b. Injection, insulin per 5 units	l. Heavy-duty wheel-chair with detachable arms
J0290	______	J2001	______	c. Rigid walker, wheeled, without seat	m. Ampicillin inj, up to 500 mg
J3420	______	L0160	______	d. Waiver of liability statement on file	n. Dimethyl sulfoxide (DMSO) inj
J1815	______	L3100-RT	______	e. Nonemergency transportation, taxi	o. Urine strips
P9010	______	A4250	______	f. Inj of colchicine	p. Vancomycin (Vancocin) inj
J1212	______	J2590	______	g. Cervical occipital/ mandibular support	q. Oxytocin (Pitocin) inj
J3370	______	A4927	______	h. Inj of lidocaine (Xylocaine)	r. Wide, heavy-duty wheelchair with detachable arms and leg rests
E1092	______	A0100	______	i. Gloves, nonsterile	s. Rt hallux valgus night splint
A4211	______	-GA	______	j. Supplies for self-administered drug injections	t. nonprescription drug

ASSIGNMENT 13.8 PROCEDURAL CODING CASE SCENARIOS

Performance Objective

Task: Locate the correct procedure code and modifier, if necessary, for each case scenario.

Conditions: Use pen or pencil and *Current Procedural Terminology* code book.

Standards: Time: ______________ minutes

Accuracy: ______________

(Note: The time element and accuracy criteria may be given by your instructor.)

Directions: Find the correct procedure codes and modifiers, if necessary, for each case scenario.

1. The physician sees Horace Hart, a 60-year-old new patient, in the office for bronchial asthma, arteriosclerotic heart disease (ASHD), and hypertension. He performs an electrocardiogram (ECG) and urinalysis (UA) without microscopy and obtains x-rays. Comprehensive metabolic and lipid panels and a complete blood count (CBC) are done by an outside laboratory.

Code Number	*Description*
Physician's bill:	
a. ______________	Initial OV, comprehensive history & examination, high-complexity decision making
b. ______________	ECG with interpret and report
c. ______________	UA, routine, nonautomated
d. ______________	Chest x-ray, two views
e. ______________	Routine venipuncture for handling of specimen
f. ______________	Handling of specimen
Laboratory's bill:	
g. ______________	Comprehensive metabolic panel: albumin, bilirubin, calcium, carbon dioxide, chloride, creatinine, glucose, phosphatase (alkaline), potassium, protein, sodium, ALT, AST, and urea nitrogen
h. ______________	Lipid panel
i. ______________	CBC, completely automated with complete automated differential

If the doctor decides to have the chest x-rays interpreted by a radiologist, the procedural code billed by the radiologist would be ______________.

2. Mr. Hart is seen again in the office on May 12. On May 25, he is seen at home at 2 AM with asthma exacerbation, possible myocardial infarct, and congestive heart failure. The doctor consulted with a thoracic cardiovascular surgeon by telephone. He also called to make arrangements for hospitalization. To complete the patient care, these services required 2 hours and 40 minutes of non–face-to-face time in addition to the time spent examining the patient during the house call.

Code Number	*Description*
a. ______________	OV, problem-focused history & examination, straightforward decision making
b. ______________	Home visit, detailed interval history & examination, high- complexity decision making
c. ______________	Detention time, prolonged (list time required)

3. On June 9, Horace Hart is seen again in the hospital. The thoracic cardiovascular surgeon who was telephoned the previous day was called in for consultation to formally examine the patient and says that surgery is necessary, which is scheduled the following day. The patient's physician sees the patient for his asthmatic condition and acts as assistant surgeon. The surgeon does the follow-up care and assumes care in the case.

Code Number	*Description*
Primary care physician/assistant surgeon's bill:	
a. ______________	Hospital visit, problem-focused history & examination, low-complexity decision making
b. ______________	Pericardiotomy
Thoracic cardiovascular surgeon's bill:	
c. ______________	Consultation, comprehensive history & examination, moderate-complexity decision making
d. ______________	Pericardiotomy

ASSIGNMENT 13.9 CASE SCENARIO FOR CRITICAL THINKING

Performance Objective

Task: Locate the correct procedure code and modifier, if necessary, for each case scenario.

Conditions: Use pen or pencil and *Current Procedural Terminology* code book.

Standards: Time: ______________ minutes

Accuracy: ______________

(Note: The time element and accuracy criteria may be given by your instructor.)

Directions: Read through this progress note on Roy A. Takashima. Abstract information from the note about the subjective symptoms, objective findings, and diagnoses. List the diagnostic and procedure codes you think this case would warrant.

Takashima, Roy A.
October 5, 20xx

Patient presents with many things going on. First, he's had no difficulties after the feral cat bite, and the cat was normal on quarantine.

He seemed to be recovering from the flu but is plagued with a persistent cough and pain down the center of his chest attributed to bronchitis without fever or grossly discolored phlegm.

Physical examination shows expiratory rhonchi and gross exacerbation of his cough on forced expiration. Spirometry before and after bronchodilator was remarkably good; he is symptomatically improved with a Proventil inhaler, which he is given as a sample. I don't think other antibiotics would help.

His reflux is under good control with proprietary antacids with a clear examination.

He has several areas of seborrheic keratoses on his face and head that need attention.

Finally, in follow-up, he needs a complete physical examination.

Ting Cho, MD

Diagnosis: Influenza and acute bronchitis

Subjective symptoms ____

____

Objective findings ____

____

____

Diagnosis code ______________________________ ______________

______________________________ ______________

E/M code ______________

Spirometry code ______________________________ ______________

ASSIGNMENT 13.10 CALCULATE FEES BASED ON RESOURCE-BASED RELATIVE VALUE SYSTEM

Performance Objective

Task: Calculate and insert the correct amounts for the Medicare scenario.

Conditions: Use a pen or pencil, the description of the problem and the reference material listed in the problem.

Standards: Time: ______________ minutes

Accuracy: ______________

(Note: The time element and accuracy criteria may be given by your instructor.)

Problem: In the late 1980s, Medicare's Resource-Based Relative Value System (RBRVS) became the way payment was determined each year. However, since the early 1990s, annual fee schedules have been supplied by local fiscal intermediaries, so the RBRVS has become more useful in determining practice cost to convert patients to capitation in negotiations of managed care contracts. Because physicians may request determination of fees for certain procedures to discover actual cost and what compensation ratios should be, it is important to know how Medicare fees are determined. Each year, the *Federal Register* publishes geographic practice cost indices (GPCIs) by Medicare carrier and locality, as well as relative value units (RVUs) and related information. This assignment will give you some mathematical practice in using figures for annual conversion factors to determine fees for given procedures in various regions of the United States. Refer to Figs 13.1 and 13.2, which are pages of the *Federal Register.*

a. HCPCS Code 47600: Removal of gallbladder. The medical practice is located in Phoenix, Arizona.

	Work	*Overhead*	*Malpractice*
RVUs	______________	______________	______________
GPCI	× ______________	× ______________	× ______________

\+ ______________ + ______________ + ______________ = Total adjusted RVUs

2018 conversion factor \$35.99 Total adjusted RVUs ______________ = allowed

amount \$ ______________.

b. HCPCS Code 47715: Excision of bile duct cyst. The medical practice is located in Arkansas.

	Work	*Overhead*	*Malpractice*
RVUs	______________	______________	______________
GPCI	× ______________	× ______________	× ______________

\+ ______________ + ______________ + ______________ = Total adjusted RVUs

2018 conversion factor \$35.99 Total adjusted RVUs ______________ = allowed

amount \$ ______________.

c. HCPCS Code 48146: Pancreatectomy. The medical practice is located in Fresno, California.

	Work	*Overhead*	*Malpractice*
RVUs	______________	______________	______________
GPCI	× ______________	× ______________	× ______________

\+ ______________ + ______________ + ______________ = Total adjusted RVUs

2018 conversion factor \$35.99 Total adjusted RVUs 3 = allowed

amount \$ ______________.

ADDENDUM D—GEOGRAPHIC PRACTICE COST INDICES BY MEDICARE CARRIER AND LOCALITY					
Carrier number	Locality number	Locality name	Work	Practice expense	Mal-practice
510	5	Birmingham, AL	0.981	0.913	0.824
510	4	Mobile, AL	0.964	0.911	0.824
510	2	North Central AL	0.970	0.867	0.824
510	1	Northwest AL	0.985	0.869	0.824
510	6	Rest of AL	0.975	0.851	0.824
510	3	Southeast AL	0.972	0.869	0.824
1020	1	Alaska	1.106	1.255	1.042
1030	5	Flagstaff (city), AZ	0.983	0.911	1.255
1030	1	Phoenix, AZ	1.003	1.016	1.255
1030	7	Prescott (city), AZ	0.983	0.911	1.255
1030	99	Rest of Arizona	0.987	0.943	1.255
1030	2	Tucson (city), AZ	0.987	0.989	1.255
1030	8	Yuma (city), AZ	0.983	0.911	1.255
520	13	Arkansas	0.960	0.856	0.302
2050	26	Anaheim-Santa Ana, CA	1.046	1.220	1.370
542	14	Bakersfield, CA	1.028	1.050	1.370
542	11	Fresno/Madera, CA	1.006	1.009	1.370
542	13	Kings/Tulare, CA	0.999	1.001	1.370
2050	18	Los Angeles, CA (1st of 8)	1.060	1.196	1.370
2050	19	Los Angeles, CA (2nd of 8)	1.060	1.196	1.370

Fig. 13.1

ADDENDUM B—RELATIVE VALUE UNITS (RVUs) AND RELATED INFORMATION

HCPCS[1]	MOD	Status	Description	Work RVUs	Practice expense RVUs[2]	Mal-practice RVUs	Total	Global period	Update
47399	....	C	Liver surgery procedure	0.00	0.00	0.00	0.00	YYY	S
47400	....	A	Incision of liver duct	19.11	8.62	1.38	29.11	090	S
47420	....	A	Incision of bile duct	15.48	9.59	2.01	27.08	090	S
47425	....	A	Incision of bile duct	14.95	11.84	2.48	29.27	090	S
47440	....	A	Incision of bile duct	18.51	10.61	2.23	31.35	090	S
47460	....	A	Incision of bile duct sphincter	14.57	15.71	1.84	32.12	090	N
47480	....	A	Incision of gallbladder	8.14	7.68	1.61	17.43	090	S
47490	....	A	Incision of gallbladder	6.11	3.61	0.38	10.10	090	N
47500	....	A	Injection for liver x-rays	1.98	1.53	0.14	3.65	000	N
47505	....	A	Injection for liver x-rays	0.77	1.34	0.14	2.25	000	N
47510	....	A	Insert catheter, bile duct	7.47	2.90	0.25	10.62	090	N
47511	....	A	Insert bile duct drain	10.02	2.90	0.25	13.17	090	N
47525	....	A	Change bile duct catheter	5.47	1.61	0.16	7.24	010	N
47530	....	A	Revise, reinsert bile tube	5.47	1.53	0.19	7.19	090	N
47550	....	A	Bile duct endoscopy	3.05	1.58	0.35	4.98	000	S
47552	....	A	Biliary endoscopy, thru skin	6.11	1.38	0.21	7.70	000	S
47553	....	A	Biliary endoscopy, thru skin	6.42	3.84	0.63	10.89	000	N
47554	....	A	Biliary endoscopy, thru skin	9.16	3.97	0.68	13.81	000	S
47555	....	A	Biliary endoscopy, thru skin	7.64	2.66	0.30	10.60	000	N
47556	....	A	Biliary endoscopy, thru skin	8.66	2.66	0.30	11.62	000	N
47600	....	A	Removal of gallbladder	10.80	7.61	1.60	20.01	090	S
47605	....	A	Removal of gallbladder	11.66	8.23	1.77	21.66	090	S
47610	....	A	Removal of gallbladder	14.01	9.47	2.02	25.50	090	S
47612	....	A	Removal of gallbladder	14.91	14.39	3.08	32.38	090	S
47620	....	A	Removal of gallbladder	15.97	11.35	2.39	29.71	090	S
47630	....	A	Removal of bile duct stone	8.40	3.79	0.40	12.59	090	N
47700	....	A	Exploration of bile ducts	13.90	7.71	1.60	23.21	090	S
47701	....	A	Bile duct revision	26.87	8.30	1.92	37.09	090	S
47710	....	A	Excision of bile duct tumor	18.64	12.19	2.49	33.32	090	S
47715	....	A	Excision of bile duct cyst	14.66	8.31	1.73	24.70	090	S
47716	....	A	Fusion of bile duct cyst	12.67	6.63	1.55	20.85	090	S
47720	....	A	Fuse gallbladder and bowel	12.03	9.26	1.95	23.34	090	S
47721	....	A	Fuse upper gi structures	14.57	11.55	2.50	28.62	090	S
47740	....	A	Fuse gallbladder and bowel	14.08	10.32	2.16	26.56	090	S
47760	....	A	Fuse bile ducts and bowel	20.15	11.74	2.56	34.45	090	S
47765	....	A	Fuse liver ducts and bowel	19.25	14.77	3.00	37.02	090	S
47780	....	A	Fuse bile ducts and bowel	20.63	13.22	2.76	36.61	090	S
47800	....	A	Reconstruction of bile ducts	17.91	13.37	2.46	33.74	090	S
47801	....	A	Placement, bile duct support	11.41	5.54	0.82	17.77	090	S
47802	....	A	Fuse liver duct and intestine	16.19	10.38	1.77	28.34	090	S
47999	....	C	Bile tract surgery procedure	0.00	0.00	0.00	0.00	YYY	S
48000	....	A	Drainage of abdomen	13.25	7.13	1.42	21.80	090	S
48001	....	A	Placement of drain, pancreas	15.71	8.22	1.91	25.84	090	S
48005	....	A	Resect/debride pancreas	17.77	9.29	2.16	29.22	090	S
48020	....	A	Removal of pancreatic stone	13.12	6.86	1.59	21.57	090	S
48100	....	A	Biopsy of pancreas	10.30	4.26	0.80	15.36	090	S
48102	....	A	Needle biopsy, pancreas	4.48	2.44	0.25	7.17	010	N
48120	....	A	Removal of pancreas lesion	12.93	9.83	2.09	24.85	090	S
48140	....	A	Partial removal of pancreas	18.47	13.44	2.86	34.77	090	S
48145	....	A	Partial removal of pancreas	19.30	15.88	3.20	38.38	090	S
48146	....	A	Pancreatectomy	21.97	16.67	1.94	40.58	090	S
48148	....	A	Removal of pancreatic duct	14.57	8.32	1.70	24.59	090	S
48150	....	A	Partial removal of pancreas	34.55	22.79	4.80	62.14	090	S
48151	....	D	Partial removal of pancreas	0.00	0.00	0.00	0.00	090	0
48152	....	A	Pancreatectomy	31.33	22.79	4.80	58.92	090	S
48153	....	A	Pancreatectomy	34.55	22.79	4.80	62.14	090	S
48154	....	A	Pancreatectomy	31.33	22.79	4.80	58.92	090	S
48155	....	A	Removal of pancreas	19.65	20.63	4.31	44.59	090	S
48160	....	N	Pancreas removal, transplant	0.00	0.00	0.00	0.00	XXX	0
48180	....	A	Fuse pancreas and bowel	21.11	12.74	2.66	36.51	090	S
48400	....	A	Injection, intraoperative	1.97	1.04	0.24	3.25	ZZZ	S
48500	....	A	Surgery of pancreas cyst	12.17	8.62	1.68	22.47	090	S
48510	....	A	Drain pancreatic pseudocyst	11.34	7.62	1.46	20.42	090	S
48520	....	A	Fuse pancreas cyst and bowel	13.11	11.43	2.46	27.00	090	S
48540	....	A	Fuse pancreas cyst and bowel	15.95	12.80	2.68	31.43	090	S
48545	....	A	Pancreatorrhaphy	14.81	7.75	1.81	24.37	090	S
48547	....	A	Duodenal exclusion	21.42	11.20	2.61	35.23	090	S

[1] All numeric CPT HCPCS Copyright 1993 American Medical Association.
[2] *Indicates reduction of Practice Expense RVUs as a result of OBRA 1993.

Fig. 13.2

14 The Paper Claim: CMS-1500

Cheryl Fassett

KEY TERMS

Your instructor may wish to select some words pertinent to this chapter for a test. For definitions of the terms, further study, and/or reference, the words, phrases, and abbreviations may be found in the glossary at the end of the Textbook. *Key terms for this chapter follow.*

Administrative Simplification Compliance Act
clean claim
deleted claim
dirty claim
durable medical equipment number
electronic claim
employer identification number
facility provider number
group National Provider Identifier (group NPI)
Health Insurance Claim Form (CMS-1500)
incomplete claim
intelligent character recognition
invalid claim
National Provider Identifier
National Uniform Claim Committee
optical character recognition
paper claim
pending claim
physically clean claim
rejected claim
Social Security number
state license number
suspended claim
taxonomy code

KEY ABBREVIATIONS

See how many abbreviations and acronyms you can translate and then use this as a handy reference list. Definitions for the key abbreviations are located near the back of the Textbook *in the glossary.*

ASCA ______________________

CMS-1500 ______________________

DME ______________________

DNA ______________________

EIN ______________________

EMG ______________________

EPSDT ______________________

ICR ______________________

LMP ______________________

MSP ______________________

NA, N/A ______________________

NPI ______________________

NUCC ______________________

OCR ______________________

SOF ______________________

SSN ______________________

PERFORMANCE OBJECTIVES

The student will be able to:

- Define and spell the key terms and key abbreviations for this chapter, given the information from the *Textbook* glossary, within a reasonable time period and with enough accuracy to obtain a satisfactory evaluation.
- After reading the chapter, answer the fill-in-the-blank, mix and match, multiple choice, and true/false review questions, with enough accuracy to obtain a satisfactory evaluation.
- Given a handwritten CMS-1500 form, type a CMS-1500 Health Insurance Claim Form and list the reasons why the claim was either rejected or delayed, within a reasonable time period and with enough accuracy to obtain a satisfactory evaluation.
- Given the patients' medical chart notes and blank insurance claim forms, complete each CMS-1500 Health Insurance Claim Form for billing, within a reasonable time period and with enough accuracy to obtain a satisfactory evaluation.

STUDY OUTLINE

The Paper Claim CMS-1500
- National Uniform Claim Committee
- History of the Paper Claim CMS-1500

Types of Submitted Claims
- Claim Status

Abstracting From Medical Records
- Cover Letter Accompanying Insurance Claims

Health Insurance Claim Form (CMS-1500)
- Basic Guidelines for Submitting a Claim
- Completion of Insurance Claim Forms

Common Reasons Why Claim Forms Are Delayed or Rejected

Claim Completion Guidelines
- Optical Character Recognition
- Do's and Don'ts for Claim Completion

Instructions for the Health Insurance Claim Form (CMS-1500)
- Block-by-Block Instructions for Completion of the CMS-1500

Insurance Program Templates

ASSIGNMENT 14.1 REVIEW QUESTIONS

Part I Fill in the Blank

Review the objectives, key terms, chapter information, glossary definitions of key terms, and figures before completing the following review questions.

1. What legislation required all claims sent to the Medicare program be submitted electronically, effective October 16, 2003?

   ____

2. State the name of the health insurance claim form that was required for use effective April 1, 2014. ____

3. Does Medicare accept the CMS-1500 claim form?

   ____

4. What is a pended claim?

   ____

5. How many days will it take to process a Medicare claim that is submitted electronically?

   ____

6. If a claim is submitted on behalf of the patient, and coverage of the services is denied, what is the most effective way to present the situation to the patient?

   ____

7. What is *dual coverage*?

   ____

8. The insurance company with the first responsibility for payment of a bill for medical services is known as the

   ____

9. The CMS-1500 claim form allows for reporting of a maximum of ______________ diagnosis codes per claim form.

10. What internet resource can be used to find physician provider numbers?

    ____

11. For electronic submission of claims, what allows the physician's name to be printed in the signature block where it would normally be signed?

    ____

12. When preparing a claim that is to be optically scanned, birth dates are keyed in with how many digits?

    ____

13. If circumstances make it impossible to obtain a signature each time a paper claim is submitted, the patient's signature may be obtained and maintained in the patient's medical record. The claim block should be completed with ______________________ or ______________________, thus indicating the signature is on file.

Part II Mix and Match

14. Match the types of claims listed in the right column with their descriptions and fill in the blanks with the appropriate letters.

_______ Claim missing required information

_______ Phrase used when a claim is held back from payment

_______ Claim that is submitted and then optically scanned by the insurance carrier and converted to electronic form

_______ Claim that needs manual processing because of errors or to solve a problem

_______ Claim that needs clarification and answers to some questions

_______ Claim that is canceled or voided if the incorrect claim form is used or itemized charges are not provided

_______ Claim that is paperless

_______ Claim that is submitted within the time limit and correctly completed

_______ Medicare claim that contains information that is complete and necessary but is illogical or incorrect

a. Clean claim
b. Paper claim
c. Invalid claim
d. Dirty claim
e. Electronic claim
f. Pending claim
g. Rejected claim
h. Incomplete claim
i. Deleted claim

15. Match the types of numbers listed in the right column with their descriptions and fill in the blanks with the appropriate letters.

_______ A number issued by the federal government to each individual for personal use

_______ A Medicare lifetime provider number

_______ A number listed on a claim when submitting insurance claims to insurance companies under a group name

_______ A number that a health care provider must obtain to practice in a state

_______ A number used when billing for supplies and equipment

_______ A number issued to a hospital

_______ An individual health care provider's federal tax identification number issued by the Internal Revenue Service

a. State license number
b. Employer identification number
c. Social Security number
d. Group national provider number
e. National Provider Identifier
f. Durable medical equipment number
g. Facility provider number

PART III MULTIPLE CHOICE

Choose the best answer.

16. The basic paper claim form currently used by health care professionals and suppliers to bill insurance carriers for services provided to patients is the:
a. UB-04 claim form.
b. CMS-1500 claim form.
c. Attending physician's statement.
d. COMB-1.

17. What is the exception to the Administrative Simplification Compliance Act's (ASCA's) requirement for providers to send claims to Medicare electronically?
a. Chiropractors
b. Providers who have more than 25 full-time employees
c. Providers with fewer than 10 full-time employees
d. Any provider who requests a financial hardship

18. Under ASCA, plans other than Medicare:
    a. may allow submission of claims on paper.
    b. will never allow submission of claims on paper.
    c. only allow submission of claims on paper.
    d. must follow the claims submission guidance of the American Medical Association (AMA).

19. The National Uniform Claim Committee (NUCC) is made up of which of the following?
    a. AMA representatives
    b. Centers for Medicare and Medicaid Services (CMS) representatives
    c. Providers
    d. All of the above

20. The most recently revised version of the 1500 Health Insurance Claim Form developed in 2012 accommodates:
    a. the change in the names of the government agency from Health Care Finance Administration to Centers for Medicare and Medicaid Services (CMS).
    b. requirements for allowing optical scanning of the claim.
    c. changes in the Electronic Claims Submission Version 5010 837P.
    d. changes to the *Current Procedural Terminology* (CPT) coding system.

21. If a patient has dual coverage:
    a. insurance information for the primary carrier should be obtained.
    b. insurance information for both the primary and the secondary carrier should be obtained.
    c. insurance information for the secondary carrier can be obtained after the primary insurance carrier processes the claim.
    d. the primary carrier has insurance information for the secondary carrier and will automatically forward the claim to the secondary carrier if necessary.

22. Health Insurance Portability and Accountability Act (HIPAA) laws require that the provider rendering the service be identified on the claim form by:
    a. reporting of the correct provider number.
    b. reporting of the correct International Classification of Diseases (ICD)-10 code.
    c. reporting of the correct CPT code.
    d. reporting of the correct facility code.

23. The Omnibus Budget Reconciliation Act (OBRA) requires Medicare administrative contractors to:
    a. deny all claims received after 1 year from date of service.
    b. pay all clean claims that are submitted within 1 year from date of service.
    c. investigate all clean claims not paid on time.
    d. pay interest on all clean claims not paid on time.

24. A claim that is investigated on a postpayment basis that is found to be "not due" will require:
    a. resubmission of a claim.
    b. manual review of the claim.
    c. refund of the monies paid.
    d. additional medical records.

25. If there is a balance remaining on a patient's account after the patient's primary insurance has paid, and the patient has secondary coverage, the billing specialist should:
    a. send a bill to the patient for the remaining balance.
    b. send a claim form to the secondary insurance for the remaining balance.
    c. send a claim form to the secondary insurance with a copy of the explanation of benefits from the primary carrier.
    d. monitor the claim to determine whether the patient has sent a claim to the secondary carrier.

26. The maximum number of diagnostic codes that can be submitted on the CMS-1500 claim form is:
    a. four.
    b. six.
    c. eight.
    d. twelve.

27. National Provider Identifier (NPI) numbers are used to report:
    a. referring physicians.
    b. ordering physicians.
    c. performing physicians.
    d. all of the above.

28. NPI numbers are assigned:
    a. each time a health care provider contracts with a new payer.
    b. annually, per health care provider.
    c. once in a lifetime, per health care provider.
    d. each time the provider moves to another state.

29. To correct a claim that has been denied because of an invalid procedure code, the billing specialist should:
    a. check the patient registration form to ensure all data were reported accurately.
    b. confirm the code in the CPT manual to ensure it is valid for the date of service.
    c. confirm the code in the ICD-10 manual to ensure it is valid for the date of service.
    d. confirm the provider's NPI number to make sure it was reported accurately.

30. To correct a claim that was denied because more than six lines were entered on the claim, the billing specialist should:
    a. readjust the printer, so all claim lines fit on the form, reprint, and send.
    b. reenter data with the appropriate code range for the dates of service and bill on one line.
    c. bill six claim lines on one claim and complete an additional paper claim for the additional claim lines.
    d. write off the additional claim lines that have been denied.

PART IV TRUE/FALSE

Write "T" or "F" in the blank to indicate whether you think the statement is true or false.

_______ 31. The insurance billing specialist does not need to know how to complete a paper claim because most claims are submitted electronically.

_______ 32. Physicians who experience downtimes of internet services that are out of their control for more than two days may submit claims to Medicare on paper.

_______ 33. The goal of the NUCC is to provide a warehouse for providers to purchase CMS-1500 claim forms.

_______ 34. Effective June 1, 2013, providers were required to use only the CMS-1500 claim form.

_______ 35. Use of the standardized CMS-1500 claim form has simplified processing of paper claims.

_______ 36. Quantities of the CMS-1500 claim form can be purchased through CMS or downloaded from the CMS website and used for submission.

_______ 37. Interest rates that apply to the Prompt Payment Interest Rate can be located on the Treasury's Financial Fiscal Service page.

_______ 38. Medicare claims that require further investigation before being processed are referred to as "other" claims.

_______ 39. A diagnosis should never be submitted without supporting documentation in the medical record.

_______ 40. Claims for dates of services in two different years may be submitted on the same claim form.

_______ 41. Services that are inclusive in the global surgical package that have no charge associated with them should not be submitted on the CMS-1500 claim form.

_______ 42. Proofreading claims before submission can prevent denials and delay of claim processing.

_______ 43. When submitting supplemental documentation for processing of a claim, the patient's name and date of service need only be on the front of a two-sided document.

_______ 44. Handwriting is permitted on optically scanned paper claims.

_______ 45. Use the abbreviation "DNA" when information is not applicable.

ASSIGNMENT 14.2 COMPLETE A HEALTH INSURANCE CLAIM FORM FOR A PRIVATE CASE

Performance Objective

Task: Complete a health insurance claim form

Conditions: Use Merry M. McLean's patient record, one health insurance claim form, a computer or pen.

Standards: Claim Productivity Measurement

Time: ________________ minutes

Accuracy: ________________

(Note: The time element and accuracy criteria may be given by your instructor.)

Directions:

1. Complete the Health Insurance Claim Form, using NUCC guidelines, and send the form to the Prudential Insurance Company for Mrs. Merry M. McLean by referring to the patient record. Date the claim June 15 of the current year. Record on the financial account record/statement when you have billed the insurance company.

2. A Performance Evaluation Checklist may be reproduced from the "Instruction Guide to the Workbook" in a section before Chapter 1 if your instructor wishes you to submit it to assist with scoring and comments.

After the instructor has returned your work to you, either make the necessary corrections and place your work in a three-ring notebook for future reference, or, if you received a high score, place it in your portfolio for reference when applying for a job.

COLLEGE CLINIC
4567 Broad Avenue, Woodland Hills, XY 12345-0001
(555)-486-9002
Fax: (555) 487-8976
NPI: 3664021CC

PATIENT INFORMATION:		INSURANCE INFORMATION:	
Name:	Merry M. McLean	Primary:	Prudential Insurance 5621 Wilshire Blvd. Merck, XY 12346 (555) 664-9023
Address:	4919 Dolphin Way Woodland Hills, XY 12345		
Telephone:	(555) 486-1859		
Date of Birth:	02/02/1948	Policy Number:	459-XX-9989
Social Security:	459-XX-9989	Group Number:	8832
Occupation:	SECRETARY	Subscriber:	Harry L. McLean
Employer:	Porter Company 5490 Wilshire Blvd. Merck, XY 12346	Secondary:	None
Status:	Married		
Spouse:	Harry L. McLean		

DIAGNOSIS INFORMATION

1. N32.0	Vesicle fistula, not otherwise specified	5.	
2. R32	Urinary incontinence, unspecified	6.	
3.		7.	
4.		8.	

PROCEDURE INFORMATION

Description	Date	Code	Charge
1. Office visit, new patient	05/06/20XX	99203	70.92
2. Urinalysis	05/06/20XX	81000	8.00
3. Cystoscopy	05/10/20XX	52000	167.05
4. Initial hospital care	05/16/20XX	99221	73.00
5. Repair vesicovaginal fistula	05/17/20XX	51900	1196.82
6. Hospital visit	05/18/20XX	99024	N/C
7. Hospital visit	05/19/20XX	99024	N/C
8. Hospital visit	05/20/20XX	99024	N/C
9. Hospital visit	05/21/20XX	99024	N/C
10. Discharge	05/22/20XX	99024	N/C
11. Follow-up office visit	06/05/20XX	99024	N/C

NOTES: Referred by: Emdee Fine, MD, 5000 Wilshire Blvd., Merck, XY 12346
NPI: 73027175XX
Treating MD: Gene Ulibarri, MD
NPI: 25678831XX
Place of service: College Clinic for 5/6–5/10, 6/5
College Hospital for 5/16–5/22
4500 Broad Avenue, Woodland Hills, XY 12345
NPI: X950731067

ASSIGNMENT 14.3 COMPLETE ONE HEALTH INSURANCE CLAIM FORM FOR A PRIVATE CASE

Performance Objective

Task: Complete one health insurance claim form.

Conditions: Use Walter J. Stone's E/M patient record, one health insurance claim form, a computer or pen.

Standards: Claim Productivity Measurement

Time: ________________ minutes

Accuracy: ________________

(Note: The time element and accuracy criteria may be given by your instructor.)

Directions: You will be billing for all services listed on the patient's progress notes for Dr. Clarence Cutler.

1. Complete one Health Insurance Claim Form, addressing it to Travelers Insurance Company for Mr. Walter J. Stone by referring to patient record. Date the claim May 5 of the current year. Use NUCC guidelines.

2. A Performance Evaluation Checklist may be reproduced from the "Instruction Guide to the Workbook" that appears in a section before Chapter 1 if your instructor wishes you to submit it to assist with scoring and comments.

After the instructor has returned your work to you, either make the necessary corrections and place your work in a three-ring notebook for future reference or, if you received a high score, place it in your portfolio for reference when applying for a job.

COLLEGE CLINIC
4567 Broad Avenue, Woodland Hills, XY 12345-0001
(555)-486-9002
Fax: (555) 487-8976
NPI: 3664021CC

PATIENT INFORMATION:		INSURANCE INFORMATION:	
Name:	Walter J. Stone	Primary:	Travelers Insurance
Address:	2008 Converse Street		5460 Olympic Blvd.
	Woodland Hills, XY 12345		Woodland Hills, XY 12345
Telephone:	(555) 345-0776	Policy Number:	456-XX-9989
Date of Birth:	03/14/1949	Group Number:	6754
Social Security:	456-XX-9989	Subscriber:	Walter J. Stone
Occupation:	ADVERTISING AGENT	Secondary:	None
Employer:	RV Black and Associates		
	1267 Broad Street		
	Woodland Hills, XY 12345		
Status:	Widowed		
Spouse:			

DIAGNOSIS INFORMATION

1. K25.0 Acute gastric ulcer with hemorrhage
2. K80.18 Calculus of gallbladder and bile duct with cholecystitis, unspecified, without obstruction
3. K92.2 Gastrointestinal hemorrhage, unspecified
4. I10 Essential hypertension, benign

PROCEDURE INFORMATION

Description	Date	Code	Charge
1. Initial hospital care	05/03/20XX	99222	120.80
2. Cholecystectomy	05/04/20XX	43255	741.99
3. Endoscopy	05/04/20XX	43255-51-59-99	281.51

NOTES: Referred by: Gaston Input, MD, College Hospital
NPI: 32783127XX
Treating MD: Clarence Cutler, MD
NPI: 43050047XX
Place of service: College Hospital
4500 Broad Avenue, Woodland Hills, XY 12345
NPI: X950731067

ASSIGNMENT 14.4 LOCATE ERRORS ON A COMPLETED HEALTH INSURANCE CLAIM FORM

Performance Objective

Task: Locate errors on a completed health insurance claim form and post the information to the patient's ledger card.

Conditions: Use Tom N. Parkinson's completed insurance claim (Fig. 14.1), one health insurance claim form, a computer or pen.

Standards: Time: ________________ minutes

Accuracy: ________________

(Note: The time element and accuracy criteria may be given by your instructor.)

Guidance: To alleviate frustration and ease the process of completing a claim form for the first time, you will be editing a claim and then taking the correct information and inserting it on a blank CMS-1500 form. Refer to Chapter 14 in the Textbook for block-by-block private payer instructions for completing the CMS-1500 insurance claim form. Refer to Fig. 14.3 in the Textbook for visual placement of data.

Directions: Study the completed claim form (Fig. 14.1) and search for missing or incorrect information. If possible, verify all information. Highlight or circle in red all incorrect or missing information. Insert the correct information on the claim form. Now transfer all the data to a blank CMS-1500 claim form. If mandatory information is missing, insert the word "NEED" in the corresponding block of the claim form.

A Performance Evaluation Checklist may be reproduced from the "Instruction Guide to the Workbook" that appears in a section before Chapter 1 if your instructor wishes you to submit it to assist with scoring and comments.

Optional: List, in block-by-block order, the reasons why the claim may either be rejected or delayed according to the errors found.

General Directions for Claim Form Completion

Assume that the Health Insurance Claim Form CMS-1500 is printed in red ink for processing by optical character recognition (OCR) or intelligent character recognition (ICR). Complete the form using NUCC guidelines and send it to the proper insurance carrier. Refer to Chapter 14 in the Textbook for block instructions. Claim form templates have been completed to use as visual examples for placement of data; they may be found at the end of Chapter 14 in the Textbook. Screened areas on each form do not apply to the insurance program example shown and should be left blank.

All physicians in College Clinic accept assignment of benefits for all types of insurance that you will be billing for; indicate this by checking "yes" in Block 27. For each claim completed, be sure to insert your initials at the lower left corner of the claim form.

DRAFT - NOT FOR OFFICIAL USE

HEALTH INSURANCE CLAIM FORM

APPROVED BY NATIONAL UNIFOR MCLAIM COMMITTEE (NUCC) 02/12

PICA | PICA

CARRIER

1. MEDICARE (Medicare#) / MEDICAID (Medicaid#) / TRICARE (ID#DoD#) / CHAMPVA (Member ID#) / GROUP HEALTH PLAN (ID#) / FECA BLK LUNG (ID#) / OTHER (ID#)	GROUP HEALTH PLAN: X
1a. INSURED'S I.D. NUMBER (For Program in Item 1)	PX4278A
2. PATIENT'S NAME (Last Name, First Name, Middle Initial)	Parkinson, Tom, N
3. PATIENT'S BIRTH DATE MM DD YY / SEX	04 06 1993 / M X
4. INSURED'S NAME (Last Name, First Name, Middle Initial)	Parkinson, Jamie, B
5. PATIENT'S ADDRESS (No., Street)	4510 South A Street
6. PATIENT RELATIONSHIP TO INSURED (Self / Spouse / Child / Other)	Child X
7. INSURED'S ADDRESS (No., Street)	4510 South A Street
CITY / STATE	Woodland Hills / XY
8. RESERVED FOR NUCC USE	
CITY / STATE (Insured)	Woodland Hills / XY
ZIP CODE / TELEPHONE (Include Area Code)	12345-0000 / (555) 7421560
ZIP CODE / TELEPHONE (Include Area Code) (Insured)	12345-0000 / (555) 7421560
9. OTHER INSURED'S NAME (Last Name, First Name, Middle Initial)	
10. IS PATIENT'S CONDITION RELATED TO:	
11. INSURED'S POLICY GROUP OR FECA NUMBER	
a. OTHER INSURED'S POLICY OR GROUP NUMBER	
a. EMPLOYMENT? (Current or Previous) YES / NO	NO X
a. INSURED'S DATE OF BIRTH MM DD YY / SEX M / F	
b. RESERVED FOR NUCC USE	
b. AUTO ACCIDENT? YES / NO / PLACE (State)	NO X
b. OTHER CLAIM ID (Designated by NUCC)	
c. RESERVED FOR NUCC USE	
c. OTHER ACCIDENT? YES / NO	NO X
c. INSURANCE PLAN NAME OR PROGRAM NAME	
d. INSURANCE PLAN NAME OR PROGRAM NAME	
10d. CLAIM CODES (Designated by NUCC)	
d. IS THERE ANOTHER HEALTH BENEFIT PLAN? YES / NO *If yes*, complete items 9, 9a, and 9d.	NO X

READ BACK OF FORM BEFORE COMPLETING & SIGNING THIS FORM.

12. PATIENT'S OR AUTHORIZED PERSON'S SIGNATUREI authorize the release of any medical or other information necessary to process this claim. I also request payment of government benefits either to myself or to the party who accepts assignment below.

SIGNED ______ DATE ______

13. INSURED'S OR AUTHORIZED PERSON'S SIGNATURE I authorize payment of medical benefits to the undersigned physician or supplier for services described below.

SIGNED ______

PATIENT AND INSURED INFORMATION

14. DATE OF CURRENT: ILLNESS, INJURY, or PREGNANCY(LMP) MM DD YY QUAL.	
15. OTHER DATE QUAL. MM DD YY	
16. DATES PATIENT UNABLE TO WORK IN CURRENT OCCUPATION FROM / TO	
17. NAME OF REFERRING PROVIDER OR OTHER SOURCE	
17a. / 17b. NPI	
18. HOSPITALIZATION DATES RELATED TO CURRENT SERVICES FROM / TO	
19. ADDITIONAL CLAIM INFORMATION (Designated by NUCC)	
20. OUTSIDE LAB? YES / NO / $ CHARGES	NO X
21. DIAGNOSIS OR NATURE OF ILLNESS OR INJURY Relate A-L to service line below (24E) ICD Ind.	0
A. B. C. D. E. F. G. H. I. J. K. L.	
22. RESUBMISSION CODE / ORIGINAL REF. NO.	
23. PRIOR AUTHORIZATION NUMBER	

	24. A. DATE(S) OF SERVICE From MM DD YY	To MM DD YY	B. PLACE OF SERVICE	C. EMG	D. PROCEDURES, SERVICES, OR SUPPLIES (Explain Unusual Circumstances) CPT/HCPCS	MODIFIER	E. DIAGNOSIS POINTER	F. $ CHARGES	G. DAYS OR UNITS	H. EPSDT Family Plan	I. ID. QUAL.	J. RENDERING PROVIDER ID. #
1	07 14 20XX				99242			80 24	1		NPI	
2	07 14 20XX				71020		A	38 96	1		NPI	4627889700
3											NPI	
4											NPI	
5											NPI	
6											NPI	

25. FEDERAL TAX I.D. NUMBER SSN EIN	7034597
26. PATIENT'S ACCOUNT NO.	
27. ACCEPT ASSIGNMENT? (For govt. claims, see back) YES / NO	YES X
28. TOTAL CHARGE	$ 119 20
29. AMOUNT PAID	$
30. Rsvd for NUCC Use	$
31. SIGNATURE OF PHYSICIAN OR SUPPLIER INCLUDING DEGREES OR CREDENTIALS (I certify that the statements on the reverse apply to this bill and are made a part thereof.)	Gerald Practon 071420XX SIGNED *Gerald Practon* DATE
32. SERVICE FACILITY LOCATION INFORMATION	a. NPI b.
33. BILLING PROVIDER INFO & PH #	(555) 4869002 College Clinic 4567 Broad Avenue Woodland Hills XY 12345-0001 a. 3664021CC b.

PHYSICIAN OR SUPPLIER INFORMATION

NUCC Instruction Manual available at: www.nucc.org *PLEASE PRINT OR TYPE* OMB APPROVAL PENDING

ASSIGNMENT 14.5 COMPLETE A CLAIM FORM FOR A MEDICARE/MEDICAID CASE

Performance Objective

Task: Complete a CMS-1500 claim form for a Medicare/Medicaid case.

Conditions: Use Helen P. Nolan's patient record, one health insurance claim form, a pen or pencil.

Standards: Claim Productivity Measurement

Time: ____________________ minutes

Accuracy: ____________________

(Note: The time element and accuracy criteria may be given by your instructor.)

Directions:

1. Complete the CMS-1500 claim form, using NUCC guidelines for a Medicare/Medicaid case. If your instructor wants you to direct it to your local Medicare fiscal intermediary, obtain the name and address by going to the internet. Refer to Mrs. Helen P. Nolan's patient record for information. Date the claim May 31 of the current year.

2. Refer to Chapter 14 and Fig. 14.5 of the textbook for instructions on how to complete the CMS-1500 claim form.

3. A Performance Evaluation Checklist may be reproduced from the "Instruction Guide to the Workbook" that appears in a section before Chapter 1 if your instructor wishes you to submit it to assist with scoring and comments.

After the instructor has returned your work to you, either make the necessary corrections and place your work in a three-ring notebook for future reference or, if you received a high score, place it in your portfolio for reference when applying for a job.

COLLEGE CLINIC
4567 Broad Avenue, Woodland Hills, XY 12345-0001
(555)-486-9002
Fax: (555) 487-8976
NPI: 3664021CC

PATIENT INFORMATION:		INSURANCE INFORMATION:	
Name:	Helen P. Nolan	Primary:	Medicare
Address:	2588 Cedar Street Woodland Hills, XY 12345		
Telephone:	(555) 660-9878	Policy Number:	632XX3209D
Date of Birth:	05/10/37	Group Number:	
Social Security:	732-XX-1573	Subscriber:	
Occupation:	HOMEMAKER	Secondary:	Medicaid
Employer:		Policy Number:	1960235894901XX
Status:	Widowed	Group Number:	
Spouse:			

DIAGNOSIS INFORMATION

1. I84.131 Internal and external bleeding hemorrhoids
2. K60.5 Anorectal fistula
3.
4.

PROCEDURE INFORMATION

Description	Date	Code	Charge
1. Office visit, new patient	05/01/20XX	99203-25	64.92
2. Diagnostic proctoscopy	05/01/20XX	46614	166.68
3. Hemorrhoidectomy with fistulectomy	05/08/20XX	46258	582.17

NOTES:
Referred by: James B. Jeffers, MD, 100 S. Broadway, Woodland Hills, XY 12345
NPI: 12345069XX
Treating MD: Rex Rumsey, MD
NPI: 19999047XX
Place of service: 5/1 College Clinic
5/8 College Hospital
4500 Broad Avenue, Woodland Hills, XY 12345
NPI: X950731067

ASSIGNMENT 14.6 COMPLETE A CLAIM FORM FOR A MEDICARE CASE

Performance Objective

Task: Complete a CMS-1500 claim form for a Medicare case.

Conditions: Use Elsa M. Mooney's patient record, one health insurance claim form, a pen or pencil.

Standards: Claim Productivity Measurement

Time: ____________________ minutes

Accuracy: ____________________

(Note: The time element and accuracy criteria may be given by your instructor.)

Directions:

1. Complete the CMS-1500 claim form, using National Uniform Claim Committee (NUCC) guidelines for a Medicare case. If your instructor wants you to direct it to your local fiscal intermediary, obtain the name and address by going to the internet. Refer to Mrs. Elsa M. Mooney's patient record for information. Date the claim December 21 of the current year. Dr. Cardi is a participating physician who is accepting assignment.

2. Refer to Chapter 14 (Fig. 14.4) of the textbook for instructions on how to complete this claim form and a Medicare template.

3. A Performance Evaluation Checklist may be reproduced from the "Instruction Guide to the Workbook" that appears in a section before Chapter 1 if your instructor wishes you to submit it to assist with scoring and comments.

After the instructor has returned your work to you, either make the necessary corrections and place your work in a three-ring notebook for future reference or, if you received a high score, place it in your portfolio for reference when applying for a job.

COLLEGE CLINIC
4567 Broad Avenue, Woodland Hills, XY 12345-0001
(555)-486-9002
Fax: (555) 487-8976
NPI: 3664021CC

PATIENT INFORMATION:		INSURANCE INFORMATION:	
Name:	Elsa M. Mooney	Primary:	Medicare
Address:	5750 Canyon Road		
	Woodland Hills, XY 12345	Policy Number:	321XX2653A
Telephone:	(555) 452-4968	Group Number:	
Date of Birth:	02/06/1930	Subscriber:	
Social Security:	321-XX-2653	Secondary:	none
Occupation:	RETIRED SECRETARY	Policy Number:	
Employer:		Group Number:	
		Subscriber:	
Status:	Widowed		
Spouse:			

DIAGNOSIS INFORMATION

1. I25.119 Atherosclerotic heart disease of native coronary artery with unspecified angina pectoris
2.
3.
4.

PROCEDURE INFORMATION

Description	Date	Code	Charge
1. Initial office visit, new pt	12/15/20XX	99203	64.92
2. ECG with interpret & report	12/15/20XX	93000	31.36

NOTES:

Referred by: George Gentle, MD, 1000 N. Main St., Woodland Hills, XY 12345
NPI: 40213102XX

Treating MD: Perry Cardi, MD
NPI: 67805027XX

Place of service: College Clinic
4500 Broad Avenue, Woodland Hills, XY 12345
NPI: X950731067

ASSIGNMENT 14.7 COMPLETE A CLAIM FORM FOR A MEDICAID CASE

Performance Objective

Task: Complete a CMS-1500 claim form.

Conditions: Use Rose Clarkson's patient record, one health insurance claim form, a pen or pencil.

Standards: Claim Productivity Measurement

Time: ________________ minutes

Accuracy: ________________

(Note: The time element and accuracy criteria may be given by your instructor.)

Directions:

1. Using National Uniform Claim Committee (NUCC) guidelines, complete the Health Insurance Claim Form and direct it to Medicaid for Rose Clarkson by referring to her patient record. Date the claim September 6 of the current year. If your instructor wants you to insert the name and address of your Medicaid fiscal agent on the claim, obtain the address by going to the internet.

2. Refer to Chapter 14 (Fig. 14.3) in the *Textbook* for instructions on how to complete this claim form and a Medicaid template.

3. A Performance Evaluation Checklist may be reproduced from the "Instruction Guide to the Workbook" in the section before Chapter 1 if your instructor wishes you to submit it to assist with scoring and comments.

After the instructor has returned your work to you, either make the necessary corrections and place your work in a three-ring notebook for future reference or, if you received a high score, place it in your portfolio for reference when applying for a job.

COLLEGE CLINIC
4567 Broad Avenue, Woodland Hills, XY 12345-0001
(555)-486-9002
Fax: (555) 487-8976
NPI: 3664021CC

PATIENT INFORMATION:		INSURANCE INFORMATION:	
Name:	Rose Clarkson	Primary:	Medicaid
Address:	3408 Jackson Street Hempstead, XY 11551-0300	Policy Number:	CC99756329346X
Telephone:	(555) 487-2209	Group Number:	
Date of Birth:	03/09/1954	Subscriber:	
Social Security:	030-XX-9543	Secondary:	none
Occupation:	UNEMPLOYED	Policy Number:	
Employer:		Group Number:	
		Subscriber:	
Status:			
Spouse:			

DIAGNOSIS INFORMATION

1. I50.9 Congestive heart failure
2. I34.1 Nonrheumatic mitral valve prolapse
3.
4.

PROCEDURE INFORMATION

Description	Date	Code	Charge
1. Initial office visit, new pt	09/04/20XX	99203	70.92
2. 12 lead ECG	09/04/20XX	93000	34.26
3. Echocardiogram with Doppler	09/04/20XX	99306	250.73
4. Chest x-ray	09/04/20XX	71010	31.95

NOTES:
Referred by: James Jackson, MD, 100 N. Main St., Hempstead, XY 11551
NPI: 72011337XX
Treating MD: Perry Cardi, MD
NPI: 67805027XX
Place of service: College Clinic
4500 Broad Avenue, Woodland Hills, XY 12345
NPI: X950731067

ASSIGNMENT 14.8 COMPLETE A CLAIM FORM FOR A MEDICAID CASE

Performance Objective

Task: Complete a CMS-1500 claim form for a Medicaid case

Conditions: Use Stephen M. Drake's patient record, one health insurance claim form, a pen or pencil.

Standards: Claim Productivity Measurement

Time: ________________ minutes

Accuracy: ________________

(Note: The time element and accuracy criteria may be given by your instructor.)

Directions:

1. Using NUCC guidelines, complete the Health Insurance Claim Form and direct it to Medicaid for Stephen M. Drake by referring to his patient record. Date the claim May 26 of the current year. If your instructor wants you to insert the name and address of your Medicaid fiscal agent on the claim, obtain it by going to the internet. Do not list services not charged for (N/C) on the claim form. Remember that the physician must always sign all forms on Medicaid cases; stamped signatures are not allowed.

2. Refer to Chapter 14 (Fig. 14.3) in the Textbook for instructions on how to complete this claim form and a Medicaid template.

3. A Performance Evaluation Checklist may be reproduced from the "Instruction Guide to the Workbook" that appears in the section before Chapter 1 if your instructor wishes you to submit it to assist with scoring and comments.

After the instructor has returned your work to you, either make the necessary corrections and place your work in a three-ring notebook for future reference or, if you received a high score, place it in your portfolio for reference when applying for a job.

COLLEGE CLINIC
4567 Broad Avenue, Woodland Hills, XY 12345-0001
(555)-486-9002
Fax: (555) 487-8976
NPI: 3664021CC

PATIENT INFORMATION:		INSURANCE INFORMATION:	
Name:	Stephen M. Drake	Primary:	Medicaid
Address:	2317 Charnwood Avenue Woodland Hills, XY 12345	Policy Number:	197152403316X
Telephone:	(555) 277-5831	Group Number:	
Date of Birth:	04/03/1991	Subscriber:	
Social Security:	566-XX-0081	Secondary:	none
Occupation:	STUDENT	Policy Number:	
Employer:		Group Number:	
		Subscriber:	
Status:			
Spouse:			

DIAGNOSIS INFORMATION

1. J03.90	Acute tonsillitis, unspecified
2. J35.03	Chronic tonsillitis and adenoiditis
3. J02.0	Streptococcal sore throat
4.	

PROCEDURE INFORMATION

Description	Date	Code	Charge
1. Initial office visit, new pt	05/01/20XX	99203	70.92
2. Strep culture	05/01/20XX	87081	25.00
3. Injection, antibiotic	05/01/20XX	90772	5.22
4. Bicillin	05/01/20XX	J0540	10.00
5. Follow-up office visit	05/08/20XX	99212-57	28.55
6. Remove tonsils and adenoids	05/09/20XX	42821	410.73
7. Post-op office visit	05/17/20XX	99024	N/C

NOTES:
Referred by: James Jeffers, MD, 100 S. Broadway, Hempstead, XY 12345
NPI: 12345069XX
Treating MD: Gerald Practon, MD
NPI: 46278897XX
Place of service: College Clinic for 5/1–5/8, 5/17
College Hospital for 5/9
4500 Broad Avenue, Woodland Hills, XY 12345
NPI: X950731067

ASSIGNMENT 14.9 COMPLETE A CLAIM FORM FOR A TRICARE STANDARD CASE

Performance Objective

Task: Complete a CMS-1500 claim form for a TRICARE Standard case.

Conditions: Use Rosa M. Sandoval's patient record, one health insurance claim form, a pen or pencil.

Standards: Claim Productivity Measurement

Time: ________________ minutes

Accuracy: ____________________

(Note: The time element and accuracy criteria may be given by your instructor.)

Directions:

1. Using National Uniform Claim Committee (NUCC) guidelines, complete the CMS-1500 claim form. Refer to Miss Rosa M. Sandoval's patient record for information. Date the claim May 31 of the current year. Dr. Atrics is not accepting assignment on this TRICARE Standard case but is completing the claim for the patient's convenience.

2. Refer to Chapter 14 (Fig. 14.8) of the Textbook for instructions on how to complete this claim form and to view a TRICARE template.

3. A Performance Evaluation Checklist may be reproduced from the "Instruction Guide to the Workbook" chapter if your instructor wishes you to submit it to assist with scoring and comments.

After the instructor has returned your work to you, either make the necessary corrections and place your work in a three-ring notebook for future reference or, if you received a high score, place it in your portfolio for reference when applying for a job.

COLLEGE CLINIC
4567 Broad Avenue, Woodland Hills, XY 12345-0001
(555)-486-9002
Fax: (555) 487-8976
NPI: 3664021CC

PATIENT INFORMATION:		INSURANCE INFORMATION:	
Name:	Rosa Sandoval	Primary:	Tricare Standard PO Box 1234 West End, YZ 01222
Address:	209 West Maple St Woodland Hills, XY 12345		
Telephone:	(555) 456-3322	Policy Number:	886-XX-0999
Date of Birth:	11/01/1991	Group Number:	
Social Security:	994-XX-1164	Subscriber:	Herman J. Sandoval (DOB 2/10/70)
Guarantor:	Herman J. Sandoval (Father)		
		Secondary:	none
		Policy Number:	
		Group Number:	
		Subscriber:	

DIAGNOSIS INFORMATION

1. H66.001 Acute suppurative otitis media without spontaneous rupture of ear drum, right ear
2. H66.3x1 Chronic suppurative otitis media, NOS, right ear
3.
4.

PROCEDURE INFORMATION

Description	Date	Code	Charge
1. Initial office visit, new pt	05/01/20XX	99202-25	51.91
2. Myringotomy	05/01/20XX	69420-RT	97.76
3. Post-op visit	05/03/20XX	99024	N/C
4. Post-op visit	05/08/20XX	99024	N/C

NOTES:
Referred by: mother
Treating MD: Pedro Atrics, MD
NPI: 137640017XX
Place of service: College Clinic
4500 Broad Avenue, Woodland Hills, XY 12345
NPI: X950731067

ASSIGNMENT 14.10 COMPLETE A CLAIM FORM FOR A TRICARE EXTRA CASE

Performance Objective

Task: Complete a CMS-1500 claim form for a TRICARE Extra case.

Conditions: Use Darlene B. Drew's patient record, one health insurance claim form, a pen or pencil.

Standards: Claim Productivity Measurement

Time: ________________ minutes

Accuracy: ______________________

(Note: The time element and accuracy criteria may be given by your instructor.)

Directions:

1. Using NUCC guidelines, complete the CMS-1500 claim form. Refer to Mrs. Darlene B. Drew's patient record for information and post to the financial statement. Date the claim February 3 of the current year. Assume that the No Availability Statement (NAS) has been transmitted electronically so that the physician can treat the patient at College Hospital. Dr. Ulibarri is accepting assignment on this TRICARE Extra case.

2. Refer to Chapter 14 (Fig. 14.8) of the Textbook for instructions on how to complete this claim form and to view a TRICARE template.

3. A Performance Evaluation Checklist may be reproduced from the "Instruction Guide to the Workbook" shown in the section before Chapter 1 if your instructor wishes you to submit it to assist with scoring and comments.

After the instructor has returned your work to you, either make the necessary corrections and place your work in a three-ring notebook for future reference or, if you received a high score, place it in your portfolio for reference when applying for a job.

COLLEGE CLINIC
4567 Broad Avenue, Woodland Hills, XY 12345-0001
(555)-486-9002
Fax: (555) 487-8976
NPI: 3664021CC

PATIENT INFORMATION:		INSURANCE INFORMATION:	
Name:	Darlene Drew	Primary:	Tricare Extra PO Box 1234 West End, YZ 01222
Address:	720 Ganley Street Woodland Hills, XY 12345		
Telephone:	(555) 466-1002	Policy Number:	67531
Date of Birth:	12/22/1951	Effective date:	1/1/1980
Social Security:	450-XX-3762	Subscriber:	Harry M. Drew Service# 221XX0711 DOB 4/15/1937
Occupation:	SEAMSTRESS		
Employer:	J. B. Talon Company 2111 Ventura Blvd. Merck, XY 12346	Secondary:	none
Status:	Married		
Spouse:	Harry M. Drew		

DIAGNOSIS INFORMATION

1. N34.0 Abscess of urethral gland
2. B96.5 Pseudomonas (aeruginosa)
3.
4.

PROCEDURE INFORMATION

Description	Date	Code	Charge
1. Initial office visit, new pt	01/13/20XX	99203-25	70.92
2. Urinalysis	01/13/20XX	81000	8.00
3. Drainage of Skene's gland abscess	01/13/20XX	53060	147.95
4. Handling/transport culture specimen	01/13/20XX	99000	5.00
5. Office visit	01/18/20XX	99212	28.55
6. Excision of Skene's gland	01/24/20XX	53270-58	184.39
7. Post-op visit	01/27/20XX	99024	n/c

NOTES: Referred by: James B. Jeffers, MD, 100 S. Broadway, Woodland Hills, XY 12345
NPI: 12345069XX
Treating MD: Gene Ulibarri, MD
NPI: 25678831XX
Place of service: College Clinic for 1/13–18, 1/27
College Hospital for 1/24
4500 Broad Avenue, Woodland Hills, XY 12345
NPI: X950731067

ASSIGNMENT 14.11 COMPLETE A CLAIM FORM FOR A WORKERS' COMPENSATION CASE

Performance Objectives

Task: Complete a CMS-1500 claim form for a workers' compensation case.

Conditions: Use Glen M. Hiranuma's patient record, a CMS-1500 claim form, a pen or pencil.

Standards: Claim Productivity Measurement

Time: ________________ minutes

Accuracy: ____________________

(Note: The time element and accuracy criteria may be given by your instructor.)

Directions:

1. Using National Uniform Claim Committee (NUCC) guidelines, complete a CMS-1500 claim form and direct it to the proper workers' compensation carrier. Refer to Mr. Glen M. Hiranuma's patient record for information. As a result of this work-related injury, the patient was unable to work on 5/22 through the returning date of 6/5. Date the claim May 24 of the current year.

2. Refer to Chapter 14 (Fig. 14.10) of the Textbook for instructions on how to complete this claim form and to view a workers' compensation template.

3. A Performance Evaluation Checklist may be reproduced from the "Instruction Guide to the Workbook" that appears in the section before Chapter 1 if your instructor wishes you to submit it to assist with scoring and comments.

After the instructor has returned your work to you, either make the necessary corrections and place your work in a three-ring notebook for future reference or, if you received a high score, place it in your portfolio for reference when applying for a job.

COLLEGE CLINIC
4567 Broad Avenue, Woodland Hills, XY 12345-0001
(555)-486-9002
Fax: (555) 487-8976
NPI: 3664021CC

PATIENT INFORMATION:		INSURANCE INFORMATION:	
Name:	Glen Hiranuma	Primary:	State Insurance Fund
Address:	4372 Hanley Avenue		14156 Magnolia Blvd.
	Woodland Hills, XY 12345		Torres, XY 12349
Telephone:	(555) 467-3383	Policy Number:	016-2432-211
Date of Birth:	12/24/1955	Date of Injury:	05/22/20XX
Social Security:	558-XX-9960	Subscriber:	
Occupation:	HOUSE PAINTER	Secondary:	none
Employer:	Pittsburgh Paint Company	Policy Number:	
	3725 Bonfield Avenue	Group Number:	
	Woodland Hills, XY 12345	Subscriber:	
Status:	Married		
Spouse:	Esme M. Hiranuma		

DIAGNOSIS INFORMATION

1. S06.0x1 Concussion with loss of consciousness of 30 minutes or less
2. S43.92 Unspecified sprain of left shoulder girdle
3. S70.212 Abrasion of left hip
4. S80.812 Abrasion left lower leg
5. W11.xxxA Fall on and from ladder, initial encounter

PROCEDURE INFORMATION

Description	Date	Code	Charge
1. Hospital admit	05/22/20XX	99222	120.80
2. WC Report	05/22/20XX	99080	50.00
3. Discharge	05/23/20XX	99238	65.26

NOTES:
Referred by: Pittsburgh Pain Company
Treating MD: Gerald Practon, MD
NPI: 46278897XX
Place of service: College Hospital
4500 Broad Avenue, Woodland Hills, XY 12345
NPI: X950731067
Patient unable to work from 5/23/20xx to 06/05/20xx

ASSIGNMENT 14.12 COMPLETE A CLAIM FORM FOR A WORKERS' COMPENSATION CASE

Performance Objective

Task: Complete a CMS-1500 claim form for a workers' compensation case.

Conditions: Use Carlos A. Giovanni's patient record, a CMS-1500 claim form, a pen or pencil.

Standards: Claim Productivity Measurement

Time: ___________________ minutes

Accuracy: _______________

(Note: The time element and accuracy criteria may be given by your instructor.)

Directions:

1. Using NUCC guidelines, complete a CMS-1500 claim form for November dates of service and direct it to the correct workers' compensation carrier for this workers' compensation claim. Refer to Mr. Carlos A. Giovanni's patient record for information to record on the claim. Date the claim November 30 of the current year. Note: A progress report is being submitted with this claim; complete a separate CMS-1500 for services for December.

2. Refer to Chapter 14 (Fig. 14.10) of the textbook for instructions on how to complete this claim form and to view a workers' compensation template.

3. A Performance Evaluation Checklist may be reproduced from the "Instruction Guide to the Workbook" that appears in a section before Chapter 1 if your instructor wishes you to submit it to assist with scoring and comments.

After the instructor has returned your work to you, either make the necessary corrections and place your work in a three-ring notebook for future reference or, if you received a high score, place it in your portfolio for reference when applying for a job.

COLLEGE CLINIC
4567 Broad Avenue, Woodland Hills, XY 12345-0001
(555)-486-9002
Fax: (555) 487-8976
NPI: 3664021CC

PATIENT INFORMATION:		INSURANCE INFORMATION:	
Name:	Carlos A. Giovanni	Primary:	State Compensation Ins Fund
Address:	89 Beaumont Court Woodland Hills, XY 12345		600 S. Lafayette Park Place Ehrlich, XY 12350
Telephone:	(555) 677-3485		
Date of Birth:	10/24/1955	Policy Number:	57780
Social Security:	556-XX-9699	Date of Injury:	11/11/20XX
Occupation:	TV REPAIRMAN	Subscriber:	
Employer:	Giant Television Company 8764 Ocean Avenue Woodland Hills, XY 12345	Secondary:	none
		Policy Number:	
		Group Number:	
Status:	Married	Subscriber:	
Spouse:	Maria Giovanni		

DIAGNOSIS INFORMATION

1. S02.91xA Fracture of skull and facial bones, initial encounter for closed fracture
2. S06.0x1 Concussion with loss of consciousness of 30 minutes or less
3. W13.xxxA Fall from, out of or through building or structure

PROCEDURE INFORMATION

Description	Date	Code	Charge
1. Hospital admit	11/11/20XX	99223-57	152.98
2. WC Report	11/11/20XX	99080	50.00
3. Craniotomy	11/12/20XX	61314	2548.09
4. Hospital visits	11/13-29/20XX	99024	N/C
5. Discharge	11/30/20XX	99024	N/C
6. Office visit	12/07/20XX	99024	N/C
7. Office visit	12/21/20XX	99024	N/C
8. Office visit	12/29/20XX	99024	N/C
9. Medical report	12/29/20XX	99080	50.00

NOTES:
Referred by: Giant Television Company
Treating MD: Astro Parkinson, MD
NPI: 46789377XX
Place of service: College Clinic for 12/7–12/29
College Hospital for 11/11–11/30
4500 Broad Avenue, Woodland Hills, XY 12345
NPI: X950731067
Patient unable to work from 11/12/20xx–01/14/20xx

15 The Electronic Claim

Cheryl Fassett

KEY TERMS

Your instructor may wish to select some words pertinent to this chapter for a test. For definitions of the terms, further study, and/or reference, the words, phrases, and abbreviations may be found in the glossary at the end of the Textbook. *Key terms for this chapter follow.*

Accredited Standards Committee X12
Accredited Standards Committee X12 Version 5010
Administrative Simplification Enforcement Tool
American National Standards Institute
application service provider
audit trail
batch
business associate agreement
cable modem
claim attachments
clearinghouse
code sets
covered entity
data elements
digital subscriber line
direct data entry
electronic data interchange
electronic funds transfer
electronic remittance advice
encoder
encryption
HIPAA Transaction and Code Set Rule
National Standard Format
real time
standard transactions
T-1
taxonomy codes
trading partner
trading partner agreement

KEY ABBREVIATIONS

See how many abbreviations and acronyms you can translate, and then use this as a handy reference list. Definitions for the key abbreviations are located near the back of the Textbook *in the glossary.*

ANSI ________________________________

ASC X12 ________________________________

ASET ________________________________

ASP ________________________________

ATM ________________________________

DDE ________________________________

DHHS ________________________________

DSL ________________________________

EDI ________________________________

EFT ________________________________

EHR ________________________________

EMC ________________________________

EOMB ________________________________

ERA ________________________________

HPID ________________________________

IRS ________________________________

MAC ________________________________

NDC ________________________________

NSF ________________________________

PMS ________________________________

TCS rule ________________________________

PERFORMANCE OBJECTIVES

The student will be able to:

- Define and spell the key terms and key abbreviations for this chapter, given the information from the textbook glossary, within a reasonable time period and with enough accuracy to obtain a satisfactory evaluation.
- After reading the chapter, answer the fill-in-the-blank, multiple choice, and true/false review questions with enough accuracy to obtain a satisfactory evaluation.
- Decide whether keyed medical and nonmedical data elements are required, situational, or not used when electronically submitting the 837P health care claim.
- State which medical and nonmedical code sets for 837P electronic claims are required, situational, or not used.
- Input data into the element for place of service codes for 837P electronic claims submission.
- Indicate the patient's relationship to the insured by using the individual relationship code numbers for 837P electronic claims submission.
- Select the correct taxonomy codes for the specialists for submission of 837P electronic claims submission.
- Locate errors, given computer-generated insurance forms, within a reasonable time period and with enough accuracy to obtain a satisfactory evaluation.
- Fill in the correct meaning of each abbreviation, given a list of common medical abbreviations and symbols that appear in chart notes, with enough accuracy to obtain a satisfactory evaluation.

STUDY OUTLINE

Electronic Data Interchange
Electronic Claims
Advantages of Electronic Claim Submission
Clearinghouses
Transaction and Code Set Regulations: Streamlining Electronic Data Interchange
- Transaction and Code Set Standards

Electronic Standard HIPAA 837P
- Levels of Information for 837P Standard Transaction Format
- Accredited Standards Committee X12 Version 5010

Claims Attachments Standards
Standard Unique Identifiers
- Standard Unique Employer Identifier
- Standard Unique Health Care Provider Identifier
- Standard Unique Health Plan Identifier
- Standard Unique Patient Identifier

Practice Management System
Building the Claim
- Encounter or Multipurpose Billing Forms
- Keying Insurance Data for Claim Transmission
- Encoder
- Clean Electronic Claims Submission

Putting HIPAA Standard Transactions to Work
- Interactive Transactions
- Electronic Funds Transfer
- Electronic Remittance Advice

Methods for Sending Claims
Computer Claims Systems
- Carrier-Direct
- Clearinghouses

Transmission Reports
- Electronic Processing Problems
- Solutions to Electronic Processing Problems
- Billing and Account Management Schedule
- Administrative Simplification Enforcement Tool

ASSIGNMENT 15.1 REVIEW QUESTIONS

Part I Fill in the Blank

Review the objectives, key terms, glossary definitions of key terms, chapter information, and figures before completing the following review questions.

1. Exchange of data in a standardized format through computer systems is a technology known as ______________________________.

2. The act of converting computerized data into a code so that unauthorized users are unable to read it is a security system known as ______________________.

3. Payment to the provider of service of an electronically submitted insurance claim may be received in approximately ______________________________.

4. Medical practices that do not use the services of clearinghouses submit claims through a ______________________________ to the insurance company.

5. Refer to Table 15.1 in the *textbook* to list benefits of using Health Insurance Portability and Accountability Act (HIPAA) standard transactions and code sets.

   a. ______________________________

   b. ______________________________

   c. ______________________________

   d. ______________________________

   e. ______________________________

   f. ______________________________

6. Dr. Morgan has 10 or more full-time employees and submits insurance claims for his Medicare patients. Is his medical practice subject to the HIPAA transaction rules?

   ____

7. Dr. Maria Montez does not submit insurance claims electronically and has five full-time employees. Is she required to abide by HIPAA transaction rules?

   ____

8. Refer to Table 15.2 in the *textbook* to name the standard code sets used for the following:

   a. Physician services ______________________________

   b. Diseases and injuries ______________________________

   c. Pharmaceuticals and biologics ______________________________

9. Refer to Table 15.3 in the *textbook* to complete these statements.

   a. The staff at College Clinic submit professional health care claims for each of their providers and must use the industry standard electronic format called ______________________________ to transmit them electronically.

   b. The billing department at College Hospital must use the industry standard electronic format called ______________________ to transmit health care claims electronically.

c. The Medicare fiscal intermediary (insurance carrier) uses the industry standard electronic format called ______________________ to transmit payment information to the College Clinic and College Hospital.

d. It has been three weeks since Gordon Marshall's health care claim was transmitted to the XYZ insurance company, and you wish to inquire about the status of the claim. The industry standard electronic format that must be used to transmit this inquiry is called ______________________.

e. Dr. Practon's insurance billing specialist must use the industry standard electronic format called __________ to obtain information about Beatrice Garcia's health policy benefits and coverage from the insurance plan.

10. The family practice taxonomy code is ______________________.

11. The American National Standards Institute formed the ______________________, which developed the electronic data exchange standards.

12. Refer to Table 15.4 in the textbook to name the levels for data collected to construct and submit an electronic claim.

a. ______________________

b. ______________________

c. ______________________

d. ______________________

e. ______________________

f. ______________________

13. HIPAA electronic standards for claim submission were upgraded to Version ____________, and all providers, payers, and clearinghouses were required to use it effective January 1, 2012.

14. The Claims Attachments Standards have not yet been adopted; however, it was mandated for compliance as of ______________________, as required under the Affordable Care Act.

15. The ________________ is an all numeric 10-character number assigned to each provider and required for all transactions with health plans effective May 23, 2007.

16. The most important function of a practice management system is ________________.

17. To look for and correct all errors before the health claim is transmitted to the insurance carrier, you ______________________ or ______________________.

18. Much of the patient and insurance information required to complete the CMS-1500 form can be found on the ______________________ that is used to post charges.

19. Add-on software to a practice management system that can reduce the time it takes to build or review a claim before batching is known as a/an ______________________.

20. Many insurance companies, such as Medicare, provide instant access to information about pending claims through online ______________________________.

21. An electronic funds transfer (EFT) agreement may allow for health plans to ______________ overpayments from a provider's bank account.

22. The Medicare electronic remittance advice was previously referred to as a/an ____.

23. On completion of a signed agreement and approval of enrollment with a third-party payer for electronic claims submission, the provider will be assigned a/an ______________________ number.

24. When computer software is upgraded, the health care organization must submit a batch of _____________ to the insurance carrier to determine whether claims can be transmitted successfully.

25. Under HIPAA transaction standard Accredited Standards Committee (ASC) X12 Version 5010, a _________________________ digit ZIP code is required to report service facility locations.

26. The ____________________________________ is an electronic tool that enables organizations to file a complaint against a noncompliant covered entity that is negatively affecting the efficient processing of claims.

Part II Multiple Choice

Choose the best answer.

27. Electronic claims are submitted by means of:
    a. the US Postal Service.
    b. fax transmission.
    c. phone transmission.
    d. electronic data interchange (EDI).

28. Today, most claims are submitted by means of:
    a. the US Postal Service.
    b. fax transmission.
    c. phone transmission.
    d. EDI.

29. The online error-edit process allows providers to:
    a. correct claim errors before transmission of the claim.
    b. decrease labor costs by freeing staff to do other duties.
    c. reduce postage fees and trips to the post office.
    d. reduce storage of claims.

30. Under HIPAA, data elements that are used uniformly to document why patients are seen (diagnosis) and what is done to them during their encounter (procedure) are known as:
    a. medical code sets.
    b. information elements.
    c. transaction and code set (TCS) standards.
    d. National Standard Format (NSF).

31. The standard transaction that replaces the paper CMS-1500 claim form and more than 400 versions of the electronic NSF is called the:
    a. 270.
    b. 837I.
    c. 837P.
    d. 837D.

32. The next version of the electronic claims submission that will be proposed for consideration once lessons are learned from implementation of Version 5010 will be:
    a. Version 5011.
    b. Version 5012.
    c. Version 6001.
    d. Version 7030.

33. A standard unique number that will be assigned to identify individual health plans under the Affordable Care Act is referred to as a/an:
    a. employer identification number (EIN).
    b. electronic remittance advice (ERA).
    c. health plan identifier (HPID).
    d. National Provider Identifier (NPI).

34. Uniform patient identifiers:
    a. were required on all claims effective May 23, 2007.
    b. were required on all claims effective October 1, 2012.
    c. were required on all claims effective October 1, 2014.
    d. are not yet required, and the proposal is on hold for implementation of the standard.

35. An authorization and assignment of benefits signature for a patient who was treated in the hospital but has never been to the provider's office:
    a. should be obtained by the provider when he or she sees the patient in the hospital.
    b. must be mailed to the patient for signature before submission of a claim.
    c. can be obtained from the patient at his or her first office visit.
    d. is not required; the authorization obtained by the hospital applies to that provider's claim filing.

36. A paperless computerized system that enables payments to be transferred automatically to a physician's bank account by a third-party payer may be done via:
    a. electronic savings account.
    b. ERA.
    c. EFT.
    d. EDI.

37. An electronic Medicare remittance advice that takes the place of a paper Medicare explanation of benefits (EOB) is referred to as:
    a. American National Standards Institute (ANSI) 277.
    b. ANSI 820.
    c. ANSI 830.
    d. ANSI 835.

38. A method for submitting claims electronically by keying information into the payer system for processing is accomplished through use of:
    a. a clearinghouse.
    b. carrier direct entry.
    c. an application service provider.
    d. digital subscriber line (DSL).

39. A report that is generated by a payer and sent to the provider to show how many claims were received as electronic claims and how many of the claims were automatically rejected and will not be processed is called a:
    a. send-and-receive file report.
    b. scrubber report.
    c. transaction transmission summary.
    d. rejection analysis report.

40. The HIPAA transaction standard ASC X12 Version 5010 requires that anesthesia services be reported:
    a. per day.
    b. per unit.
    c. per second.
    d. per minute.

Part III True/False

Write "T" or "F" in the blank to indicate whether you think the statement is true or false.

_______ 41. Like paper claims, electronic claims require the performing physician's signature.

_______ 42. Claims can be submitted to various insurance payers in a single-batch electronic transmission.

_______ 43. Under HIPAA, insurance payers can require health care providers to use the payer's own version of local code sets.

_______ 44. As *International Classification of Diseases* (ICD) and *Current Procedural Terminology* (CPT) codes are deleted and become obsolete, they should immediately be removed from the practice's computer system.

_______ 45. HIPAA has brought forth electronic formats for determination of eligibility for a health insurance plan.

_______ 46. HIPAA's electronic standard transactions are identified by a four-digit number that precedes "ASC X12N."

_______ 47. Implementation of ICD-10 resulted in the upgrade to HIPAA transaction standard ASC X12 Version 6020.

_______ 48. HIPAA requires that the NPI number be used to identify employers rather than inputting the actual name of the company when submitting claims.

_______ 49. HIPAA limits how computer systems may transmit data and formats for storage of data.

_______ 50. A paper remittance advice is generated by Medicare when using ANSI 835 Version 5010.

_______ 51. HIPAA transaction standard ASC X12 Version 5010 allows employer identification numbers to be used to report as a primary identifier.

_______ 52. When transmitting electronic claims, inaccuracies that violate the HIPAA standard transaction format are known as *syntax errors*.

_______ 53. An organization may file a complaint online against someone whose actions affect the ability of a transaction to be accepted or efficiently processed by using the Administration Simplification Enforcement Tool (ASET).

ASSIGNMENT 15.2 CRITICAL THINKING FOR MEDICAL AND NONMEDICAL CODE SETS FOR 837P ELECTRONIC CLAIMS SUBMISSION

Performance Objective

Task: Decide whether keyed medical and nonmedical data elements are required, situational, or not used when electronically submitting the 837P health care claim.

Conditions: List of keyed data elements (Table 15.5 in Textbook) and pen or pencil.

Standards: Time: __________ minutes

Accuracy: __________

(Note: The time element and accuracy criteria may be given by your instructor.)

Directions: When submitting the 837P health care claim, supporting code sets of medical and nonmedical data are composed of "Required" and "Situational" data elements. Read each keyed data element and answer whether you think it is **R** for required, **S** for situational, or **N** for not used.

a. Patient's type of insurance ____________________

b. Patient's ZIP code ____________________

c. Insured's name ____________________

d. Principal diagnosis code ____________________

e. Referring provider's NPI ____________________

f. Procedure code ____________________

g. Provider's signature ____________________

h. Date of service ____________________

i. Place of service ____________________

j. Procedure modifier ____________________

ASSIGNMENT 15.3 INPUT DATA INTO ELEMENT FOR PLACE OF SERVICE CODES FOR 837P ELECTRONIC CLAIMS SUBMISSIONS

Performance Objective

Task: Insert the correct place of service code for each location description where the medical professional service was rendered.

Conditions: Place of service codes reference (Fig. 15.1), list of places where medical care was rendered, and pen or pencil.

Standards: Time: __________ minutes

Accuracy: __________

(Note: The time element and accuracy criteria may be given by your instructor.)

Directions: When submitting the 837P electronic claim, place of service codes must be entered in data element 1331. Refer to the place of service codes reference list and insert the correct code for each place of service for the following locations.

a. Inpatient psychiatric facility __________

b. Physician's office __________

c. Outpatient hospital __________

d. Intermediate nursing facility __________

e. Independent clinic __________

f. Independent laboratory __________

g. Birthing center __________

h. End-stage renal disease treatment facility __________

i. Inpatient hospital __________

j. Hospice __________

PLACE OF SERVICE CODES	
Codes	**Place of Service**
01	Pharmacy
00-02	Unassigned
03	School
04	Homeless shelter
05	Indian health service free-standing facility
06	Indian health service provider-based facility
07	Tribal 638 free-standing facility
08	Tribal 638 provider-based facility
09	Prison/correctional facility
10	Unassigned
11	Doctor's office
12	Patient's home
13	Assisted living facility
14	Group home
15	Mobile unit
16	Temporary lodging
17-19	Unassigned
20	Urgent care facility
21	Inpatient hospital
22	Outpatient hospital or urgent care center
23	Emergency department—hospital
24	Ambulatory surgical center
25	Birthing center
26	Military treatment facility/uniformed service treatment facility
27-30	Unassigned
31	Skilled nursing facility (swing bed visits)
32	Nursing facility (intermediate/long-term care facilities)
33	Custodial care facility (domiciliary or rest home services)
34	Hospice (domiciliary or rest home services)
35-40	Unassigned
41	Ambulance—land
42	Ambulance—air or water
43-48	Unassigned
49	Independent clinic
50	Federally qualified health center
51	Inpatient psychiatric facility
52	Psychiatric facility—partial hospitalization
53	Community mental health care (outpatient, twenty-four-hours-a-day services, admission screening, consultation, and educational services)
54	Intermediate care facility/mentally retarded
55	Residential substance abuse treatment facility
56	Psychiatric residential treatment center
57	Nonresidential substance abuse treatment facility
58-59	Unassigned
60	Mass immunization center
61	Comprehensive inpatient rehabilitation facility
62	Comprehensive outpatient rehabilitation facility
63-64	Unassigned
65	End-stage renal disease treatment facility
66-70	Unassigned
71	State or local public health clinic
72	Rural health clinic
73-80	Unassigned
81	Independent laboratory
82-98	Unassigned
99	Other unlisted facility

Fig. 15.1

ASSIGNMENT 15.4 SELECT THE CORRECT INDIVIDUAL RELATIONSHIP CODE NUMBER FOR 837P ELECTRONIC CLAIMS SUBMISSION

Performance Objective

Task: Insert the correct individual relationship code for the patient's relationship to the insured.

Conditions: Individual relationship code number reference (Fig. 15.2), list of individuals or entities, and pen or pencil.

Standards: Time: ______________ minutes

Accuracy: ______________

(Note: The time element and accuracy criteria may be given by your instructor.)

Directions: Refer to the individual relationship code number list, choose the correct code for the patient's relationship to the insured for the following persons, and insert it on the lines.

a. Mother ______________________________

b. Spouse ______________________________

c. Child ______________________________

d. Father ______________________________

e. Stepdaughter ______________________________

f. Emancipated minor ______________________________

g. Adopted child ______________________________

h. Handicapped dependent ______________________________

i. Stepson ______________________________

j. Sponsored dependent ______________________________

Individual Relationship Code	
Code	**Relationship**
01	Spouse
04	Grandfather or grandmother
05	Grandson or granddaughter
07	Nephew or niece
09	Adopted child
10	Foster child
15	Ward
17	Stepson or stepdaughter
19	Child
20	Employee
21	Unknown
22	Handicapped dependent
23	Sponsored dependent
24	Dependent of a minor dependent
29	Significant other
32	Mother
33	Father
34	Other adult
36	Emancipated minor
39	Organ donor
40	Cadaver donor
41	Injured plaintiff
43	Child where insured has no financial responsibility
53	Life partner
G8	Other relationship

Fig. 15.2

ASSIGNMENT 15.5 SELECT THE CORRECT TAXONOMY CODES FOR MEDICAL SPECIALISTS FOR 837P ELECTRONIC CLAIMS SUBMISSION

Performance Objective

Task: Choose the correct taxonomy code for each specialist for submission of 837P electronic claims by referring to the Health Care Provider Taxonomy code list.

Conditions: Health Care Provider Taxonomy code list (Fig. 15.3), list of providers of service, and pen or pencil.

Standards: Time: ______________ minutes

Accuracy: ______________

(Note: The time element and accuracy criteria may be given by your instructor.)

Directions: Refer to the Health Care Provider Taxonomy code list, choose the correct code for each of the following specialists, and insert the code numbers on the lines.

a. Raymond Skeleton, MD, orthopedist ______________________

b. Gaston Input, MD, gastroenterologist ______________________

c. Vera Cutis, MD, dermatologist ______________________

d. Gene Ulibarri, MD, urologist ______________________

e. Bertha Caesar, MD, obstetrician/gynecologist ______________________

f. Gerald Practon, MD, general practitioner ______________________

g. Pedro Atrics, MD, pediatrician ______________________

h. Astro Parkinson, MD, neurosurgeon ______________________

i. Brady Coccidioides, MD, pulmonary disease ______________________

j. Max Gluteus, RPT, physical therapist ______________________

College Clinic Staff		
Health Care Provider Taxonomy Codes		
Name	**Specialty**	**Taxonomy Code**
Concha Antrum, MD	Otolaryngologist	207Y00000X
Pedro Atrics, MD	Pediatrician	208000000X
Bertha Caesar, MD	Obstetrician/Gynecologist	207V00000X
Perry Cardi, MD	Cardiologist	207RC0000X
Brady Coccidioides, MD	Pulmonary disease	207RP1001X
Vera Cutis, MD	Dermatologist	207N00000X
Clarence Cutler, MD	General surgeon	208600000X
Dennis Drill, DDS	Dentist	122300000X
Max Gluteus, RPT	Physical therapist	208100000X
Cosmo Graff, MD	Plastic surgeon	208200000X
Malvern Grumose, MD	Pathologist	207ZP0105X
Gaston Input, MD	Gastroenterologist	207RG0100X
Adam Langerhans, MD	Endocrinologist	207RE0101X
Cornell Lenser, MD	Ophthalmologist	207W00000X
Michael Menter, MD	Psychiatrist	2084P0800X
Arthur O. Dont, DDS	Orthodontist	1223X0400X
Astro Parkinson, MD	Neurosurgeon	207T00000X
Nick Pedro, MD	Podiatrist	213E00000X
Gerald Practon, MD	General practitioner	208D00000X
Walter Radon, MD	Radiologist	2085R0202X
Rex Rumsey, MD	Proctologist	208C00000X
Sensitive E. Scott, MD	Anesthesiologist	207L00000X
Raymond Skeleton, MD	Orthopedist	207X00000X
Gene Ulibarri, MD	Urologist	208800000X

Fig. 15.3

ASSIGNMENT 15.6 PROOFREAD A COMPUTER-GENERATED HEALTH INSURANCE CLAIM FORM AND LOCATE INCORRECT AND MISSING DATA

Performance Objective

Task: Locate and designate blocks on the computer-generated insurance claim form that have incorrect or missing information; correct or add data before submission to the insurance company.

Conditions: Use Brad E. Diehl's patient record (Fig. 15.4), completed insurance claim (Fig. 15.5), a highlighter, and a red-ink pen.

Standards: Time: ______________ minutes

Accuracy: ______________

(Note: The time element and accuracy criteria may be given by your instructor.)

Directions: Proofread the insurance claim form (see Fig. 15.5) and locate blocks that need correction or completion before submission to the insurance company. Highlight all errors you discover. Refer to the patient's record (see Fig. 15.4) to verify pertinent demographic and insurance information. Refer to the progress notes to verify procedures and determine diagnoses. Verify all entries on the claim form, including dates, codes, rounded-out fees, and physician identification numbers. Insert all corrections and missing information in red. If you cannot locate the necessary information but know it is mandatory, write "NEED" in the corresponding block.

Optional: Retype a blank CMS-1500 claim form with all corrections and changes.

Additional Coding

1. Assume that Mr. Diehl followed Dr. Input's treatment plan. Refer to his record, abstract information, and locate procedure codes that would be billed by providers outside of the office.

Site	*Description of Service*	*Code*
a. ABC Radiology	______________	______________
b. College Hospital	______________	______________
c. Surgeon	______________	______________

2. Code the symptoms Mr. Diehl was complaining about when he presented for the January 6, 20xx, office visit.

Symptom	*ICD-10-CM Code*
a. ______________	______________
b. ______________	______________
c. ______________	______________
d. ______________	______________
e. ______________	______________

PATIENT RECORD NO. 8-6

LAST NAME	FIRST NAME	MIDDLE NAME	BIRTH DATE	SEX	HOME PHONE
Diehl	Brad	E.	09-21-46	M	555-222-0123

ADDRESS	CITY	STATE	ZIP CODE
3975 Hills Road	Woodland Hills	XY	12345

CELL PHONE	PAGER NO.	FAX NO.	E-MAIL ADDRESS
555-703-6600	555-321-0988	555-222-0123	Diehl@WB.net

PATIENT'S SOC. SEC. NO.	DRIVER'S LICENSE
561-XX-1501	M0983457

PATIENT'S OCCUPATION	NAME OF COMPANY
radio advertising salesman	KACY Radio

ADDRESS OF EMPLOYER	PHONE
4071 Mills Road, Woodland Hills, XY 12335	555-201-6666

SPOUSE OR PARENT	OCCUPATION
Tak E. Diehl (birthdate 4-7-45)	legal secretary

EMPLOYER	ADDRESS	PHONE
Attys. Dilman, Forewise & Gilson,	12 West Dix Street, Woodland Hills, XY 12345	555-222-6432

NAME OF INSURANCE	INSURED OR SUBSCRIBER
Aetna Insurance Co., 2412 Main Street, Woodland Hills, XY 12345	Brad E. Diehl

POLICY/CERTIFICATE NO.	GROUP NO.
403119	

REFERRED BY: Raymond Skeleton, MD

DATE	PROGRESS NOTES No. 8-7
1-6-20xx	NP pt comes in complaining of coughing and sneezing; some difficulty breathing. Occasional dizziness and epigastric abdominal pain with cramping. Symptoms started in July of last year. Performed a detailed history and physical examination with low complexity medical decision making. AP & lat chest x-rays taken; neg findings. BP 178/98. Pt to have cholecystography with oral contrast at ABC Radiology. Diagnostic colonoscopy (flexible) to be scheduled at College Hospital. Dx: hypertension and respiratory distress; R/O irritable colon. No disability at this time.
	GI/IIf Gaston Input, MD
1-20-xx	Pt retns for a EPF hx/exam LC MDM. Oral cholecystography reveals a single 1.5 cm radiolucent calculus within the cholecyst. Colonoscopy confirmed irritable bowel syndrome. Blood drawn and CBC (auto with diff) performed in office indicates WBC 10,000. DX: cholecystitis with cholelithiasis. Adv. cholecystectomy (abdominal approach) as soon as possible; to be scheduled at College Hospital.
	GI/IIf Gaston Input, MD

Fig. 15.4

DRAFT - NOT FOR OFFICIAL USE

HEALTH INSURANCE CLAIM FORM

APPROVED BY NATIONAL UNIFOR MCLAIM COMMITTEE (NUCC) 02/12

PICA PICA

CARRIER

1. MEDICARE (Medicare#) [ ] MEDICAID (Medicaid#) [ ] TRICARE (ID#DoD#) [ ] CHAMPVA (Member ID#) [ ] GROUP HEALTH PLAN (ID#) [X] FECA BLK LUNG (ID#) [ ] OTHER (ID#) [ ]

1a. INSURED'S I.D. NUMBER (For Program in Item 1): 403119

2. PATIENT'S NAME (Last Name, First Name, Middle Initial): Diehl, Brad, E

3. PATIENT'S BIRTH DATE MM DD YY: 09 21 1946 SEX M [ ] F [ ]

4. INSURED'S NAME (Last Name, First Name, Middle Initial): Same

5. PATIENT'S ADDRESS (No., Street): 3975 Hills Road

6. PATIENT RELATIONSHIP TO INSURED: Self [X] Spouse [ ] Child [ ] Other [ ]

7. INSURED'S ADDRESS (No., Street):

CITY: Woodland Hills STATE: XY

8. RESERVED FOR NUCC USE

CITY STATE

ZIP CODE: 12345-0000 TELEPHONE (Include Area Code): (555) 2220123

ZIP CODE TELEPHONE (Include Area Code) ( )

9. OTHER INSURED'S NAME (Last Name, First Name, Middle Initial)

10. IS PATIENT'S CONDITION RELATED TO:

11. INSURED'S POLICY GROUP OR FECA NUMBER

a. OTHER INSURED'S POLICY OR GROUP NUMBER

a. EMPLOYMENT? (Current or Previous) [ ] YES [X] NO

a. INSURED'S DATE OF BIRTH MM DD YY SEX M [ ] F [ ]

b. RESERVED FOR NUCC USE

b. AUTO ACCIDENT? [ ] YES [X] NO PLACE (State)

b. OTHER CLAIM ID (Designated by NUCC)

c. RESERVED FOR NUCC USE

c. OTHER ACCIDENT? [ ] YES [X] NO

c. INSURANCE PLAN NAME OR PROGRAM NAME

d. INSURANCE PLAN NAME OR PROGRAM NAME

10d. CLAIM CODES (Designated by NUCC)

d. IS THERE ANOTHER HEALTH BENEFIT PLAN? [ ] YES [X] NO *If yes,* complete items 9, 9a, and 9d.

READ BACK OF FORM BEFORE COMPLETING & SIGNING THIS FORM.

12. PATIENT'S OR AUTHORIZED PERSON'S SIGNATUREI authorize the release of any medical or other information necessary to process this claim. I also request payment of government benefits either to myself or to the party who accepts assignment below.

SIGNED Signature on file DATE

13. INSURED'S OR AUTHORIZED PERSON'S SIGNATURE I authorize payment of medical benefits to the undersigned physician or supplier for services described below.

SIGNED Signature on file

PATIENT AND INSURED INFORMATION

14. DATE OF CURRENT: ILLNESS, INJURY, or PREGNANCY(LMP) MM DD YY QUAL.

15. OTHER DATE QUAL. MM DD YY

16. DATES PATIENT UNABLE TO WORK IN CURRENT OCCUPATION FROM MM DD YY TO MM DD YY

17. NAME OF REFERRING PROVIDER OR OTHER SOURCE: DN Raymond Skeleton MD

17a.

17b. NPI 12678547XX

18. HOSPITALIZATION DATES RELATED TO CURRENT SERVICES FROM MM DD YY TO MM DD YY

19. ADDITIONAL CLAIM INFORMATION (Designated by NUCC)

20. OUTSIDE LAB? [ ] YES [ ] NO $ CHARGES

21. DIAGNOSIS OR NATURE OF ILLNESS OR INJURY Relate A-L to service line below (24E) ICD Ind. 0

A. R06.00 B. I1O C. K80.60 D.

E. F. G. H.

I. J. K. L.

22. RESUBMISSION CODE ORIGINAL REF. NO.

23. PRIOR AUTHORIZATION NUMBER

	24. A. DATE(S) OF SERVICE From MM DD YY	To MM DD YY	B. PLACE OF SERVICE	C. EMG	D. PROCEDURES, SERVICES, OR SUPPLIES (Explain Unusual Circumstances) CPT/HCPCS	MODIFIER	E. DIAGNOSIS POINTER	F. $ CHARGES	G. DAYS OR UNITS	H. EPSDT Family Plan	I. ID. QUAL.	J. RENDERING PROVIDER ID. #
1	01 06 20XX		11		99203		A,B	70 92	1		NPI	32783127XX
2	01 06 20XX		11		71020		A	40 97	1		NPI	32783127XX
3	01 20 20XX		11		99213		C	40 20	1		NPI	32783127XX
4	01 20 20XX		11		85025		C	25 00	1		NPI	32783127XX
5	01 20 20XX		11				C		1		NPI	32783127XX
6											NPI	

25. FEDERAL TAX I.D. NUMBER SSN EIN [ ] [ ]

26. PATIENT'S ACCOUNT NO.: 8

27. ACCEPT ASSIGNMENT? (For govt. claims, see back) [X] YES [ ] NO

28. TOTAL CHARGE $

29. AMOUNT PAID $

30. Rsvd for NUCC Use $

31. SIGNATURE OF PHYSICIAN OR SUPPLIER INCLUDING DEGREES OR CREDENTIALS (I certify that the statements on the reverse apply to this bill and are made a part thereof.)

012520XX

SIGNED DATE

32. SERVICE FACILITY LOCATION INFORMATION

Same

a. NPI b.

33. BILLING PROVIDER INFO & PH # (555) 4869002

College Clinic
4567 Broad Avenue
Woodland Hills XY 12345-0001

a. 3664021CC b.

PHYSICIAN OR SUPPLIER INFORMATION

NUCC Instruction Manual available at: www.nucc.org *PLEASE PRINT OR TYPE* OMB APPROVAL PENDING

Fig. 15.5

ASSIGNMENT 15.7 PROOFREAD A COMPUTER-GENERATED HEALTH INSURANCE CLAIM FORM AND LOCATE INCORRECT AND MISSING DATA

Performance Objective

Task: Locate and designate blocks on the computer-generated insurance claim form that have incorrect information or need completion; correct or add data before submission to the insurance company.

Conditions: Use Evert I. Strain's patient record (Fig. 15.6), completed insurance claim (Fig. 15.7), a highlighter, and a red-ink pen.

Standards: Time: ______________ minutes

Accuracy: ______________

(Note: The time element and accuracy criteria may be given by your instructor.)

Directions: Proofread the insurance claim form (see Fig. 15.7) and locate blocks that need correction or completion before submission to the insurance company. Highlight all errors you discover. Refer to the patient's record (see Fig. 15.6) to verify pertinent demographic and insurance information. Refer to the progress notes to verify procedures and determine diagnoses. Verify all entries on the claim form, including dates, codes, rounded-out fees, and physician identification numbers. Insert all corrections and missing information in red. If you cannot locate the necessary information but know it is mandatory, write "NEED" in the corresponding block.

Optional: Retype a blank CMS-1500 claim form with all corrections and changes.

Additional Coding

1. Refer to Mr. Strain's medical record, abstract information, and code procedures that would be billed by outside providers.

Site	*Description of Service*	*Code*
a. ABC Laboratory	______________	______________
b. ABC Radiology	______________	______________

PATIENT RECORD NO. 8-7

LAST NAME	FIRST NAME	MIDDLE NAME	BIRTH DATE	SEX	HOME PHONE
Strain	Evert	I	09-11-46	M	555-678-0211

ADDRESS	CITY	STATE	ZIP CODE
7650 None Such Road	Woodland Hills	XY	12345

CELL PHONE	PAGER NO.	FAX NO.	E-MAIL ADDRESS
555-430-2101	555-320-9980	555-678-0211	Strain@WB.net

PATIENT'S SOC. SEC. NO.	DRIVER'S LICENSE
453-XX-4739	Y0923658

PATIENT'S OCCUPATION	NAME OF COMPANY
mechanical engineer	R & R Company

ADDRESS OF EMPLOYER	PHONE
2400 Davon Road, Woodland Hills, XY 12345	555-520-8977

SPOUSE OR PARENT	OCCUPATION
Ester I. Strain (wife)	administrative assistant

EMPLOYER	ADDRESS	PHONE
University College	4021 Book Road, Woodland Hills, XY 12345	555-450-9908

NAME OF INSURANCE	INSURED OR SUBSCRIBER
ABC Insurance Co., P.O. Box 130, Woodland Hills, XY 12345	Evert I. Strain

POLICY/CERTIFICATE NO.	GROUP NO.
453-XX-4739	96476A

REFERRED BY: Gerald C. Jones, MD, 1403 Haven Street, Woodland Hills, XY 12345 NPI # 54754966XX

DATE	PROGRESS NOTES No. 8-8
1-8-20xx	Est pt comes in complaining of frequent urination, headaches, polyphagia; unable to
	remember current events. These problems have been present for almost a year.
	A comprehensive history is taken and compared to his last H & P 2 years ago.
	A com PX is performed. BP 160/110; pt was prescribed antihypertensive medication but
	discontinued it when the prescription ran out. Lab report, hand carried by pt from an
	urgent care center, indicates SGOT in normal range and cholesterol elevated. Fasting blood
	sugar extremely high. Dx: diabetes mellitus, malignant hypertensive, and ASCVD.
	Pt to have 3 hour GTT tomorrow a.m. at ABC laboratory. STAT CT scan of head s̄ contrast
	ordered at ABC radiology to follow lab work. Arrangement will be made for pt to be
	admitted to College Hospital. Disability 1/9 through 1/31.
	GI/llf Gerald Practon, MD
1-9-xx	Admit to College Hospital (C hx/exam MC MDM).
	GI/llf Gerald Practon, MD
1-10-xx	Hosp visit (PF hx/exam SF MDM). CT scan of head reviewed, neg. findings. Pt alert and
	comfortable. If blood sugar and BP remain stable, discharge planned for tomorrow.
	BP 130/85.
	GI/llf Gerald Practon, MD
1-11-xx	DC from hosp. Pt to be seen in one week in ofc.
	GI/llf Gerald Practon, MD

Fig. 15.6

CARRIER

HEALTH INSURANCE CLAIM FORM

APPROVED BY NATIONAL UNIFOR MCLAIM COMMITTEE (NUCC) 02/12

PICA | PICA

1. MEDICARE (Medicare#) ☐ MEDICAID (Medicaid#) ☐ TRICARE (ID#DoD#) ☐ CHAMPVA (Member ID#) ☐ GROUP HEALTH PLAN (ID#) ☒ FECA BLK LUNG (ID#) ☐ OTHER (ID#) ☐

1a. INSURED'S I.D. NUMBER (For Program in Item 1): 453 XX 4739 96476A

2. PATIENT'S NAME (Last Name, First Name, Middle Initial): Strain, Evert, I

3. PATIENT'S BIRTH DATE MM DD YY: 09 21 1946 SEX M ☒ F ☐

4. INSURED'S NAME (Last Name, First Name, Middle Initial): Same

5. PATIENT'S ADDRESS (No., Street): 7650 None Such Road

6. PATIENT RELATIONSHIP TO INSURED: Self ☒ Spouse ☐ Child ☐ Other ☐

7. INSURED'S ADDRESS (No., Street)

CITY: Woodland Hills STATE: XY

8. RESERVED FOR NUCC USE

CITY STATE

ZIP CODE TELEPHONE (Include Area Code) ( )

ZIP CODE TELEPHONE (Include Area Code) ( )

9. OTHER INSURED'S NAME (Last Name, First Name, Middle Initial)

10. IS PATIENT'S CONDITION RELATED TO:

11. INSURED'S POLICY GROUP OR FECA NUMBER

a. OTHER INSURED'S POLICY OR GROUP NUMBER

a. EMPLOYMENT? (Current or Previous) ☐ YES ☒ NO

a. INSURED'S DATE OF BIRTH MM DD YY SEX M ☐ F ☐

b. RESERVED FOR NUCC USE

b. AUTO ACCIDENT? ☐ YES ☒ NO PLACE (State)

b. OTHER CLAIM ID (Designated by NUCC)

c. RESERVED FOR NUCC USE

c. OTHER ACCIDENT? ☐ YES ☒ NO

c. INSURANCE PLAN NAME OR PROGRAM NAME

d. INSURANCE PLAN NAME OR PROGRAM NAME

10d. CLAIM CODES (Designated by NUCC)

d. IS THERE ANOTHER HEALTH BENEFIT PLAN? ☐ YES ☐ NO *If yes,* complete items 9, 9a, and 9d.

READ BACK OF FORM BEFORE COMPLETING & SIGNING THIS FORM.

12. PATIENT'S OR AUTHORIZED PERSON'S SIGNATUREI authorize the release of any medical or other information necessary to process this claim. I also request payment of government benefits either to myself or to the party who accepts assignment below.

SIGNED Signature on file DATE

13. INSURED'S OR AUTHORIZED PERSON'S SIGNATURE I authorize payment of medical benefits to the undersigned physician or supplier for services described below.

SIGNED Signature on file

PATIENT AND INSURED INFORMATION

14. DATE OF CURRENT: ILLNESS, INJURY, or PREGNANCY(LMP) MM DD YY QUAL.

15. OTHER DATE QUAL. MM DD YY

16. DATES PATIENT UNABLE TO WORK IN CURRENT OCCUPATION FROM MM DD YY TO MM DD YY

17. NAME OF REFERRING PROVIDER OR OTHER SOURCE: DN Gerald C Jones

17a. 17b. NPI 54754966XX

18. HOSPITALIZATION DATES RELATED TO CURRENT SERVICES: FROM 01 09 20XX TO 01 11 20XX

19. ADDITIONAL CLAIM INFORMATION (Designated by NUCC)

20. OUTSIDE LAB? ☐ YES ☒ NO $ CHARGES

21. DIAGNOSIS OR NATURE OF ILLNESS OR INJURY Relate A-L to service line below (24E) ICD Ind. 0

A. E11.9 B. I10 C. I25.10 D.
E. F. G. H.
I. J K. L.

22. RESUBMISSION CODE ORIGINAL REF. NO.

23. PRIOR AUTHORIZATION NUMBER

	24. A. DATE(S) OF SERVICE From MM DD YY	To MM DD YY	B. PLACE OF SERVICE	C. EMG	D. PROCEDURES, SERVICES, OR SUPPLIES (Explain Unusual Circumstances) CPT/HCPCS	MODIFIER	E. DIAGNOSIS POINTER	F. $ CHARGES	G. DAYS OR UNITS	H. EPSDT Family Plan	I. ID. QUAL.	J. RENDERING PROVIDER ID. #
1	01 08 20XX		11		99215			96 97	1		NPI	46278897XX
2	01 09 20XX		21		99222			120 80	1		NPI	46278897XX
3	1 10 20XX		21		99231			37 74	1		NPI	46278897XX
4	01 11 20XX		21		99231			65 26	1		NPI	46278897XX
5											NPI	
6											NPI	

25. FEDERAL TAX I.D. NUMBER: 7034597 SSN ☐ EIN ☒

26. PATIENT'S ACCOUNT NO.: 8-7

27. ACCEPT ASSIGNMENT? (For govt. claims, see back) ☒ YES ☐ NO

28. TOTAL CHARGE $ 320 77

29. AMOUNT PAID $

30. Rsvd for NUCC Use $

31. SIGNATURE OF PHYSICIAN OR SUPPLIER INCLUDING DEGREES OR CREDENTIALS (I certify that the statements on the reverse apply to this bill and are made a part thereof.)

Gerald Practon MD 012520XX

SIGNED Gerald Practon MD DATE

32. SERVICE FACILITY LOCATION INFORMATION: Same

a. NPI b.

33. BILLING PROVIDER INFO & PH # (555) 4869002

College Clinic
4567 Broad Avenue
Woodland Hills XY 12345-0001

a. 3664021CC b.

PHYSICIAN OR SUPPLIER INFORMATION

NUCC Instruction Manual available at: www.nucc.org *PLEASE PRINT OR TYPE* OMB APPROVAL PENDING

Fig. 15.7

ASSIGNMENT 15.8 DEFINE PATIENT RECORD ABBREVIATIONS

Performance Objective

Task: Insert definitions of abbreviations.

Conditions: Use pencil or pen.

Standards: Time: ______________ minutes

Accuracy: ______________

(Note: The time element and accuracy criteria may be given by your instructor.)

Directions: After completing the assignments in this chapter, you will be able to define the abbreviations shown here.

Abbreviations pertinent to the record of Brad E. Diehl:

NP ______________________

LC ______________________

pt ______________________

MDM ______________________

AP ______________________

cm ______________________

lat ______________________

neg ______________________

BP ______________________

CBC ______________________

R/O ______________________

auto ______________________

retn ______________________

diff ______________________

EPF ______________________

WBC ______________________

hx ______________________

DX ______________________

exam ______________________

adv ______________________

Abbreviations pertinent to the record of Evert I. Strain:

est ______________________

CT ______________________

pt ______________________

C ______________________

H & P ______________________

hx ______________________

comp ______________________

exam ______________________

PX ______________________

MC ______________________

BP ______________________

MDM ______________________

lab ______________________

hosp ______________________

SGOT ______________________

PF ______________________

Dx ______________________

SF ______________________

ASCVD ______________________

neg ______________________

GTT ______________________

DC ______________________

STAT ______________________

ofc ______________________

16 Receiving Payments and Insurance Problem Solving

Linda M. Smith

KEY TERMS

Your instructor may wish to select some words pertinent to this chapter for a test. For definitions of the terms, further study, and/or reference, the words, phrases, and abbreviations may be found in the glossary at the end of the textbook. *Key terms for this chapter follow.*

Administrative Law Judge hearing
aging report
appeal
claim denial management
delinquent claim
denied claim
explanation of benefits
inquiry
insurance payment poster
insurance payment posting
lost claim
medical necessity
overpayment
peer review
Qualified Independent Contractor
rebill (resubmit)
rejected claim
reimbursement
remittance advice
revenue cycle management
review
suspended claim
suspense
tracer

KEY ABBREVIATIONS

See how many abbreviations and acronyms you can translate, and then use this as a handy reference list. Definitions for the key abbreviations are located near the back of the textbook *in the glossary.*

ALJ ____________________

CMS ____________________

DAB ____________________

EOB ____________________

HIPAA ____________________

NPI ____________________

QIC ____________________

RA ____________________

RCM ____________________

PERFORMANCE OBJECTIVES

The student will be able to:

- Define and spell the key terms and key abbreviations for this chapter, given the information from the *textbook* glossary, within a reasonable time period and with enough accuracy to obtain a satisfactory evaluation.
- After reading the chapter, answer the fill-in-the-blank, multiple choice, and true/false review questions with enough accuracy to obtain a satisfactory evaluation.

- Review an aging report to determine the method of follow-up needed to zero out all patient accounts.
- Locate the errors on each claim, given three returned insurance claims, within a reasonable time period and with enough accuracy to obtain a satisfactory evaluation.
- Complete form CMS-1965, Request for Medicare Hearing by an Administrative Law Judge, Part B, Medicare Claim, within a reasonable time period and with enough accuracy to obtain a satisfactory evaluation.
- File an appeal by composing and printing a letter with envelope, within a reasonable time period and with enough accuracy to obtain a satisfactory evaluation.

STUDY OUTLINE

Revenue Cycle Management
Response From a Submitted Claim
Claim Policy Guidelines
- Insured
- Electronic Claims Submission
- Contracts and Fee Schedules
- Reimbursement Time Frames

Explanation of Benefits
- Components of an Explanation of Benefits
- Interpreting an Explanation of Benefits
- Posting an Explanation of Benefits
- Secondary Insurance
- EOB Management

Claim Management Techniques
- Insurance Claims Register
- Purging Paid Files
- Aging Reports

Claim Inquiries
Problem Claims
- Types of Problems

Rebilling
Review and Appeal Process
Filing an Appeal
- Medicare Review and Redetermination Process
- TRICARE Review and Appeal Process

State Insurance Commissioner
- Commission Objectives
- Types of Problems

Commission Inquiries
Claim Denial Management

ASSIGNMENT 16.1 REVIEW QUESTIONS

Part I Fill in the Blank

Review the objectives, key terms, and chapter information before completing the following review questions.

1. The process in the health care organization uses to track services provided from registration and appointment scheduling to the final payment for services is referred to as

   ________________________.

2. Once a claim has been successfully submitted to the insurance carrier, the next step in the revenue cycle is for the insurance billing specialist to _________ the claim until a response is received from the responsible party and the service has been paid in full.

3. Who dictates the guidelines for claims submission, such as which services are covered, the reimbursement rates, and time limits for claim submission and payment?

   ____

4. Time limits for filing claims promptly can be found in the __________________ or the ______________.

5. What is the purpose of prompt payment laws?

   ____

6. After an insurance claim is processed by the insurance carrier (paid, suspended, rejected, or denied), a document known as a/an __________________________ is sent to the patient and to the provider of professional medical services.

7. A claim that is processed by a third-party payer but is held in an indeterminate state is referred to as a _____________ claim.

8. Claims paid with no errors are designated as ____________________.

9. Claims that are not paid within 30 to 45 days of the service date are referred to as

   _____________________ claims.

10. A ______________ claim is a submitted claim that does not follow specific third-party payer instructions or contains technical errors.

11. A service is considered ___________________ if it is provided in accordance with the generally accepted standards of medical practice and is clinically appropriate.

12. State the solution if a claim for routine foot care has been denied as a noncovered service.

    ____

    ____

    ____

13. State the solution if a claim has been denied because the professional service rendered was for an injury that is being considered as compensable under workers' compensation.

____

____

____

14. When an insurance carrier changes the code submitted to one of lesser value and it reduces the reimbursement amount, it is referred to as ________________.

15. When an insurance carrier reimburses a service at an amount over and above the amount due, it is referred to as an ________________.

16. Patient accounts with a balance should be billed on a ______________ basis.

17. A/an __________________ is a request for a review and reconsideration of a claim that has been underpaid, incorrectly paid, or denied by an insurance company.

18. A/an ______________ is an evaluation of a denied claim performed by a group of unbiased practicing physicians or other health care professionals to judge the effectiveness and efficiency of professional care rendered and to determine if payment can be made.

19. Name the five levels for appealing a Medicare claim.

 a. ____
 b. ____
 c. ____
 d. ____
 e. ____

20. A/an ____________________is an independent contractor who conducts reconsiderations for Medicare claims going through the appeals process.

21. To pursue judicial review of a Medicare claim in federal district court, the amount of the case must meet the minimum dollar amount of __________________ in 2018.

22. A TRICARE expedited appeal must be filed within ______________ of the receipt of the initial denial.

23. A TRICARE nonexpedited appeal must be filed within ______________ of the receipt of the initial denial.

24. ______________ are public officials who regulate the Insurance Industry in their state.

25. Effective claim denial management starts with ____________ the reason for denials.

Part II Multiple Choice

Choose the best answer.

26. A written request made to an insurance company to locate the status of an insurance claim is often referred to as:
    a. an inquiry.
    b. a follow-up.
    c. a tracer.
    d. all of the above.

27. When an electronic claim is transmitted for several services and one service is rejected for incomplete information, the solution is to:
    a. resubmit a paper claim with the needed data for the rejected services only.
    b. add the required information in field 19 that it is a retransmission
    c. add the required information and retransmit the rejected claim.
    d. not transmit a rejected claim.

28. A request for payment to a third-party payer asking for a review of an insurance claim that has been denied is referred to as a/an:
    a. review.
    b. appeal.
    c. request.
    d. demand.

29. When overpayments are identified, the Office of Inspector General (OIG) strongly advises that:
    a. service providers hold it for 30 days to make sure it was not due them.
    b. service providers place in a hold account until the insurance carrier requests it.
    c. service providers return the overpayment within 180 days of receipt of payment.
    d. service providers return the overpayment promptly when the insurance poster identifies it.

30. The steps in claim denial management are:
    a. Identify, Appeal, Categorize, Measure, Strategize.
    b. Appeal, Identify, Categorize, Strategize, Measure.
    c. Strategize, Categorize, Measure, Identify, Appeal.
    d. Identify, Measure, Categorize, Appeal, Strategize.

Part III True/False

Write "T" or "F" in the blank to indicate whether you think the statement is true or false.

_______ 31. An insurance billing specialist's primary goal is to assist in management of the revenue cycle.

_______ 32. A patient's insurance card specifies the detailed benefits and coverages.

_______ 33. All health insurance companies are obligated to reimburse health care organizations promptly for services rendered.

_______ 34. The elements within a remittance advice (RA) document and an explanation of benefits (EOB) document are different.

_______ 35. There is a standard format for EOB forms that all carriers are expected to follow.

_______ 36. Due to issues concerning timely filing, it is wise to be aggressive on claims that are outstanding for more than 30 to 45 days.

_______ 37. Information collected at the front desk does not impact denials.

_______ 38. Services are considered medically necessary if they are in accordance with the generally accepted standards of medical practice.

_______ 39. If any insurance carrier has downcoded a claim, thereby reducing reimbursement, there is no other recourse than to write off the balance.

_______ 40. If a claim has not been paid within a reasonable amount of time, the most effective follow-up method is to simply rebill the claim.

ASSIGNMENT 16.2 USING AN AGING REPORT FOR FOLLOW-UP

Performance Objective

Task: Use the aging report in Fig. 16.1 to complete follow-up.

Conditions: Refer to the aging report (see Fig. 16.1) and use a pen or computer.

Standards: Time: _______________ minutes

Accuracy: _______________

(Note: The time element and accuracy criteria may be given by your instructor.)

Directions: Review the aging report in Fig. 16.1 and consider the following scenario:

The Happy Day Primary Care Office is reviewing their aging report to follow up on outstanding payments. The office charges Aetna $260 for initial office visits and $145 for established patient office visits. Electronic claims that are filed to Aetna are reimbursed within to the office within 30 days of initial electronic claim submission. Answer the following questions.

1. Who were the three patients who were most recently billed?

____

____

____

2. Do phone calls to Aetna need to be made for patients that are in the 0 to 30 days categories? Why or why not?

____

____

3. Which two patients have balances that are different from typical office visit charges submitted to Aetna?

____

____

4. What would account for the difference in the balance from the original total charges submitted to Aetna?

____

____

5. Would it be appropriate to send the patients in categories beyond 60 days to a collection agency? Why or why not?

____

____

AETNA

Patient Name	Acct #	Primary Insurance	Secondary Insurance	0–30 days	31–60 days	61–90 days	91–120 days	Over 120 days	Total Balance
Bassett, Eleanor	75846	AETNA		$145.00	$0.00	$0.00	$0.00	$0.00	$145.00
Herron, John	83029	AETNA		$0.00	$42.41	$0.00	$0.00	$0.00	$42.41
Holt, Maxine	64739	AETNA	BLUE SHIELD	$145.00	$0.00	$0.00	$0.00	$0.00	$145.00
Kellog, Keenan	24537	AETNA		$0.00	$0.00	$145.00	$0.00	$0.00	$145.00
Lincoln, Frank	85940	AETNA		$0.00	$15.00	$0.00	$0.00	$0.00	$15.00
Markham, Melanie	14263	AETNA	MEDICARE	$0.00	$0.00	$0.00	$260.00	$0.00	$260.00
McDonald, Lydia	56374	AETNA		$260.00	$0.00	$0.00	$0.00	$0.00	$260.00
McLean, Mary	24395	AETNA		$0.00	$0.00	$0.00	$0.00	$260.00	$260.00
				$550.00	**$57.41**	**$145.00**	**$260.00**	**$260.00**	**$1,272.41**

Fig. 16.1

ASSIGNMENT 16.3 POST TO A FINANCIAL ACCOUNTING RECORD (LEDGER) FROM AN EXPLANATION OF BENEFITS (EOB) DOCUMENT

Performance Objective

Task: Post data from an EOB document to a patient's financial accounting record (ledger).

Conditions: Use a blank financial accounting record (ledger) (Fig. 16.2), an EOB document (Fig. 16.3), and a pen or computer.

Standards: Time: ________________ minutes

Accuracy: ________________

(Note: The time element and accuracy criteria may be given by your instructor.)

Background: Most payments in the medical office are posted in the same practice management billing software that the electronic claims are submitted from. However, to develop the skills and understanding for payment posting, a paper financial accounting ledger has been provided.

Directions: Post in ink the payment received and preferred provider organization (PPO) adjustment to a patient's financial accounting record (ledger) (see Fig. 16.2) by referring to an EOB document (see Fig. 16.3). An EOB document is defined in Fig. 16.2 in the textbook.

After the instructor has returned your work to you, either make the necessary corrections and place your work in a three-ring notebook for future reference or, if you received a high score, place it in your portfolio for reference when applying for a job.

1. Locate patient's financial accounting record (ledger) and EOB.

2. Ledger lines 6 and 7: Insert date of service (DOS), reference (CPT code number, check number, or dates of service for posting adjustments or when insurance was billed), description of the transaction, charge amounts, payments, adjustments, and running current balance. The posting date is the actual date the transaction is recorded. If the DOS differs from the posting date, list the DOS in the reference or description column.

Acct No. 9-3

STATEMENT
Financial Account

COLLEGE CLINIC
4567 Broad Avenue
Woodland Hills, XY 12345-0001
Tel. 555-486-9002
Fax No. 555-487-8976

Mr. Jabe Bortolussi
989 Moorpark Road
Woodland Hills, XY 12345

Phone No. (H) (555) 230-8870 (W) (555) 349-6689 Birth date 04-07-71

Primary Insurance Co. ABC Insurance Company Policy/Group No. 4206/010

DATE	REFERENCE	DESCRIPTION	CHARGES		CREDITS PYMNTS.		CREDITS ADJ.		BALANCE	
	BALANCE FORWARD →									
6-3-xx	99204	E/M NP Level 4	250	00					250	00
6-3-xx	94375	Respiratory flow vol loop	40	00					290	00
6-3-xx	94060	Spirometry	75	00					365	00
6-3-xx	94664	Aerosol inhalation	50	00					415	00
6-3-xx	94760	Pulse oximetry	50	00					465	00

PLEASE PAY LAST AMOUNT IN BALANCE COLUMN

THIS IS A COPY OF YOUR FINANCIAL ACCOUNT AS IT APPEARS ON OUR RECORDS

Fig. 16.2

Claim No.:	1-00-16987087-00-zmm
Group Name:	COLLEGE CLINIC
Group No.:	010
Employee:	JABE V. BORTOLUSSI
Patient:	JABE V. BORTOLUSSI
SSN:	554-XX-8876
Plan No.:	4206
Prepared by:	M. SMITH
Prepared on:	07/04/20XX

ABC Insurance Company
P.O. Box 4300
Woodland Hills, XY 12345-0001

GERALD PRACTON MD
4567 BROAD AVENUE
WOODLAND HILLS XY 12345

Patient Responsibility	
Amount not covered:	00
Co-pay amount:	00
Deductible:	00
Co-insurance:	64.61
Patient's total responsibility:	64.61
Other insurance payment:	00

EXPLANATION OF BENEFITS

Treatment Dates	Service Code	CPT Code	Charge Amount	Not Covered	Reason Code	PPO Discount	Covered Amount	Deductible Amount	Co-pay Amount	Paid At	Payment Amount
06/03/xx	200	99204	250.00	00	48	136.00	114.00	00	00	80%	91.20
06/03/xx	540	94375	40.00	00	48	00	40.00	00	00	80%	32.00
06/03/xx	540	94060	75.00	00	48	00	75.00	00	00	80%	60.00
06/03/xx	200	94664	50.00	00	48	1.55	48.45	00	00	80%	38.76
06/03/xx	540	94760	50.00	00	48	4.40	45.60	00	00	80%	36.48
		TOTAL	465.00	00		141.95	323.05	00	00		258.44

Other Insurance Credits or Adjustments 00

Total Payment Amount 258.44

CPT Code
99204 OFFICE/OUTPT VISIT E&M NEW MOD-HI SEVERIT
94375 RESPIRATORY FLOW VOLUM LOOP
94060 BRONCHOSPSM EVAL SPIROM PRE & POST BRON
94664 AEROSOL/VAPOR INHALA; INIT DEMO & EVAL
94760 NONINVASIVE EAR/PULSE OXIMETRY-02 SAT

Reason Code
48 CON DISCOUNT/PT NOT RESPONSIBLE

Participant		Date
GERALD PRACTON MD		07-04-xx
Patient		ID Number
JABE V. BORTOLUSSI		554-XX-8876
Plan Number	Patient Number	Office No.
4206		010

GC 1234567890

258.44

PAY TO THE ORDER OF

COLLEGE CLINIC
4567 BROAD AVENUE
WOODLAND HILLS XY 12345

J M Smith

ABC Insurance Company

Fig. 16.3

ASSIGNMENT 16.4 LOCATE ERRORS ON A RETURNED INSURANCE CLAIM

Performance Objective

Task: Highlight the blocks on the insurance claim form where errors are discovered.

Conditions: Use an insurance claim form (Fig. 16.4) and a highlighter or red pen.

Standards: Time: ______________ minutes

Accuracy: ______________

(Note: The time element and accuracy criteria may be given by your instructor.)

Directions: An insurance claim (see Fig. 16.4) was returned by the Prudential Insurance Company. Highlight or circle in red all blocks on the claim form where errors are discovered.

Option 1: Retype the claim and either insert the correction, if data are available to fix the error, or insert the word "NEED" in the block of the claim form.

Option 2: On a separate sheet of paper, list the blocks from 1 to 33 and state where errors occur. A Performance Evaluation Checklist may be reproduced from the "Instruction Guide to the Workbook" chapter if your instructor wishes you to submit it to assist with scoring and comments.

After the instructor has returned your work to you, either make the necessary corrections and place your work in a three-ring notebook for future reference or, if you received a high score, place it in your portfolio for reference when applying for a job.

HEALTH INSURANCE CLAIM FORM

APPROVED BY NATIONAL UNIFOR MCLAIM COMMITTEE (NUCC) 02/12

Prudential Insurance Company
500 South Bend Street
Woodland Hills XY 12345-0001

CARRIER

PICA | PICA

1. MEDICARE (Medicare#) ☐ MEDICAID (Medicaid#) ☐ TRICARE (ID#DoD#) ☐ CHAMPVA (Member ID#) ☐ GROUP HEALTH PLAN (ID#) ☐ FECA BLK LUNG (ID#) ☐ OTHER (ID#) ☒

1a. INSURED'S I.D. NUMBER (For Program in Item 1)

2. PATIENT'S NAME (Last Name, First Name, Middle Initial): Johnson, Emily B.

3. PATIENT'S BIRTH DATE MM DD YY: 02 12 1963 SEX M ☐ F ☐

4. INSURED'S NAME (Last Name, First Name, Middle Initial): Johnson, Erron T.

5. PATIENT'S ADDRESS (No., Street): 4391 Everett Street

6. PATIENT RELATIONSHIP TO INSURED: Self ☐ Spouse ☒ Child ☐ Other ☐

7. INSURED'S ADDRESS (No., Street): Same

CITY: Woodland Hills STATE: XY

8. RESERVED FOR NUCC USE

CITY STATE

ZIP CODE: 12345-0001 TELEPHONE (Include Area Code): ( )

ZIP CODE TELEPHONE (Include Area Code): ( )

9. OTHER INSURED'S NAME (Last Name, First Name, Middle Initial)

10. IS PATIENT'S CONDITION RELATED TO:

11. INSURED'S POLICY GROUP OR FECA NUMBER

a. OTHER INSURED'S POLICY OR GROUP NUMBER

a. EMPLOYMENT? (Current or Previous) ☐ YES ☐ NO

a. INSURED'S DATE OF BIRTH MM DD YY SEX M ☐ F ☐

b. RESERVED FOR NUCC USE

b. AUTO ACCIDENT? ☐ YES ☐ NO PLACE (State)

b. OTHER CLAIM ID (Designated by NUCC)

c. RESERVED FOR NUCC USE

c. OTHER ACCIDENT? ☐ YES ☐ NO

c. INSURANCE PLAN NAME OR PROGRAM NAME

d. INSURANCE PLAN NAME OR PROGRAM NAME

10d. CLAIM CODES (Designated by NUCC)

d. IS THERE ANOTHER HEALTH BENEFIT PLAN? ☐ YES ☒ NO *If yes,* complete items 9, 9a, and 9d.

READ BACK OF FORM BEFORE COMPLETING & SIGNING THIS FORM.

12. PATIENT'S OR AUTHORIZED PERSON'S SIGNATUREI authorize the release of any medical or other information necessary to process this claim. I also request payment of government benefits either to myself or to the party who accepts assignment below.

SIGNED *Emily B. Johnson* DATE 1/4/2020

13. INSURED'S OR AUTHORIZED PERSON'S SIGNATURE I authorize payment of medical benefits to the undersigned physician or supplier for services described below.

SIGNED *Emily B. Johnson*

PATIENT AND INSURED INFORMATION

14. DATE OF CURRENT: ILLNESS, INJURY, or PREGNANCY(LMP) MM DD YY QUAL.

15. OTHER DATE QUAL. MM DD YY

16. DATES PATIENT UNABLE TO WORK IN CURRENT OCCUPATION FROM MM DD YY TO MM DD YY

17. NAME OF REFERRING PROVIDER OR OTHER SOURCE

17a.

17b. NPI 67805027XX

18. HOSPITALIZATION DATES RELATED TO CURRENT SERVICES FROM MM DD YY TO MM DD YY

19. ADDITIONAL CLAIM INFORMATION (Designated by NUCC)

20. OUTSIDE LAB? ☐ YES ☒ NO $ CHARGES

21. DIAGNOSIS OR NATURE OF ILLNESS OR INJURY Relate A-L to service line below (24E) ICD Ind. 0

A. B. C. D.
E. F. G. H.
I. J. K. L.

22. RESUBMISSION CODE ORIGINAL REF. NO.

23. PRIOR AUTHORIZATION NUMBER

	24. A. DATE(S) OF SERVICE From MM DD YY	To MM DD YY	B. PLACE OF SERVICE	C. EMG	D. PROCEDURES, SERVICES, OR SUPPLIES (Explain Unusual Circumstances) CPT/HCPCS	MODIFIER	E. DIAGNOSIS POINTER	F. $ CHARGES	G. DAYS OR UNITS	H. EPSDT Family Plan	I. ID. QUAL.	J. RENDERING PROVIDER ID. #
1	01 04 20XX		11		99213		A	125 00	1		NPI	705687717XX
2	01 04 20XX		11		99213		A	125 00			NPI	
3											NPI	
4											NPI	
5											NPI	
6											NPI	

PHYSICIAN OR SUPPLIER INFORMATION

25. FEDERAL TAX I.D. NUMBER SSN EIN: 7180561XX ☐ ☐

26. PATIENT'S ACCOUNT NO.: 237819

27. ACCEPT ASSIGNMENT? (For govt. claims, see back) ☒ YES ☐ NO

28. TOTAL CHARGE $ 250 00

29. AMOUNT PAID $ 0 00

30. Rsvd for NUCC Use $

31. SIGNATURE OF PHYSICIAN OR SUPPLIER INCLUDING DEGREES OR CREDENTIALS (I certify that the statements on the reverse apply to this bill and are made a part thereof.)

SIGNED *Vera Cutis, MD* DATE 01/06/20XX

32. SERVICE FACILITY LOCATION INFORMATION

a. NPI b.

33. BILLING PROVIDER INFO & PH # (555) 4869002
College Clinic
4567 Broad Avenue
Woodland Hills XY 12345-0001

a. 3664021CC b.

NUCC Instruction Manual available at: www.nucc.org — PLEASE PRINT OR TYPE — OMB APPROVAL PENDING

Fig. 16.4

ASSIGNMENT 16.5 LOCATE ERRORS ON A RETURNED INSURANCE CLAIM

Performance Objective

Task: Highlight the blocks on the insurance claim form where errors are discovered.

Conditions: Use an insurance claim form (Fig. 16.5) and a highlighter or red pen.

Standards: Time: ________________ minutes

Accuracy: ________________

(Note: The time element and accuracy criteria may be given by your instructor.)

Directions: An insurance claim was returned by the Healthtech Insurance Company. Highlight or circle in red all blocks on the claim form where errors are discovered.

Option 1: Retype the claim and either insert the correction if data are available to fix the error or insert the word "NEED" in the block of the claim form.

Option 2: On a separate sheet of paper, list the blocks from 1 to 33 and state where errors occur. A Performance Evaluation Checklist may be reproduced from the "Instruction Guide to the Workbook" that appears in the section before Chapter 1 if your instructor wishes you to submit it to assist with scoring and comments.

After the instructor has returned your work to you, either make the necessary corrections and place your work in a three-ring notebook for future reference or, if you received a high score, place it in your portfolio for reference when applying for a job.

DRAFT - NOT FOR OFFICIAL USE

HEALTH INSURANCE CLAIM FORM

APPROVED BY NATIONAL UNIFOR MCLAIM COMMITTEE (NUCC) 02/12

Healthtech Insurance Company
4821 West Lake Avenue
Woodland Hills XY 12345-0001

CARRIER

PICA | PICA

1. MEDICARE (Medicare#) [ ] MEDICAID (Medicaid#) [X] TRICARE (ID#DoD#) [X] CHAMPVA (Member ID#) [ ] GROUP HEALTH PLAN (ID#) [ ] FECA BLK LUNG (ID#) [ ] OTHER (ID#) [X]

1a. INSURED'S I.D. NUMBER (For Program in Item 1): 433129870ANC

2. PATIENT'S NAME (Last Name, First Name, Middle Initial): Dugan, Charles C

3. PATIENT'S BIRTH DATE MM DD YY: 12 24 1968 SEX M [X] F [ ]

4. INSURED'S NAME (Last Name, First Name, Middle Initial): Same

5. PATIENT'S ADDRESS (No., Street): 5900 Elm Street

6. PATIENT RELATIONSHIP TO INSURED: Self [X] Spouse [ ] Child [ ] Other [ ]

7. INSURED'S ADDRESS (No., Street): Same

CITY: Woodland Hills STATE: XY

8. RESERVED FOR NUCC USE

CITY STATE

ZIP CODE: 12345-0001 TELEPHONE (Include Area Code): (555) 5593300

ZIP CODE TELEPHONE (Include Area Code) ( )

9. OTHER INSURED'S NAME (Last Name, First Name, Middle Initial)

10. IS PATIENT'S CONDITION RELATED TO:

11. INSURED'S POLICY GROUP OR FECA NUMBER

a. OTHER INSURED'S POLICY OR GROUP NUMBER

a. EMPLOYMENT? (Current or Previous) [ ] YES [X] NO

a. INSURED'S DATE OF BIRTH MM DD YY SEX M [ ] F [ ]

b. RESERVED FOR NUCC USE

b. AUTO ACCIDENT? [ ] YES [X] NO PLACE (State)

b. OTHER CLAIM ID (Designated by NUCC)

c. RESERVED FOR NUCC USE

c. OTHER ACCIDENT? [ ] YES [X] NO

c. INSURANCE PLAN NAME OR PROGRAM NAME

d. INSURANCE PLAN NAME OR PROGRAM NAME

10d. CLAIM CODES (Designated by NUCC)

d. IS THERE ANOTHER HEALTH BENEFIT PLAN? [ ] YES [ ] NO *If yes*, complete items 9, 9a, and 9d.

READ BACK OF FORM BEFORE COMPLETING & SIGNING THIS FORM.

12. PATIENT'S OR AUTHORIZED PERSON'S SIGNATUREI authorize the release of any medical or other information necessary to process this claim. I also request payment of government benefits either to myself or to the party who accepts assignment below.

SIGNED ____ DATE ____

13. INSURED'S OR AUTHORIZED PERSON'S SIGNATURE I authorize payment of medical benefits to the undersigned physician or supplier for services described below.

SIGNED ____

PATIENT AND INSURED INFORMATION

14. DATE OF CURRENT: ILLNESS, INJURY, or PREGNANCY(LMP) MM DD YY QUAL.

15. OTHER DATE QUAL. MM DD YY

16. DATES PATIENT UNABLE TO WORK IN CURRENT OCCUPATION FROM MM DD YY TO MM DD YY

17. NAME OF REFERRING PROVIDER OR OTHER SOURCE

17a.
17b. NPI 67805027XX

18. HOSPITALIZATION DATES RELATED TO CURRENT SERVICES FROM MM DD YY TO MM DD YY

19. ADDITIONAL CLAIM INFORMATION (Designated by NUCC)

20. OUTSIDE LAB? [ ] YES [X] NO $ CHARGES

21. DIAGNOSIS OR NATURE OF ILLNESS OR INJURY Relate A-L to service line below (24E) ICD Ind. 0

A. S51.801 B. C. D.
E. F. G. H.
I. J. K. L.

22. RESUBMISSION CODE ORIGINAL REF. NO.

23. PRIOR AUTHORIZATION NUMBER

	24. A. DATE(S) OF SERVICE From MM DD YY	To MM DD YY	B. PLACE OF SERVICE	C. EMG	D. PROCEDURES, SERVICES, OR SUPPLIES (Explain Unusual Circumstances) CPT/HCPCS	MODIFIER	E. DIAGNOSIS POINTER	F. $ CHARGES	G. DAYS OR UNITS	H. EPSDT Family Plan	I. ID. QUAL.	J. RENDERING PROVIDER ID. #
1	09 55 20XX		11		99203		A	70 92	1		NPI	46278897XX
2	09 55 20XX		11		12001		A				NPI	46278897XX
3											NPI	
4											NPI	
5											NPI	
6											NPI	

PHYSICIAN OR SUPPLIER INFORMATION

25. FEDERAL TAX I.D. NUMBER: 7034597XX SSN [ ] EIN [X]

26. PATIENT'S ACCOUNT NO.: 238293

27. ACCEPT ASSIGNMENT? (For govt. claims, see back) [X] YES [ ] NO

28. TOTAL CHARGE $

29. AMOUNT PAID $

30. Rsvd for NUCC Use $

31. SIGNATURE OF PHYSICIAN OR SUPPLIER INCLUDING DEGREES OR CREDENTIALS (I certify that the statements on the reverse apply to this bill and are made a part thereof.)

SIGNED *Gerald Practon, MD* DATE 09/30/20XX

32. SERVICE FACILITY LOCATION INFORMATION
College Hospital
4500 Broad Avenue
Woodland Hills XY 12345-0001

a. 937310XX b.

33. BILLING PROVIDER INFO & PH # (555) 4869002
College Clinic
4567 Broad Avenue
Woodland Hills XY 12345-0001

a. 3664021CC b.

NUCC Instruction Manual available at: www.nucc.org *PLEASE PRINT OR TYPE* OMB APPROVAL PENDING

Fig. 16.5

ASSIGNMENT 16.6 LOCATE ERRORS ON A RETURNED INSURANCE CLAIM

Performance Objective

Task: Highlight the blocks on the insurance claim form where errors are discovered.

Conditions: Use an insurance claim form (Fig. 16.6) and a highlighter or red pen.

Standards: Time: ________________ minutes

Accuracy: ________________

(Note: The time element and accuracy criteria may be given by your instructor.)

Directions: An insurance claim (see Fig. 16.6) was returned by an insurance plan. Highlight or circle in red all blocks on the claim form where errors are discovered.

Option 1: Retype the claim and either insert the correction if data are available to fix the error or insert the word "NEED" in the block of the claim form.

Option 2: On a separate sheet of paper, list the blocks from 1 to 33 and state where errors occur. A Performance Evaluation Checklist may be reproduced from the "Instruction Guide to the Workbook" that appears in the section before Chapter 1 if your instructor wishes you to submit it to assist with scoring and comments.

After the instructor has returned your work to you, either make the necessary corrections and place your work in a three-ring notebook for future reference or, if you received a high score, place it in your portfolio for reference when applying for a job.

DRAFT - NOT FOR OFFICIAL USE

HEALTH INSURANCE CLAIM FORM

APPROVED BY NATIONAL UNIFOR MCLAIM COMMITTEE (NUCC) 02/12

American Insurance Company
509 Main Street
Woodland Hills XY 12345-0001

CARRIER

PICA ☐☐☐ PICA ☐☐☐

PATIENT AND INSURED INFORMATION

1. MEDICARE ☐ (Medicare#) MEDICAID ☐ (Medicaid#) TRICARE ☐ (ID#DoD#) CHAMPVA ☐ (Member ID#) GROUP HEALTH PLAN ☐ (ID#) FECA BLK LUNG ☐ (ID#) OTHER [X] (ID#)

1a. INSURED'S I.D. NUMBER (For Program in Item 1)

2. PATIENT'S NAME (Last Name, First Name, Middle Initial): Mary T Avery

3. PATIENT'S BIRTH DATE MM DD YY: 05 07 1980 SEX M ☐ F ☐

4. INSURED'S NAME (Last Name, First Name, Middle Initial): Same

5. PATIENT'S ADDRESS (No., Street): 4309 Main Street

6. PATIENT RELATIONSHIP TO INSURED: Self [X] Spouse ☐ Child ☐ Other ☐

7. INSURED'S ADDRESS (No., Street)

CITY: Woodland Hills STATE: XY

8. RESERVED FOR NUCC USE

CITY STATE

ZIP CODE: 12345-0001 TELEPHONE (Include Area Code): (555) 4509899

ZIP CODE TELEPHONE (Include Area Code) ( )

9. OTHER INSURED'S NAME (Last Name, First Name, Middle Initial)

10. IS PATIENT'S CONDITION RELATED TO:

11. INSURED'S POLICY GROUP OR FECA NUMBER

a. OTHER INSURED'S POLICY OR GROUP NUMBER

a. EMPLOYMENT? (Current or Previous) ☐ YES [X] NO

a. INSURED'S DATE OF BIRTH MM DD YY SEX M ☐ F ☐

b. RESERVED FOR NUCC USE

b. AUTO ACCIDENT? ☐ YES [X] NO PLACE (State)

b. OTHER CLAIM ID (Designated by NUCC)

c. RESERVED FOR NUCC USE

c. OTHER ACCIDENT? ☐ YES [X] NO

c. INSURANCE PLAN NAME OR PROGRAM NAME

d. INSURANCE PLAN NAME OR PROGRAM NAME

10d. CLAIM CODES (Designated by NUCC)

d. IS THERE ANOTHER HEALTH BENEFIT PLAN? ☐ YES ☐ NO *If yes*, complete items 9, 9a, and 9d.

READ BACK OF FORM BEFORE COMPLETING & SIGNING THIS FORM.

12. PATIENT'S OR AUTHORIZED PERSON'S SIGNATUREI authorize the release of any medical or other information necessary to process this claim. I also request payment of government benefits either to myself or to the party who accepts assignment below.

SIGNED *Mary T. Avery* DATE 11/20/2007

13. INSURED'S OR AUTHORIZED PERSON'S SIGNATURE I authorize payment of medical benefits to the undersigned physician or supplier for services described below.

SIGNED *Mary T. Avery*

PHYSICIAN OR SUPPLIER INFORMATION

14. DATE OF CURRENT: ILLNESS, INJURY, or PREGNANCY(LMP) MM DD YY QUAL.

15. OTHER DATE QUAL. MM DD YY

16. DATES PATIENT UNABLE TO WORK IN CURRENT OCCUPATION MM DD YY FROM 11 09 20XX TO 11 30 20XX

17. NAME OF REFERRING PROVIDER OR OTHER SOURCE: Gerald Practon MD

17a. 17b. NPI

18. HOSPITALIZATION DATES RELATED TO CURRENT SERVICES MM DD YY FROM 11 11 20XX TO 11 12 20XX

19. ADDITIONAL CLAIM INFORMATION (Designated by NUCC)

20. OUTSIDE LAB? ☐ YES [X] NO $ CHARGES

21. DIAGNOSIS OR NATURE OF ILLNESS OR INJURY Relate A-L to service line below (24E) ICD Ind. 0

A. J03.90 B. C. D.
E. F. G. H.
I. J. K. L.

22. RESUBMISSION CODE ORIGINAL REF. NO.

23. PRIOR AUTHORIZATION NUMBER

	24. A. DATE(S) OF SERVICE From MM DD YY	To MM DD YY	B. PLACE OF SERVICE	C. EMG	D. PROCEDURES, SERVICES, OR SUPPLIES (Explain Unusual Circumstances) CPT/HCPCS	MODIFIER	E. DIAGNOSIS POINTER	F. $ CHARGES	G. DAYS OR UNITS	H. EPSDT Family Plan	I. ID. QUAL.	J. RENDERING PROVIDER ID. #
1	11 10 20XX		11		99203		A	50 00	1		NPI	43050047XX
2	11 11 20XX		21		99222		A	120 80			NPI	43050047XX
3	11 11 20XX		21		42821		A	410 73			NPI	43050047XX
4	11 22 20XX		21		99231		A	20 00			NPI	
5											NPI	
6											NPI	

25. FEDERAL TAX I.D. NUMBER: 715737291XX SSN ☐ EIN [X]

26. PATIENT'S ACCOUNT NO.: 456273

27. ACCEPT ASSIGNMENT? (For govt. claims, see back) ☐ YES ☐ NO

28. TOTAL CHARGE $ 29. AMOUNT PAID $ 30. Rsvd for NUCC Use $

31. SIGNATURE OF PHYSICIAN OR SUPPLIER INCLUDING DEGREES OR CREDENTIALS (I certify that the statements on the reverse apply to this bill and are made a part thereof.)

SIGNED DATE 11/15/20XX

32. SERVICE FACILITY LOCATION INFORMATION
College Hospital
4500 Broad Avenue
Woodland Hills XY 12345-0001

a. X950731067 b.

33. BILLING PROVIDER INFO & PH # (555) 4869002
College Clinic
4567 Broad Avenue
Woodland Hills XY 12345-0001

a. 3664021CC b.

NUCC Instruction Manual available at: www.nucc.org PLEASE PRINT OR TYPE OMB APPROVAL PENDING

Fig. 16.6

ASSIGNMENT 16.7 REQUEST FOR MEDICARE HEARING BY AN ADMINISTRATIVE LAW JUDGE

Performance Objective

Task: Insert information on a Request for Medicare Hearing by an Administrative Law Judge (Form OMHA-100)

Conditions: Request for Medicare Hearing by an Administrative Law Judge (Form OMHA-100) (Fig. 16.7), and a computer with printer.

Standards: Time: ________________ minutes

Accuracy: ________________

(Note: The time element and accuracy criteria may be given by your instructor.)

Directions: You receive a Medicare EOB and payment check for the patient Bill Hutch, but the amount is incorrect because of an excessive reduction in the allowed payment. An appeal was made in September and denied; the document control number assigned by Medicare Blue Shield is 240-577-9008. Dr. Brady Coccidioides believes that a mistake has been made and wishes to request a hearing.

Complete the Request for Medicare Hearing by an Administrative Law Judge (Form OMHA-100) for this case (see Fig. 16.7 in the textbook). Mr. Hutch's e-mail address is bhutch@gmail.net. Complete the form as the appellant and do not fill in the representative's portion. The Health Insurance Claim Number is the patient's Medicare identification number, Block 1a. No additional evidence is to be presented; the doctor does not wish to appear for the hearing. Date the form December 5, 20xx. The beneficiary has assigned his appeal rights to the provider.

After the instructor has returned your work to you, either make the necessary corrections and place your work in a three-ring notebook for future reference or, if you received a high score, place it in your portfolio for reference when applying for a job.

DEPARTMENT OF HEALTH AND HUMAN SERVICES
Office of Medicare Hearings and Appeals

REQUEST FOR ADMINISTRATIVE LAW JUDGE (ALJ) HEARING OR REVIEW OF DISMISSAL

Section 1: Which Medicare Part are you appealing (if known)? (*Check one*)

☐ Part A ☐ Part B ☐ Part C (*Medicare Advantage*) or Medicare Cost Plan ☐ Part D (*Prescription Drug Plan*)

Section 2: Which party are you, or which party are you representing? (*Check one*)

☐ The Medicare beneficiary or enrollee, or a successor (such as an estate), who received or requested the items or services being appealed, or is appealing a Medicare Secondary Payer issue.

☐ The provider or supplier that furnished the items or services to the Medicare beneficiary or enrollee, a Medicaid State agency, or an applicable plan appealing a Medicare Secondary Payer issue.

☐ Other. *Please explain*:

Section 3: What is your (the appealing party's) information? (*Representative information in next section*)

Name (*First, Middle Initial, Last*)		Firm or Organization (*if applicable*)	
Address where appeals correspondence should be sent	City	State	ZIP Code
Telephone Number	Fax Number	E-Mail	

Section 4: What is the representative's information? (*Skip if you do not have a representative*)

Name		Firm or Organization (*if applicable*)	
Mailing Address	City	State	ZIP Code
Telephone Number	Fax Number	E-Mail	

Did you file an appointment of representation (form CMS-1696) or other documents authorizing your representation at a prior level of appeal?

☐ No. *Please file the document(s) with this request.*
☐ Yes

Section 5: What is being appealed? *Submit a separate request for each Reconsideration or Dismissal that you wish to appeal. If the appeal involves multiple beneficiaries or enrollees, use the multiple claim attachment (OMHA-100A).*

Name of entity that issued the Reconsideration or Dismissal (*or attach a copy of the Reconsideration or Dismissal*)		Reconsideration (Medicare Appeal or Case) Number (*or attach a copy of the Reconsideration or Dismissal*)	
Beneficiary or Enrollee Name		Health Insurance Claim Number	
Beneficiary or Enrollee Mailing Address	City	State	ZIP Code
What item(s) or service(s) are you appealing? (*N/A if appealing a Dismissal*)		Date(s) of service being appealed (*if applicable*)	
Supplier or Provider Name (*N/A for Part D appeals*)		Supplier or Provider Telephone Number (*N/A for Part D appeals*)	
Supplier or Provider Mailing Address (*N/A for Part D appeals*)	City	State	ZIP Code

Section 6: For appeals of prescription drugs ONLY (*Skip for all other appeals*)

Part D Prescription Drug Plan Name	What drug(s) are you appealing?

Are you requesting an expedited hearing?
(*An expedited hearing is only available if your appeal is not solely related to payment (for example, you do not have the drug) and applying the standard time frame for a decision (90 days) may jeopardize your health, life, or ability to regain maximum function*)

☐ No. ☐ Yes. *On a separate sheet, please explain or have your prescriber explain why applying the standard time frame for a decision (90 days) may jeopardize your health, life, or ability to regain maximum function.*

OMHA-100 (03/17) **PAGE 1 OF 2** PSC Publishing Services (301) 443-6740. EF

Fig. 16.7 (From Department of Health and Human Services, Office of Medicare Hearings and Appeals.)

Section 7: Why do you disagree with the Reconsideration or Dismissal being appealed? *(Attach a continuation sheet if necessary)*

Section 8: Are you submitting evidence with this request, or do you plan to submit evidence?

☐ I am not planning to submit evidence at this time. *(Skip to Section 9, below)*

☐ I am submitting evidence with this request.

☐ I plan to submit evidence. Indicate what you plan to submit and when you plan to submit it:

Was the evidence already submitted for the matter that you are appealing?	☐ No. *Part A and Part B appeals only. If you are a provider or supplier, or a provider or supplier that is representing a beneficiary, you must include a statement explaining why the evidence is being submitted for the first time and was not submitted previously.* ☐ Yes.

Section 9: Is there other information about your appeal that we should know?

Are you aggregating claims to meet the amount in controversy requirement? *(If yes, attach your aggregation request. See 42 C.F.R. § 405.1006(e) and (f), and 423.1979(c) for request requirements.)*	☐ No	☐ Yes
Are you waiving the oral hearing before an ALJ and requesting a decision based on the record? *(If yes, attach a completed form OMHA-104 or other explanation. N/A if requesting review of a dismissal.)*	☐ No	☐ Yes
Does the request involve claims that were part of a statistical sample? *(If yes, please explain the status of any appeals for claims in the sample that are not included in this request.)*	☐ No	☐ Yes

Section 10: Certification of copies sent to other parties *(Part A and Part B appeals only)*

If another party to the claim or issue that you are appealing was sent a copy of the Reconsideration or Dismissal, you must send a copy of your request for an ALJ hearing or review of dismissal to that party.

Indicate the party (or their representative) to whom and address where you are sending a copy of the request, and when the copy will be sent *(attach a continuation sheet if there are multiple parties).*

Name of Recipient		
Mailing Address		
City	State	ZIP Code
Date of Mailing		

☐ Check here if no other parties were sent a copy of the Reconsideration or Dismissal.

Section 11: Filing instructions

Your appealed claim must meet the current amount in controversy requirement to file an appeal. See the Reconsideration or Dismissal or visit www.hhs.gov/omha for information on the current amount in controversy. Send this request form to the entity in the appeal instructions that came with your reconsideration (for example, requests for hearing following a Part C reconsideration are generally sent to the entity that conducted the reconsideration). If instructed to send to OMHA, use the addresses below.

Beneficiaries and enrollees, send your request to:	**For expedited Part D appeals, send your request to:**	**All other appellants, send your request to:**
OMHA Centralized Docketing Attn: Beneficiary Mail Stop 200 Public Square, Suite 1260 Cleveland, Ohio 44114-2316	OMHA Centralized Docketing Attn: Expedited Part D Mail Stop 200 Public Square, Suite 1260 Cleveland, Ohio 44114-2316	OMHA Centralized Docketing 200 Public Square, Suite 1260 Cleveland, Ohio 44114-2316

We must receive this request within 60 calendar days after you received the Reconsideration or Dismissal that you are appealing. We will assume that you received the Reconsideration or Dismissal 5 calendar days after the date of the Reconsideration or Dismissal, unless you provide evidence to the contrary. *If you are filing this request late, attach a completed form OMHA-103 or other explanation for the late filing.*

PRIVACY ACT STATEMENT

The legal authority for the collection of information on this form is authorized by the Social Security Act (section 1155 of Title XI and sections 1852(g)(5), 1860D-4(h)(1), 1869(b)(1), and 1876 of Title XVIII). The information provided will be used to further document your appeal. Submission of the information requested on this form is voluntary, but failure to provide all or any part of the requested information may affect the determination of your appeal. Information you furnish on this form may be disclosed by the Office of Medicare Hearings and Appeals to another person or governmental agency only with respect to the Medicare Program and to comply with Federal laws requiring the disclosure of information or the exchange of information between the Department of Health and Human Services and other agencies.

If you need large print or assistance, please call 1-855-556-8475

OMHA-100 (03/17)

PAGE 2 OF 2

Fig. 16.7, cont'd

ASSIGNMENT 16.8 FILE AN APPEAL

Performance Objective

Task: Compose, format, key, proofread, and print a letter of appeal, and attach to this document photocopies of information to substantiate reimbursement requested.

Conditions: Computer, printer, letterhead paper, envelope, attachments, thesaurus, English dictionary, medical dictionary, and pen or pencil.

Standards: Time: ________________ minutes

Accuracy: ________________

(Note: The time element and accuracy criteria may be given by your instructor.)

Scenario: After retyping and resubmitting Mary T. Avery's insurance claim in Assignment 16.7 (see Fig. 16.6), the insurance company sends an EOB/RA (health insurance claim number 123098) with a check in the amount of $300 to the College Clinic for payment of the claim. Dr. Cutler wishes an appeal to be made for an increase of the payment of an additional $100. (Note: This patient's marital status is single, and the insured's identification number is T45098.)

Directions: Use the retyped claim to Assignment 16.7 for Mary T. Avery. Follow these basic step-by-step procedures.

1. Compose, format, key, proofread, and print a letter.
2. Include the beneficiary's name, health insurance claim number, dates of service in question, and items or services in question with name, address, and signature of the provider.
3. Compose a letter with an introduction that stresses the medical practice's qualifications, the physician's commitment to complying with regulations and providing appropriate services, and the importance of the practice to the payer's panel of physicians or specialists.
4. Provide a detailed account of the necessity of the treatment given and its relationship to the patient's problems and chief complaint. You might cross-reference the medical record and emphasize parts of it that the reviewer may have missed.
5. Explain the reason why the provider does not agree with the payment. Use a blank sheet, labeling it "Explanation of Benefits," because you do not have this printed document to attach.
6. Abstract excerpts from the coding resource book if necessary.
7. Direct the correspondence to Mr. Donald Pearson, a claims adjuster at the American Insurance Company, 509 Main Street, Woodland Hills, XY 12345.
8. Address an envelope for the letter.
9. Retain copies of all data sent for the physician's files.

17 Collection Strategies

Linda M. Smith

KEY TERMS

Your instructor may wish to select some words pertinent to this chapter for a test. For definitions of the terms, further study, and/or reference, the words, phrases, and abbreviations may be found in the glossary at the end of the textbook. *Key terms for this chapter follow.*

accounts receivable
age analysis
automatic stay
balance
bankruptcy
bonding
cash flow
collateral
collection ratio
credit
credit card
creditor
cycle billing
debit card
debt
debtor
discount
dun messages
embezzlement
estate administrator
estate executor
fee schedule
financial accounting record
garnishment
itemized statement
lien
netback
no charge
nonexempt assets
professional courtesy
secured debt
skip
statute of limitations
unsecured debt
write-off

KEY ABBREVIATIONS

See how many abbreviations and acronyms you can translate and then use this as a handy reference list. Definitions for the key abbreviations are located near the back of the textbook *in the glossary.*

A/R ______________________

ATM ______________________

e-check ______________________

ERISA ______________________

FACT ______________________

FCBA ______________________

FCRA ______________________

FDCPA ______________________

FEHBA ______________________

FTC ______________________

N/A ______________________

NC ______________________

NSF ______________________

TILA ______________________

W2 ______________________

PERFORMANCE OBJECTIVES

The student will be able to:

- Define and spell the key terms and key abbreviations for this chapter, given the information from the *textbook* glossary, within a reasonable time period and with enough accuracy to obtain a satisfactory evaluation.
- After reading the chapter, answer the fill-in-the-blank, mix and match, multiple choice, and true/false review questions with enough accuracy to obtain a satisfactory evaluation.
- Select an appropriate dun message for a patient's bill, given a patient's ledger/statement, within a reasonable time period and with enough accuracy to obtain a satisfactory evaluation.
- Post a courtesy adjustment, given a patient's ledger/statement, within a reasonable time period and with enough accuracy to obtain a satisfactory evaluation.
- Post a patient's charges and payment to the patient's financial accounting record, within a reasonable time period and with enough accuracy to obtain a satisfactory evaluation.
- Compose a collection letter for a delinquent account, given letterhead stationery, within a reasonable time period and with enough accuracy to obtain a satisfactory evaluation.
- Complete a financial agreement, given a patient's ledger/statement, within a reasonable time period and with enough accuracy to obtain a satisfactory evaluation.

STUDY OUTLINE

Collection Strategies
Accounts Receivable
Patient Education
- Patient Registration Form

Fees
- Fee Schedule
- Missed Appointments
- Fee Adjustments
- Discussing Fees
- Collecting Fees

Credit and Collection Laws
- Statute of Limitations

The Collection Process
- Telephone Collection Procedures
- Collection Letters
- Insurance Collection
- Collection Agencies
- Small Claims Court
- Tracing a Skip
- Special Collection Issues

ASSIGNMENT 17.1 REVIEW QUESTIONS

Part I Fill in the Blank

Review the objectives, key terms, chapter information, glossary definitions of key terms, and figures before completing the following review questions.

1. Third-party payers who generate a large percentage of reimbursement to health care organizations are composed of

   a. ____________________

   b. ____________________

   c. ____________________

   d. ____________________.

2. The unpaid balance due from patients for professional services rendered is known as a/an

   ____________________.

3. An important document that provides demographic and identifying data for each patient and assists in billing and collection is called a/an

   ____________________.

4. A term preferable to "write-off" when used in a medical practice is ____________________.

5. To verify a check, ask the patient for a/an ____________________

   and ____________________.

6. The procedure of systematically arranging the accounts receivable, by age, from the date of service is called ____________________.

7. Write the formula for calculating the office accounts receivable (A/R) ratio.

   ____

   ____

   ____

8. What is the collection rate if a total of $40,300 was collected for the month and the total of the accounts receivable is $50,670? ____________________

9. Patient accounts that are open to charges made from time to time are referred to as

   ____

10. A court order attaching a debtor's property or wages to pay off a debt is known as

    ____________________.

11. An individual who owes on an account and moves, leaving no forwarding address, is called a/an ____________________.

12. Translate these credit and collection abbreviations.

NSF ______________________ T ______________________

WCO ______________________ SK ______________________

PIF ______________________ FN ______________________

NLE ______________________ UE ______________________

13. A straight petition in bankruptcy or absolute bankruptcy is also known as a/an ______________________.

14. A wage earner's bankruptcy is sometimes referred to as a/an ______________________.

15. State three bonding methods.

a. ______________________

b. ______________________

c. ______________________

16. A system of billing accounts at spaced intervals during the month on the basis of a breakdown of accounts by alphabet, account number, insurance type, or date of service is known as ______________________.

Part II Mix and Match

17. Match the credit and collection terms in the right column with the descriptions, and fill in the blank with the appropriate letter.

_______ Reductions of the normal fee based on a specific amount of money or a percentage of the charge

_______ Phrase to remind a patient about a delinquent account

_______ Item that permits bank customers to withdraw cash at any hour from an automated teller machine

_______ Individual owing money

_______ Claim on the property of another as security for a debt

_______ Individual record indicating charges, payments, adjustments, and balances owed for services rendered

_______ Detailed summary of all transactions of a creditor's account

_______ Person to whom money is owed

_______ Listing of accepted charges or established allowances for specific medical procedures

a. debtor

b. itemized statement

c. fee schedule

d. discounts

e. financial account record (ledger)

f. creditor

g. dun message

h. debit card

i. lien

18. Match the following federal acts with their descriptions, and fill in the blank with the appropriate letter.

_______ Law stating that a person has 60 days to complain about an error from the date that a statement is mailed	a. Equal Credit Opportunity Act
_______ Consumer protection act that applies to anyone who charges interest or agrees on payment of a bill in more than four installments, excluding a down payment	b. Fair Credit Reporting Act
_______ Regulates collection practices of third-party debt collectors and attorneys who collect debts for others	c. Fair Credit Billing Act
_______ Federal law prohibiting discrimination in all areas of granting credit	d. Truth in Lending Act
_______ Regulates agencies that issue or use credit reports on consumers	e. Fair Debt Collection Practices Act

Part III Multiple Choice

Choose the best answer.

19. Signing another person's name on a check to obtain money or pay off a debt without permission is called:
    a. embezzlement.
    b. stealing.
    c. garnishing.
    d. forgery.

20. When sending monthly statements to patients for balances due, the postal service can forward mail if the addressed envelopes contain the statement:
    a. "Please Forward."
    b. "Forwarding Service Requested."
    c. "Forwarding and Return Receipt Requested."
    d. "Send Forward."

21. When accepting a credit card as payment on an account, the proper guideline(s) to follow is/are to:
    a. ask for photo identification.
    b. accept a card only from the person whose name is on the card.
    c. get approval from the credit card company.
    d. all of the above.

22. A service offered by a nonprofit agency assisting people in paying off their debts is known as:
    a. credit counseling.
    b. debt solutions.
    c. grant-in-aid under the Hill-Burton Act.
    d. small claims court.

23. Insurance payment checks should be stamped in the endorsement area on the back "For Deposit Only," which is called a/an:
    a. conditional endorsement.
    b. qualified endorsement.
    c. special endorsement.
    d. restrictive endorsement.

Part IV True/False

Write "T" or "F" in the blank to indicate whether you think the statement is true or false.

_______ 24. Insurance companies and the federal government do not recommend waiving copayments to patients.

_______ 25. Regulation Z of the Truth in Lending Consumer Credit Cost Disclosure law applies if the patient is making three payments.

_______ 26. Most state collection laws allow telephone calls to the debtor between 8 AM and 9 PM.

_______ 27. When a patient has declared bankruptcy, it is permissible to continue to send monthly statements for a balance due.

_______ 28. A collection agency must follow all the laws stated in the Fair Debt Collection Practices Act.

ASSIGNMENT 17.2 SELECT A DUN MESSAGE

Performance Objective

Task: Select an appropriate dun message and insert it on a patient's financial accounting record (ledger card).

Conditions: Use the patient's financial accounting record (Fig. 17.1), computer, and a printer.

Standards: Time: ________________ minutes

Accuracy:________________

(Note: The time element and accuracy criteria may be given by your instructor.)

Background: Most patient account activities are recorded in the medical billing software. However, to develop the skills and understanding for payment posting, a paper financial accounting statement has been provided.

Directions: Read the scenario and refer to the patient's financial accounting record (see Fig. 17.1). Select appropriate dun messages for each month the patient has been billed. You may wish to refer to Fig. 17.5 in the textbook.

Scenario: Carrie Jones was on vacation in June and July and did not pay on her account. It is August (current year).

June 1, 20XX, dun message ____

July 1, 20XX, dun message ____

August 1, 20XX, dun message ____

After the instructor has returned your work to you, either make the necessary corrections and place your work in a three-ring notebook for future reference or, if you received a high score, place it in your portfolio for reference when applying for a job.

Acct No. 10-2

STATEMENT
Financial Account
COLLEGE CLINIC
4567 Broad Avenue
Woodland Hills, XY 12345-0001
Tel. 555-486-9002
Fax No. 555-487-8976

Carrie Jones
15543 Dean Street
Woodland Hills, XY 12345

Phone No. (H) (555) 439-8800 (W) (555) 550-8706 Birth date 05-14-72

Primary Insurance Co. Prudential Insurance Company Policy/Group No. 450998

	REFERENCE	DESCRIPTION	CHARGES		CREDITS PYMNTS.		CREDITS ADJ.		BALANCE	
								BALANCE FORWARD →	20	00
4-16–xx	99215	C hx/exam HC DM DX 582							154	99
4-17–xx		Prudential billed (4-16-xx)							154	99
5-27–xx		Rec'd insurance ck #435			30	00			124	99
6-1-xx		Billed pt							124	99
7-1-xx		Billed pt							124	99
8-1-xx		Billed pt							124	99

PLEASE PAY LAST AMOUNT IN BALANCE COLUMN

THIS IS A COPY OF YOUR FINANCIAL ACCOUNT AS IT APPEARS ON OUR RECORDS

Fig. 17.1

ASSIGNMENT 17.3 MANUALLY POST A COURTESY ADJUSTMENT

Performance Objective

Task: Post a courtesy adjustment to a patient's financial accounting record (ledger card).

Conditions: Use the patient's financial accounting record (Fig. 17.2) and a pen.

Standards: Time: ________________ minutes

Accuracy: ________________

(Note: The time element and accuracy criteria may be given by your instructor.)

Background: Most patient account activities are recorded in the medical billing software. However, to develop the skills and understanding for payment posting, a paper financial accounting statement has been provided.

Directions: Read the case scenario and refer to the patient's financial accounting record (see Fig. 17.2). You may wish to refer to Fig. 17.5 in the textbook. Post a courtesy adjustment to her financial accounting record.

Scenario: Maria Smith recently lost her job and is raising two children as a single parent. It is September 1 (current year). A discussion with Dr. Gerald Practon leads to a decision to write off the balance of the current charges on the account but not the balance forward.

After the instructor has returned your work to you, either make the necessary corrections and place your work in a three-ring notebook for future reference or, if you received a high score, place it in your portfolio for reference when applying for a job.

Acct No. 10-3

STATEMENT
Financial Account

COLLEGE CLINIC
4567 Broad Avenue
Woodland Hills, XY 12345-0001
Tel. 555-486-9002
Fax No. 555-487-8976

Ms. Maria Smith
3737 Unser Road
Woodland Hills, XY 12345

Phone No. (H) (555) 430-8877 (W) (555) 908-1233 Birth date 06-11-80

Primary Insurance Co. Metropolitan Insurance Company Policy/Group No. 4320870

	REFERENCE	DESCRIPTION	CHARGES		CREDITS PYMNTS.		CREDITS ADJ.		BALANCE	
		BALANCE FORWARD →							20	00
5-19-xx	99214	OV DX 582	61	51					81	51
5-20-xx		Metropolitan billed (5-19-xx)							81	51
6-20-xx		Rec'd ins ck #6778			25	00			56	51
7-1-xx		Pt billed							56	51
8-1-xx		Pt billed							56	51

PLEASE PAY LAST AMOUNT IN BALANCE COLUMN

THIS IS A COPY OF YOUR FINANCIAL ACCOUNT AS IT APPEARS ON OUR RECORDS

Fig. 17.2

ASSIGNMENT 17.4 MANUALLY POST A PATIENT'S CHARGES AND PAYMENT

Performance Objective

Task: Post a payment to a patient's financial accounting record (ledger card).

Conditions: Use the patient's financial accounting record (Fig. 17.3), and a pen.

Standards: Time: ________________ minutes

Accuracy: ________________

(Note: The time element and accuracy criteria may be given by your instructor.)

Background: Most patient account activities are recorded in the medical billing software. However, to develop the skills and understanding for payment posting, a paper financial accounting statement has been provided.

Directions: Read the case scenario; refer to the patient's financial accounting record (see Fig. 17.3). You may wish to refer to Fig. 17.5 in the textbook. Post the charges for the services rendered and payment to the patient's financial accounting record.

Scenario:
Date of service: October 12 (current year)
Patient: Kenneth Brown; 8896 Aster Drive; Woodland Hills, XY, 12345
Patient Phone: 555-760-5211 (home) 555-987-3855 (work)
Date of birth: 1/15/82
Insurance: None
Service Provided: EKG (CPT 93000) fee = $34.26
Service Provided: New patient visit level III (CPT 99203) fee = $70.92
Patient paid by personal check: $50.00 (check #3421)

After the instructor has returned your work to you, either make the necessary corrections and place your work in a three-ring notebook for future reference or, if you received a high score, place it in your portfolio for reference when applying for a job.

Acct No. 10-4

STATEMENT

Financial Account
COLLEGE CLINIC
4567 Broad Avenue
Woodland Hills, XY 12345-0001
Tel. 555-486-9002
Fax No. 555-487-8976

Mr. Kenneth Brown
8896 Aster Drive
Woodland Hills, XY 12345

Phone No. (H) (555) 760-5211 (W) (555) 987-3355 Birth date 01-15-82

Primary Insurance Co. none Policy/Group No.

	REFERENCE	DESCRIPTION	CHARGES	CREDITS PYMNTS.	CREDITS ADJ.	BALANCE
			BALANCE FORWARD →			

PLEASE PAY LAST AMOUNT IN BALANCE COLUMN

THIS IS A COPY OF YOUR FINANCIAL ACCOUNT AS IT APPEARS ON OUR RECORDS

Fig. 17.3

ASSIGNMENT 17.5 COMPOSE A COLLECTION LETTER

Performance Objective

Task: Compose a letter for the physician's signature and post the entry on the patient's financial accounting record (ledger card).

Conditions: Use the patient's financial accounting record (Fig. 17.4), one sheet of letterhead paper (Fig. 17.5), a number 10 envelope, English dictionary, thesaurus, medical dictionary, computer, printer, and pen.

Standards: Time: _______________ minutes

Accuracy: _______________

(Note: The time element and accuracy criteria may be given by your instructor.)

Background: Most patient account activities are recorded in the medical billing software. However, to develop the skills and understanding for payment posting, a paper financial accounting statement has been provided.

Directions: Read the case scenario, refer to the patient's financial accounting record (see Fig. 17.4), and compose a collection letter, using your signature and requesting payment. Print on letterhead stationery in full block format (paragraphs to left margin). Include a paragraph stating that a copy of the delinquent statement is enclosed. You may wish to refer to Fig. 17.16 in the textbook. Post an entry on the patient's financial accounting record.

Scenario: It is December 1 (current year), and you have sent Mr. Ron Kelsey two statements with no response. You have tried to reach him by telephone without success and have decided to send him a collection letter (see Fig. 17.5).

After the instructor has returned your work to you, either make the necessary corrections and place your work in a three-ring notebook for future reference or, if you received a high score, place it in your portfolio for reference when applying for a job.

Acct No. 10-5

STATEMENT
Financial Account

COLLEGE CLINIC
4567 Broad Avenue
Woodland Hills, XY 12345-0001
Tel. 555-486-9002
Fax No. 555-487-8976

Mr. Ron Kelsey
6321 Ocean Street
Woodland Hills, XY 12345

Phone No. (H) (555) 540-9800 (W) (555) 890-7766 Birth date 03-25-75

Primary Insurance Co. XYZ Insurance Company Policy/Group No. 8503Y

	REFERENCE	DESCRIPTION	CHARGES		CREDITS PYMNTS.		CREDITS ADJ.		BALANCE	
		BALANCE FORWARD →								
07-09-xx	99283	ER new pt EPF hx/exam MC DM	66	23					66	23
07-10-xx		XYZ Insurance billed (3-9-xx)							66	23
09-20-xx		EOB rec'd pt has not met deductible							66	23
10-01-xx		Billed pt							66	23
11-01-xx		Billed pt							66	23

PLEASE PAY LAST AMOUNT IN BALANCE COLUMN

THIS IS A COPY OF YOUR FINANCIAL ACCOUNT AS IT APPEARS ON OUR RECORDS

Fig. 17.4

COLLEGE CLINIC
4567 Broad Avenue
Woodland Hills, XY 12345-0001
Tel. (555) 486-9002
FAX (555) 487-8976

Fig. 17.5

ASSIGNMENT 17.6 ACCEPTING CREDIT CARD PAYMENTS

Performance Objective

Task: Accept a credit card payment through various tools and post the credit entry on the patient's ledger.

Conditions: Use a credit card terminal, credit card reader attachment, or secured online web portal for credit card payments and credit card receipts, and pen or pencil.

Standards: Time: ________________ minutes

Accuracy: ________________

(Note: The time element and accuracy criteria may be given by your instructor.)

Background: The medical office has many different tools to accept credit card payments, such as:

- *Credit card terminal payment:* These lightweight devices use an internet connection to complete the payment transaction. The terminal can scan the credit card data including the cardholder's name, credit card number, and expiration date, through a swipe. The terminal also can process credit card transactions in which the user manually enters credit card information; in this scenario, the transaction requires the credit card number, the expiration date, the card security code (CVV), and the patient's billing ZIP code. Both transactions, the swipe method and the manual method, cause the terminal to typically print out two receipts per transaction, one for the medical office and one for the patient. If the credit card is swiped, the patient signs the medical office receipt because it states their name in the transaction. When manually entering the credit card data, the receipt will not print the patient's name, so the medical assistant must document the patient name, date of service, and/or medical record number on the receipt. Renting a credit card terminal can be costly, so smaller medical offices prefer to use other credit card accepting options.
- *Credit card reader payment:* A smaller medical office might choose a pay-for-use credit card that accepts software packages. The package includes a tablet or smartphone attachment device for scanning credit cards and a downloadable application (Fig. 17.11 in the textbook). The application is user friendly and is able to send the patient a receipt via email or by text message. There is a minimal fee per transaction ($0.25 to $0.30) and a percent charged based on the total amount.
- *Online credit card payment:* Some medical offices use an online merchant service to accept patient credit card payments. Through a secure web portal, patients can view their medical bills online and make payments by credit card or through a service such as PayPal. The transaction receipt is emailed to the patient and to the medical office. When the medical assistant receives the transaction via email, he or she updates the patient's account to reflect the current balance. There is a per transaction cost for this service similar to other credit card acceptance applications.

Directions: Read each case scenario, review the accompanying figures, and answer the following questions:

A. Kevin Long is attending the College Clinic on May 26 (current year) for an office visit and needs to pay for his $30 copay. He presents a credit card for payment (Fig. 17.6A).

1. What should the medical assistant do to verify Kevin Long's identity before accepting the credit card for payment?

____

2. Which tool can be used to accept Kevin Long's payment?

____

3. Will the credit card receipt have Kevin's name printed? Why or why not?

____

4. Does the medical office credit card receipt require the patient's signature? Why or why not?

____

5. Was the expiration date or CVV needed for this transaction? Why or why not?

____

B. It is November 6 (current year), and you receive a phone call at the College Clinic. It is Kevin Long, who has an unpaid balance of $24.32, and it is up to you to discuss this delinquency with Mr. Long and come to an agreement on how the account can be paid. After discussion, Mr. Long decides to pay the total balance due by credit card, giving you his authorization (Fig. 17.6B).

1. Which tool can be used to accept Kevin Long's payment?

___

2. Will the credit card receipts have Kevin's name printed? Why or why not?

___

3. What must a medical assistant do to the receipt if the patient's name is not printed?

___

4. Was the CVV needed for this transaction?

___

5. How can a credit card receipt be sent to the patient?

___

C. Kevin Long received a statement from the College Clinic for an outstanding balance of $63.52 from a date of service December 12 (current year). He notices that the clinic allows him to log in to pay online. He visits the medical office's website and clicks the "Pay Your Bill" feature. The secure online web portal asks Kevin to complete a form requests his name, billing address, an email address, the credit card number, expiration date, and CVV (Fig. 17.6C). Prior to submitting the online form, Kevin notices the following statement: "By clicking this box, the user agrees to the terms of this transaction." Kevin checks the box and clicks submit to send his credit card payment electronically. A receipt for the transaction is emailed to Kevin.

1. Which tool can be used to accept Kevin Long's payment?

___

2. Will the credit card receipt have Kevin's name printed? Why or why not?

___

3. Was the CVV needed for this transaction?

___

4. How is the credit card receipt sent to the patient?

___

5. What should the medical assistant do with the transaction email received?

___

After the instructor has returned your work to you, either make the necessary corrections and place your work in a three-ring notebook for future reference or, if you received a high score, place it in your portfolio for reference when applying for a job.

COLLEGE CLINIC
4567 Broad Avenue
Woodland Hills, XY 12345-0001

05/26/20XX	**09:39:14**
Merchant ID:	**00000000262026XX**
Terminal ID:	**038802XX**
0150302859XX	

CREDIT CARD

MC SALE

Name	**Kevin Long**
CARD#	**XXXXXXXXXX4021**
INVOICE	**009**
Batch #:	**00716**
Approval Code:	**4123P**
Entry Method:	**Swiped**
SALE AMOUNT	**$30.00**

Kevin Long

Customer Signature

MERCHANT COPY

Fig. 17.6

Continued

COLLEGE CLINIC
4567 Broad Avenue
Woodland Hills, XY 12345-0001

11/6 /20XX	09:39:14
Merchant ID:	00000000262026XX
Terminal ID:	038802XX
0150302859XX	

CREDIT CARD

MC SALE

CARD#	XXXXXXXXXX4021
INVOICE	009
Batch#:	00716
Approval Code:	4123P
Entry Method:	Manual Entry
Mode:	Online
SALE AMOUNT	$24.32

Approved by patient over the phone.

____

Customer Signature

MERCHANT COPY

11/6/20XX: Spoke with Kevin Long (MR 354689); he agreed to pay balance in full with a credit card over the phone. Payment for date of service 7/3/20XX. Balance paid in full.

Fig. 17.6, cont'd

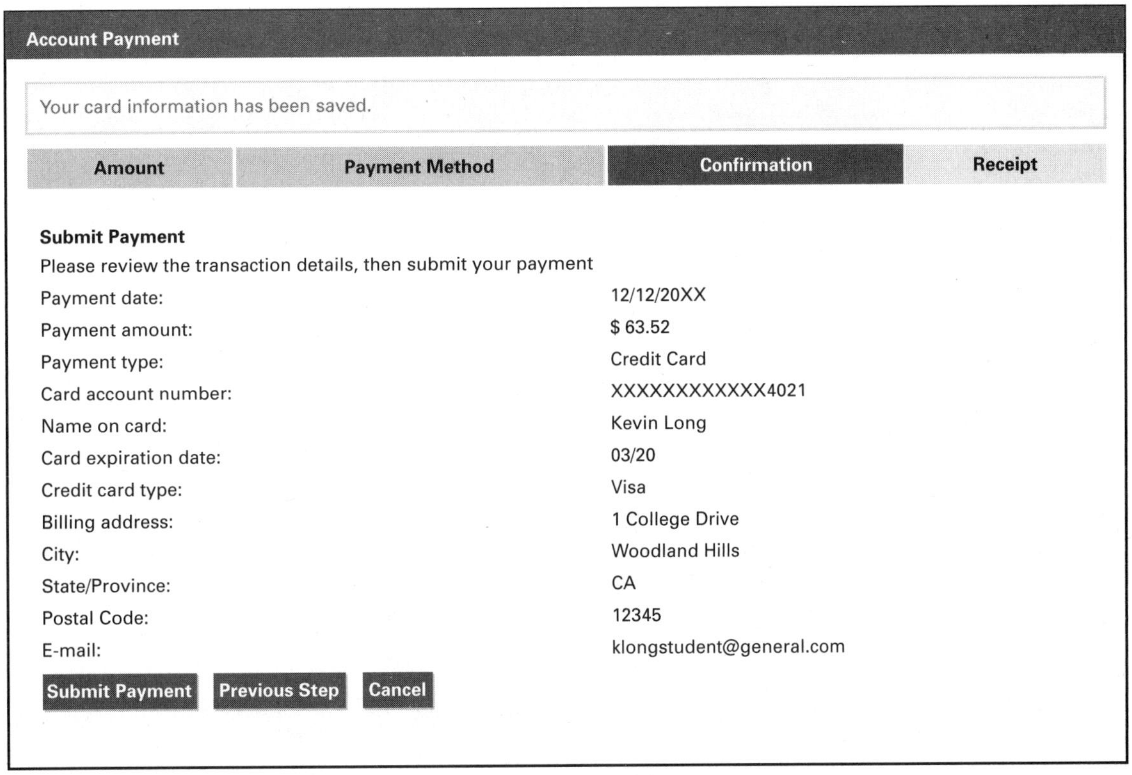

Account Payment

Your card information has been saved.

Amount	Payment Method	Confirmation	Receipt

Submit Payment

Please review the transaction details, then submit your payment

Payment date:	12/12/20XX
Payment amount:	$ 63.52
Payment type:	Credit Card
Card account number:	XXXXXXXXXXXX4021
Name on card:	Kevin Long
Card expiration date:	03/20
Credit card type:	Visa
Billing address:	1 College Drive
City:	Woodland Hills
State/Province:	CA
Postal Code:	12345
E-mail:	klongstudent@general.com

Submit Payment | Previous Step | Cancel

Fig. 17.6, cont'd

Acct No. 10-6

STATEMENT
Financial Account
COLLEGE CLINIC
4567 Broad Avenue
Woodland Hills, XY 12345-0001
Tel. 555-486-9002
Fax No. 555-487-8976

Mr. Kevin O. Long
2443 Davis Street
Woodland Hills, XY 12345

Phone No. (H) (555) 244-5600 (W) (555) 970-4466 Birth date 08-15-76

Primary Insurance Co. Blue Cross Policy/Group No. 130-XX-0987

	REFERENCE	DESCRIPTION	CHARGES		CREDITS PYMNTS.		ADJ.		BALANCE	
		BALANCE FORWARD →								
09-08-xx	99205	OV Level V DX 582	132	28					132	28
09-09-xx		Blue Cross billed (9-8-xx)							132	28
10-12-xx		BC EOB rec'd pt has not met deductible							132	28
10-23-xx		Not covered by insurance. Balance due							132	28

PLEASE PAY LAST AMOUNT IN BALANCE COLUMN

THIS IS A COPY OF YOUR FINANCIAL ACCOUNT AS IT APPEARS ON OUR RECORDS

Fig. 17.7

ASSIGNMENT 17.7 COMPLETE A FINANCIAL AGREEMENT

Performance Objective

Task: Complete a financial agreement and post an entry on the patient's ledger.

Conditions: Patient's ledger card is Fig. 17.8 and the financial agreement form is Fig. 17.9.

Standards: Time: ______________ minutes

________ Accuracy: ______________

(Note: The time element and accuracy criteria may be given by your instructor.)

Background: Most patient account activities are recorded in the medical billing software. However, to develop the skills and understanding for payment posting, a paper financial accounting statement has been provided.

Directions: Read the case scenario. Complete a financial agreement (see Fig. 17.9 by subtracting the down payment from the total debt. Refer to the patient's ledger/statement (see Fig. 17.8) and post an appropriate entry to the ledger/statement using a pen. Review the completed financial agreement with the patient (role played by another student). Ask the patient to sign the financial agreement.

Scenario: Mr. Joseph Small has a large balance due. Create a payment plan for this case. You have discussed the installment plan concerning the amount of the total debt, the down payment, amount and date of each installment, and the date of final payment. On June 1 (current year), Mr. Small is paying $500 cash as a down payment, and the balance is to be divided into five equal payments, due on the first of each month. There will be no monthly finance charge. Mr. Small's daytime telephone number is 555-760-5502. He is a patient of Dr. Brady Coccidioides.

After the instructor has returned your work to you, either make the necessary corrections and place your work in a three-ring notebook for future reference or, if you received a high score, place it in your portfolio for reference when applying for a job.

Acct No. 10-7

STATEMENT
Financial Account
COLLEGE CLINIC
4567 Broad Avenue
Woodland Hills, XY 12345-0001
Tel. 555-486-9002
Fax No. 555-487-8976

Mr. Joseph Small
655 Sherry Street
Woodland Hills, XY 12345

Phone No. (H) (555) 320-8801 (W) (555) 760-5502 Birth date 11-04-77

Primary Insurance Co. Blue Shield Policy/Group No. 870-XX-4398

	REFERENCE	DESCRIPTION	CHARGES		CREDITS PYMNTS.		CREDITS ADJ.		BALANCE	
		BALANCE FORWARD →							20	00
04-19-xx	99215	OV Level	96	97					116	97
04-30-xx	99218	Adm hosp	74	22					191	19
04-30-xx	32440	Pneumonectomy, total	1972	10					2163	29
05-20-xx		Blue Shield billed (1-19 to 30-xx)							2163	29
05-15-xx		BS EOB Pt deductible $2000 rec'd ck #544			163	29			2000	00

PLEASE PAY LAST AMOUNT IN BALANCE COLUMN

THIS IS A COPY OF YOUR FINANCIAL ACCOUNT AS IT APPEARS ON OUR RECORDS

Fig. 17.8

College Clinic
4567 Broad Avenue
Woodland Hills, XY 12345-0001
Phone: 555/486-9002
Fax: 555/487-8976

FINANCIAL PAYMENT PLAN AGREEMENT

For medical professional services rendered to:

Patient Name____________________________ Account No.__________________

Responsible Party____

Address____

____

Telephones: Home____
Mobile ____
Business____

1. Cash price of total medical treatment $____________
2. Down payment (partial payment) $____________
3. Amount covered by insurance plan $____________
4. Unpaid balance due $____________
5. **ANNUAL PERCENTAGE RATE** (interest rate) ____________%
6. **FINANCE CHARGE** ($ amt of cost to patient) $____________
7. Total amount of unpaid balance due ____________
8. Monthly payment amount $____________

TERMS:

1. ALL PAYMENTS ARE DUE ON OR BEFORE YOUR DUE DATE EACH MONTH.
2. The patient agrees to be fully responsible for the total payment of medical services performed in this office including any amounts not covered by any health insurance plan.
3. The patient has the right at any time to pay the unpaid balance due without penalty.
4. First payment due ___/___/___ and subsequent payments on the same day of each consecutive month until paid in full.

____
Signature of Patient/Responsible Party Date

____
Physician's signature or Authorized representative Date

Fig. 17.9

18 Ambulatory Surgery Centers

Rachael D'Andrea

KEY TERMS

Your instructor may wish to select some words pertinent to this chapter for a test. For definitions of the terms, further study, and/or reference, the words, phrases, and abbreviations may be found in the glossary at the end of the Textbook. *Key terms for this chapter follow.*

Accreditation Association for Ambulatory Health Care (AAAHC)
Ambulatory Payment Classification (APC) System
Ambulatory Surgery Center (ASC)
Ambulatory Surgical Unit (ASU)
Ambulatory Quality Reporting (ASCQR)
clearinghouse
CMS-1500
Current Procedural Terminology (CPT)
conversion factor (CF)
discounted fee-for-service
discounting
first listed diagnosis
geographic practice cost index (GPCI)
Health care Common Procedure Coding System (HCPCS)
International Classification of Diseases, Tenth Revision, Clinical Modification (ICD-10-CM)
local coverage determinations (LCDs)
medical necessity
Medicare Physician Provider Fee Schedule (MPFS)
modifiers
National Coverage Determinations (NCDs)
National Correct Coding Initiative (NCCI)
National Uniform Billing Committee (NUBC)
national unadjusted payment
Outpatient Prospective Payment System (OPPS)
packaged pass throughs
preadmission
preauthorization
Prospective Payment System (PPS)
Relative Value Unit (RVU)
Resource-Based Relative Value Scale (RBRVS)
revenue code
revenue cycle
Revenue Cycle Management (RCM)
status (payment) indicator
Uniform Bill 04 (UB-04)

KEY ABBREVIATIONS

AMA ______________________

APC ______________________

ASC ______________________

ASCQR ______________________

ASU ______________________

CF ______________________

CMS ______________________

CPT ______________________

ECS ______________________

EMR ______________________

GCPI ______________________

HCPCS ______________________

LCDs ______________________

MPFS ______________________

NCDs ______________________

NCCI ______________________

OPPS ______________________

PPS ______________________

RBRVS ______________________

RCM ______________________

RVU ______________________

UB-04 ______________________

PERFORMANCE OBJECTIVES

The student will be able to:

- Define and spell the key terms and key abbreviations for this chapter, given the information from the textbook glossary, within a reasonable time period and with enough accuracy to obtain a satisfactory evaluation.
- After reading the chapter, answer the multiple choice and essay questions with enough accuracy to obtain a satisfactory evaluation.

ASSIGNMENT 18.1 REVIEW QUESTIONS

Part I Multiple Choice

Choose the best answer.

1. Linking refers to which of the following?
   a. Pairing professional charges to technical charges on the claim.
   b. Substituting a HCPCS code for the appropriate CPT code
   c. Assigning a diagnosis code to a CPT code on the claim
   d. Appending modifiers to CPT/HCPCS codes

2. The function of a clearinghouse is to:
   a. transfer electronic claims to specific insurers in a secure way.
   b. confirm that the data entry is correct.
   c. manage the claims appeal process.
   d. enter and validate charges on the claims.

3. Which reimbursement methodology uses work, practice cost and malpractice cost as its variables?
   a. Capitation
   b. Standard charges
   c. Resource-Based Relative Value System
   d. Fee-for-service

4. When multiple surgical procedures are listed on the CMS-1500 claim form, the fees are listed as:
   a. a percentage of the full fee.
   b. discounted charges.
   c. sequenced by the surgeon.
   d. in numerical order.

5. The component of the RBRVS that depicts the health care professional's labor value is the:
   a. conversion factor.
   b. practice expense relative value unit.
   c. work relative value unit.
   d. work GPCI.

6. Medicare global periods define:
   a. the postoperative period for procedures.
   b. bundling.
   c. diagnosis distribution.
   d. CPT and HCPCS services.

7. Components of the Medicare global period include:
   a. preoperative visits after the decision is made to operate.
   b. intraoperative services that are part of the surgical procedure.
   c. additional surgical services required of the surgeon during the postoperative period of surgery.
   d. all of the above.

8. Level II modifiers, or HCPCS modifiers, consist of two alpha or alphanumeric characters in the sequence:
   a. –21 through –59.
   b. –01 through –99.
   c. AA through VP.
   d. A1 through XX.

9. What should be entered in field 24e of the CMS-1500 claim form to properly link the diagnosis to the service?
   a. The CPT code
   b. The ICD-10-CM code
   c. The place of service
   d. One linking reference letter from box 21

10. The fee schedule database is used to:
    a. identify the amount of revenue from each CPT code.
    b. record the transfer of claims.
    c. provide a list of all of the services performed.
    d. maintain charge information about CPT/HCPCS codes.

11. Which of the following data elements are required to calculate the Medicare approved amount? Check all that apply.
    a. RVU total value
    b. GPCI values
    c. RVU component values
    d. Conversion factor

12. The type of payment used by insurance carriers to control costs that are considered risky for the health care professional is:
    a. reimbursement.
    b. coinsurance.
    c. fee-for-service.
    d. capitation.

13. The ____________________ is the process of patient health and financial information moving into, through and out of the Ambulatory Surgery Center.
    a. revenue stream
    b. revenue cycle
    c. audit procedure
    d. managed care method

14. The term that is used to describe an insurance company that pays for the health care of the covered individual is:
    a. first party payer.
    b. second party payer.
    c. third party payer.
    d. beneficiary.

15. The specified amount of money paid to the ASC or physician, which covers the cost of the health plan member's health care services for a specific length of time is:
    a. global payment.
    b. capitation.
    c. fee-for-service.
    d. self-pay.

16. The prospective review which involves the obtaining of approval from a health insurance company prior to the health care service being rendered is the:
    a. post review audit.
    b. medical evaluation.
    c. preauthorization.
    d. precertification.

17. The payment methodology that combines the professional and technical components of a procedure is:
    a. global payment.
    b. prospective payment.
    c. retrospective payment.
    d. managed care reimbursement.

18. The verification that the patient is currently covered by the insurance plan on the date of service for the procedure is:
    a. medical necessity.
    b. medical evaluation.
    c. eligibility.
    d. predetermined rate setting.

19. The professional component of a service is the part of the service provided by:
    a. the ACS.
    b. the surgeon or physician.
    c. the hospital.
    d. none of the above.

20. The technical component of a service is the part of the service provided by (Check all that apply):
    a. the ACS.
    b. the surgeon or physician.
    c. the hospital.
    d. none of the above.

21. The ______________________ gained approval from CMS in 2018 to accredit ASCs.
    a. JCAHO
    b. AAAHC
    c. Medicare Advisory Committee
    d. AMA

22. When a hospital-based surgery center is not certified as an ASC, the _________ reimbursement rules apply.
    a. third party payer
    b. beneficiary
    c. HOPPS
    d. organization-specific

23. Which law was enacted by Congress to establish the outpatient use of the HCPCS code set?
    a. OBRA
    b. PPS
    c. HIPAA
    d. ACA

24. The HCPCS Level II codes are maintained by:
    a. AMA.
    b. CMS.
    c. Medicaid.
    d. AHIMA.

25. Medicare payment for ambulatory surgical center (ASC) services is based on rates set under:
    a. Part A.
    b. Part B.
    c. Part A and Part B.
    d. State authority.

Part II True/False

Write "T" or "F" in the blank to indicate whether you think the statement is true or false.

_______ 26. Health insurance payers have a variety of reimbursement plans and contracts with individual providers for payment. This means that the same type of service to two different patients may be paid differently depending on the type of contract or insurance that each patient has.

_______ 27. A prospective payment system is a method of reimbursement in which Medicare payment is based on a predetermined fixed amount.

_______ 28. An appeal must be filed within 6 months of a claim determination.

_______ 29. Column 1/Column 2 edits are part of the NCCI.

_______ 30. The electronic version of the CMS-1500 claim form is called the 837E.

_______ 31. A free source of information about the number of global surgical days assigned to a code is the Medicare Fee Schedule Lookup Tool.

_______ 32. The Administrative Simplification Compliance Act (ASCA) requires that claims be sent electronically to Medicare as a condition for payment.

_______ 33. The Place of Service Codes Set is required for use in the implementation guide adopted as the national standard for electronic transmission of professional health care claims under the provisions of the Health Insurance Portability and Accountability Act of 1996 (HIPAA).

_______ 34. CMS will continue to look at ASC payment reform, specifically site neutrality and efficiency of care.

_______ 35. Coverage and subsequent payment of a Medicare service depends on that service being medically necessary and medically reasonable.

_______ 36. According to Medicare, ASCs are permitted to share space with Critical Access Hospital outpatient surgery departments and with Medicare participating Independent Diagnostic Testing Facilities (IDTF).

_______ 37. The Medicare rules state that non-ASC facility services that are separately reimbursable include the physician's professional services; sale, lease, or rental of durable medical equipment for ASC patients to use at home; services performed by an independent laboratory; and hospital-based ambulance services.

_______ 38. Because an ASC bills to Part B of Medicare, the physician NCCI edits are the ones that apply.

_______ 39. The NCCI contains one table of PTP edits for physicians/practitioners and one table of PTP edits for outpatient hospital services.

_______ 40. All payers use the same modifiers.

Part III Essays

41. Discuss how correctly linking diagnoses to procedures on the CMS-1500 form can corroborate the medical necessity for a procedure that has been performed.

42. Describe how to locate the local coverage determination (LCD) for the local Medicare administrative contractor (MAC).

43. Explain the reason for assigning CPT/HCPCS modifiers.

44. If an improper payment has been paid by a third-party payer, what are the steps that should be performed prior to the appeal?

45. Define the two types of ASCs and the main differences between the billing procedures.

46. Explain three reasons for the increase in ASCs since 1970.

47. Medicare and other payers may consider a procedure to be a noncovered service when performed in an ASC for several reasons. List two.

48. For a procedure or service to be considered medically necessary, the following criteria must be met:
    - The procedure or service matches the diagnosis
    - The procedure or service is not experimental or investigational
    - The procedure or service is necessary
    - The procedure or service is provided at the most appropriate level that is safe and effective
    - The procedure or service is not elective.

    Discuss these five criteria.

49. What is the reason for the NCCI?

50. Identify two reasons for the use of the status indicator.

19 Hospital Outpatient and Inpatient Billing

Nanette Sayles

KEY TERMS

Your instructor may wish to select some words pertinent to this chapter for a test. For definitions of the terms, further study, and/or reference, the words, phrases, and abbreviations may be found in the glossary at the end of the Textbook. *Key terms for this chapter follow.*

72-hour rule
admission
admission review
against medical advice
ambulatory payment classifications
capitation
Case Mix Groups
chargemaster
concurrent review
complication
comorbidity
continued stay review
cost outlier
covered entity
diagnosis-related groups
discharge disposition
Discharge Not Final Billed
discounting
discussion
downcoding
DRG creep
gatekeeper
grouper
Health Insurance Portability and Accountability Act
hospital acquired condition
inpatient
Inpatient Prospective Payment System
Inpatient Psychiatric Facility Prospective Payment System
Inpatient Rehabilitation Facility Patient Assessment Instrument
Inpatient Rehabilitation Facility Prospective Payment System
inpatient only
International Classification of Diseases, Tenth Revision, Clinical Modification
International Classification of Diseases, Tenth Revision, Procedure Coding System
Long-Term Acute Care Hospital Prospective Payment System
major complication/comorbidity
major diagnostic categories
Medicare Administrative Contractor
observation
Outpatient Prospective Payment System
per diem
preadmission
preadmission testing
preauthorization
present on admission
principal diagnosis
prospective review
prospective payment system
Quality Improvement Organization
reason for encounter
relative weight
Resource-Based Relative Value Scale
retrospective review
revenue code
revenue cycle
Rehabilitation Impairment Category
self-pay
status indicator
swing bed
Tax Equity and Fiscal Responsibility Act of 1982
transaction set
upcoding
utilization management

KEY ABBREVIATIONS

See how many abbreviations and acronyms you can translate, and then use this as a handy reference list. Definitions for the key abbreviations are located near the back of the Textbook *in the glossary.*

ABN ____________________

AMA ____________________

ANSI ____________________

APC ____________________

ASC ____________________

CC ____________________

CE ____________________

CMG ____________________

CPT ____________________

DNFB ____________________

DRG ____________________

EMTALA ____________________

HAC ____________________

HIPAA ____________________

ICD-10-CM ____________________

ICD-10-PCS ____________________

IPO ____________________

IPF PPS ____________________

IPPS ____________________

IRF PAI ____________________

IRF PPS ____________________

LTCH ____________________

LTCH PPS ____________________

MAC ____________________

MCC ____________________

MDC ____________________

MS-DRG ____________________

OPPS ____________________

PA ____________________

PAT ____________________

POA ____________________

PPS ____________________

QIO ____________________

RBRVS ____________________

RICs ____________________

TEFRA ____________________

UB-04 ____________________

UM ____________________

PERFORMANCE OBJECTIVES

The student will be able to:

- Define and spell the key terms and key abbreviations for this chapter, given the information from the *Textbook* glossary, within a reasonable time period and with enough accuracy to obtain a satisfactory evaluation.
- After reading the chapter, answer the fill-in-the-blank, mix and match, multiple choice, and true/false review questions, with enough accuracy to obtain a satisfactory evaluation.
- Answer questions about the insurance verification process by reviewing a couple of health insurance cards within a reasonable time period and with enough accuracy to obtain a satisfactory evaluation.
- Explain the revenue cycle of hospital claims.
- Manage the Discharge Not Final Billed Report.
- Discuss the 72-hour rule.
- Explain utilization management and its role in the hospital reimbursement system.
- Explain the chargemaster.
- Explain the *International Classification of Diseases,* Tenth Revision, Procedure Coding System (ICD-10-PCS).
- Explain the role of *International Classification of Diseases,* Tenth Revision, Procedure Coding System (ICD-10-PCS) in hospital billing.
- Explain the role of Current Procedural Terminology in hospital billing.
- Explain the role of Health care Coding Procedural Coding System.
- Assign the present on admission indicator.
- Explain the reimbursement methods used when receiving reimbursement for Medicare hospital services.

STUDY OUTLINE

Revenue Cycle
- Preadmission
  - Preauthorization
  - Inpatient Only List
- Patient Care
  - Utilization Management
  - Posting Charges
  - Chargemaster
  - Discharge
- Postadmission
  - Coding
  - Health Care Claim
  - Receipt of Reimbursement
  - Hospital Acquired Conditions
  - Discharge Not Final Billed Report

Types of Reimbursement Methodologies

Medicare
- Medicare Administrative Contractor
- Quality Improvement Organizations
- Medicare Reimbursement Methodologies
- Acute Inpatient Prospective Payment System
- Hospital Outpatient Prospective Payment System
- Resource-Based Relative Value Scale
- Long Term Care Hospital Prospective Payment System
- Inpatient Rehabilitation Facility Prospective Payment System
- Psychiatric Prospective Payment System
- Ambulance Fee Schedule

ASSIGNMENT 19.1 REVIEW QUESTIONS

Part I Fill in the Blank

Review the objectives, key terms, glossary definitions of key terms, chapter information, and figures before completing the following review questions.

1. ________________ is the term used when the second procedure is paid at 50% of the APC rate.

2. In packaging, all of the supplies, medications and other services are ____________ in the APC.

3. ______________________ is coding to a lower level than deserved.

4. ______________ is the reimbursement that Medicare uses for observation services.

5. Additional reimbursement for the MS-DRG for teaching medical residents is known as a/an ____.

6. The diagnosis established after examination and listed for admission to the hospital for an illness or injury is called a/an ___________________________ diagnosis.

7. A ________________________________ is a diagnosis or condition that arises after admission that increases the patient's length of stay 75% of the time.

8. ________________________ are the basis of the IPPS.

9. ________________________ allows the hospital to bill for each service provided.

10. ________________ is important when assigning the present on admission indicator.

PART II MIX AND MATCH

1. Match the words or phrases used for managed care reimbursement methods in the left column with the definitions in the right column. Write the correct letters in the blanks.

_______ Discharge disposition	a. The basis for the OPPS
_______ Revenue cycle	b. Location where patient is going after leaving the hospital
_______ Admission review	c. When patient is formally admitted for care
_______ TEFRA	d. Timeframe when outpatient services are folded into inpatient claim
_______ Admission	e. Flat rate provided to care for patient
_______ Ambulatory payment classifications	f. Receiving reimbursement is the end result of this
_______ Observation patient	g. Code used to group charges on health care claim
_______ 72-hour rule	h. Reviews admission for appropriateness
_______ Preauthorization	i. Outpatient who stays overnight
_______ Upcoding	j. Obtaining permission from insurer before service
_______ Revenue code	k. The federal law that mandated the use of prospective payment systems for Medicare
_______ IPF PPS	l. Recertification is required at day 12 and at least every 30 days
_______ Capitation	m. Period where patient leaves hospital
_______ Interrupted stay	n. Tool used in the IRF PPS
_______ Inpatient Rehabilitation Facility Patient Assessment Instrument	o. Coding to increase reimbursement over what is deserved.

Part III Multiple Choice

Choose the best answer.

1. The result of upcoding is:
   a. downcoding.
   b. DRG creep.
   c. bundling.
   d. packaging.

2. Identify the true statement about APCS.
   a. APCs are used for inpatient claims.
   b. The hospital can receive multiple APCs for a patient visit.
   c. APCs use the fee-for-service methodology
   d. APCs use a per diem reimbursement strategy.

3. The average relative weight is:
   a. 1.
   b. 1.0000.
   c. 1.5.
   d. 1.0.

4. A preexisting condition that will, because of its effect on the specific principal diagnosis, require more intensive therapy or cause an increase in length of stay (LOS) by at least 1 day in approximately 75% of cases is called a:
   a. chronic condition.
   b. coexisting condition.
   c. comorbidity.
   d. complication.

5. A chargemaster contains:
   a. a grouper.
   b. the IRF PAI.
   c. a revenue code.
   d. the DNFB report.

Part IV True/False

Write "T" or "F" in the blank to indicate whether you think the statement is true or false.

_________ 1. A short stay outliner in the LTCH PPS is 4/5 of the length of stay.

_________ 2. 75% of the patients at an inpatient rehabilitation facility must fall into specific conditions.

_________ 3. MS-DRGs are a three-tiered system.

ASSIGNMENT 19.2 PREAUTHORIZATION

Research the internet and identify 10 procedures that frequently require preauthorization from the insurer before completion.

ASSIGNMENT 19.3 CALCULATING MS-DRG

For each of the MS-DRGs identified, complete the table. Use the most current MS-DRG tables from the Centers for Medicare and Medicaid Services website and the information therein to calculate the MS-DRG reimbursement if the facility base rate is $4,022.00 and the add-on is $340.

MS-DRG	Relative Weight	Calculations
10		
61		
101		
206		
329		

ASSIGNMENT 19.4 APC DISCOUNTING

Determine which of the following is subject to discounting.

The status indicator legend can be found at: https://med.noridianmedicare.com/web/jea/provider-types/opps/opps-payment-status-indicators

SCENARIO 1

APC	Status Indicator	Subject to Discounting Yes/No
1	C	
2	S	
3	J1	
4	T	

ASSIGNMENT 19.5 CRITIQUE OF THE INPATIENT REHABILITATION FACILITY-PATIENT ASSESSMENT INSTRUMENT (IRF-PAI)

Review the IRF-PAI document found at: https://www.cms.gov/Medicare/Medicare-Fee-for-Service-Payment/InpatientRehabFacPPS/IRFPAI.html.

Critique the assessment instrument. What do you like about it? What do you dislike? What, if anything, on the assessment instrument surprised you? Use content from the book and the IRF-PAI to support your opinions.

20 Seeking a Job and Attaining Professional Advancement

Linda M. Smith

KEY TERMS

Your instructor may wish to select some words pertinent to this chapter for a test. For definitions of the terms, further study, and/or reference, the words, phrases, and abbreviations may be found in the glossary at the end of the textbook. *Key terms for this chapter follow.*

application form
auditor
blind mailing
business associate agreement
certification
Certified Coding Specialist
Certified Coding Specialist-Physician
Certified Medical Assistant
Certified Medical Billing Specialist
Certified Professional Coder
Chargemaster Coordinator
chronologic résumé
Clinical Documentation Improvement Specialist
claims assistance professional
coding specialist
combination résumé
compliance specialist
continuing education
cover letter
employment agencies
functional résumé
immigrant
interview
mentor
National Certified Insurance and Coding Specialist
networking
portfolio
Registered Medical Assistant
Registered Medical Coder
résumé
Revenue Cycle Manager
self-employment
service contract

KEY ABBREVIATIONS

See how many abbreviations and acronyms you can translate, and then use this as a handy reference list. Definitions for the key abbreviations are located near the back of the textbook *in the glossary.*

AAPC ________________

AHIMA ________________

CAP ________________

CCAP ________________

CCS ________________

CCS-P ________________

CECP ________________

CMA ________________

CMBS ________________

CMRS ________________

CPC ________________

CPC-A ________________

CPC-H ________________

ECP ________________

EEOC ________________

HRS ________________

NCICS ________________

PAHCOM ________________

RMA ________________

RMC ________________

USCIS ________________

PERFORMANCE OBJECTIVES

The student will be able to:

- Define and spell the key terms and key abbreviations for this chapter, given the information from the *textbook* glossary, within a reasonable time period and with enough accuracy to obtain a satisfactory evaluation.
- After reading the chapter, answer the fill-in-the-blank, multiple choice, and true/false review questions with enough accuracy to obtain a satisfactory evaluation.
- Research information in preparation for creating a résumé, given a worksheet to complete, within a reasonable time period and with enough accuracy to obtain a satisfactory evaluation.
- Create an accurate résumé in a suitable font and print onto plain paper, within a reasonable time period, to obtain a satisfactory evaluation.
- Compose and print on plain paper a letter of introduction to go with the résumé and place it in a typed envelope, using one sheet of plain typing paper and a number 10 envelope, within a reasonable time period, to obtain a satisfactory evaluation.
- Complete an application form for a job, given an application for position form, within a reasonable time period and with enough accuracy to obtain a satisfactory evaluation.
- Compose and print a follow-up thank-you letter onto one sheet of plain paper. Print the address on a number 10 envelope, within a reasonable time period, to obtain a satisfactory evaluation.
- Access the internet and visit websites to research and/or obtain data, within a reasonable time period and with enough accuracy to obtain a satisfactory evaluation.

STUDY OUTLINE

Employment Opportunities
- Insurance Billing Specialist
- Advanced Job Opportunities

Professional Organizations
- Certification

Job Search
- Online Job Search
- Job Fairs
- Application
- Letter of Introduction
- Résumé
- Interview
- Follow-Up Letter

Self-Employment
- Setting Up an Office
- Finances to Consider
- Business Associate Under the Health Insurance Portability and Accountability Act
- Security and Equipment
- Marketing, Advertising, Promotion, and Public Relations
- Business Incubator
- Reassess and Continue With Success

Attaining Professional Advancement
- Networking
- Find a Mentor

Procedure 20.1: Creating an Electronic Résumé

ASSIGNMENT 20.1 REVIEW QUESTIONS

Part I Fill in the Blank

Review the objectives, key terms, glossary definitions of key terms, chapter information, and figures before completing the following review questions.

1. Name three job titles that the insurance billing specialist may find advertised.

   a. ____________________

   b. ____________________

   c. ____________________

2. A ____________ specialist works with physicians and other health care professionals to ensure that the documentation in the health record is complete and granular.

3. The process of earning a credential through a professional organization by gaining advanced education and experience is known as ____________________.

4. You have just completed a 1-year medical insurance billing course at a college. Name some preliminary job search contacts to make on campus.

   a. ____________________

   b. ____________________

   c. ____________________

   d. ____________________

5. When completing a job application form, the first step should be ______________.

   Why? ____________________

6. Name skills that may be listed on an application form or in a résumé when a person is seeking a position as an insurance billing specialist.

   a. ____________________

   b. ____________________

   c. ____________________

   d. ____________________

   e. ____________________

   f. ____________________

7. A question appears on a job application form about salary. Two ways in which to handle this question are:

   a. ____________________.

   b. ____________________.

8. State the chief purpose of a cover letter when a résumé is sent to a prospective employer.

   ____

9. What information may be omitted from a résumé, under the Civil Rights Act of 1964, informed by the EEOC?

   ____

10. A/an ______________ is a formal consultation with an employer to evaluate the qualifications of a prospective job applicant.

11. List the items to be compiled in a portfolio.

    a. ____________________

    b. ____________________

    c. ____________________

    d. ____________________

    e. ____________________

    f. ____________________

    g. ____________________

    h. ____________________

    i. ____________________

12. You are being interviewed for a job and the interviewer asks this question: "What is your religious preference?" How would you respond?

    ____

    ____

13. If a short period of time elapses after an interview and the applicant has received no word from the prospective employer, what follow-up steps may be taken?

    a. ____________________

    b. ____________________

14. If an individual creates a billing company and coding services are to be part of the offerings, the coding professional should have what type of professional status?

    ____

15. When considering self-employment, remember that the key to a successful business is to begin with a ____________________.

16. Hugh Beason was the owner of XYZ Medical Reimbursement Service. A fire occurred, damaging some of the equipment and part of the office premises requiring him to stop working for a month so that repairs could be made. What type/types of insurance would be helpful for this kind of problem?

    ____

17. A document that outlines the obligations of a billing service and a health care organization stating the responsible party for each specific duty and task is a/an ____________________.

18. List three methods a self-employed insurance billing specialist may use to price their services.

a. ____________________

b. ____________________

c. ____________________

19. A business ____________________ is an environment that grows and nurtures small businesses in their early years of existence by offering a wide range of business assistance and shared resources.

20. Gwendolyn Stevens has an insurance billing company and is attending a professional meeting where she has given business cards to a few attendees. Give two reasons for using this business marketing strategy.

a. ____________________

b. ____________________

21. Give the names of at least two national organizations that certify billers and coders.

a. ____________________

b. ____________________

Part II Multiple Choice

Choose the best answer.

22. A résumé format that emphasizes work experience dates is known as:
   a. functional.
   b. combination.
   c. business.
   d. chronologic.

23. When an individual plans to start an insurance billing company, he or she should have enough funds to operate the business for a period of:
   a. 6 months or more.
   b. 18 months or more.
   c. 1 year or more.
   d. 2 years.

24. Under Health Insurance Portability and Accountability Act (HIPAA) regulations, if a physician's insurance billing is outsourced to a person, this individual is known as a/an ____________________ because he or she uses and discloses individuals' identifiable health information.
   a. billing specialist
   b. business associate
   c. outside contractor
   d. outside vendor

25. When insurance billing is outsourced to a company, a document should be created, signed, and notarized by both parties; it is known as a:
   a. contract agreement.
   b. business agreement.
   c. service contract.
   d. legal contract.

26. A guide who offers advice, criticism, and guidance to an inexperienced person to help him or her reach a goal is known as a/an:
   a. mentor.
   b. counselor.
   c. associate.
   d. instructor.

Part III True/False

Write "T" or "F" in the blank to indicate whether you think the statement is true or false.

_______ 27. A résumé format that stresses job skills is known as functional.

_______ 28. When job applicants have similar skills and education, surveys have shown that hiring by employers has been based on bilingual skills.

_______ 29. Enhancing knowledge and keeping up-to-date are responsibilities of an insurance billing specialist.

_______ 30. Professional status of an insurance billing specialist may be obtained by passing a national examination for a Certified Medical Reimbursement Specialist (CMRS).

_______ 31. To earn the status of a claims assistance professional, this may be obtained by passing a national examination as a certified coding specialist (CCS).

ASSIGNMENT 20.2 JOB SEARCHING AND JOB SKILLS

Performance Objective

Task: Read these job advertisements. Then read the interests and abilities of the applicants to decide which job title belongs to each job hunter.

Conditions: Use the job advertisements and pen or pencil.

Standards: Time: ____________ minutes

Accuracy: ____________

(Note: The time element and accuracy criteria may be given by your instructor.)

Directions: These advertisements appeared in your local newspaper. Read the ads and then read the interests and abilities of each job applicant. Insert the job title for each applicant.

Job Titles

Insurance Biller

HS grad, computer exp, typing 40 wpm needed for busy output clinic, insurance claims knowledge

Insurance Coder

Detail-oriented individual, Dx and proc coder. 2 years exp preferred

Bilingual Collections Manager

Self-motivated individual with good communications skills. Bilingual. Enjoys working in health care.

Trudy

Trudy is bilingual in English and Spanish and enjoys working with people. She is especially good with the telephone and likes communications.

Job Title: ______________________________

Walter

Walter wants to work in the health care field. He has taken diagnostic and procedure coding classes and enjoys problem solving.

Job Title: ______________________________

Ilona

Ilona has experience with inputting patient data and transmitting insurance claims. She says she is honest and dependable.

Job Title: ______________________________

ASSIGNMENT 20.3 COMPLETE A WORKSHEET AND TYPE A RÉSUMÉ

Performance Objective

Task: Respond to a job advertisement by completing a worksheet and typing a résumé by abstracting data from your worksheet.

Conditions: Use two sheets of plain typing paper, a newspaper advertisement (Fig. 20.1), and a computer.

Standards: Time: ___________ minutes

Accuracy: ____________

(Note: The time element and accuracy criteria may be given by your instructor.)

Directions: An advertisement appeared in your local newspaper (see Fig. 20.1). You decide to apply for the position. Complete a worksheet in preparation for typing your résumé. Some of the information requested on the worksheet should not appear on the résumé but should be available if you are asked to provide it. Ask a classmate to review and comment about the information in your worksheet. Extract data that you think are relevant from the worksheet, and type a rough draft of your résumé. Ask the instructor for suggestions to improve the rough draft. Refer to Chapter 20 and Fig. 20.6 in the textbook to help organize your résumé into an attractive format before you type the final copy.

1. Insert title of personal data sheet from worksheet.

2. Insert heading: name, address, telephone number, and so on.

3. Select one of three formats for data.

4. Insert heading and data for education information.

5. Insert heading and data for skill information.

6. Insert heading and data for employment information.

7. Insert reference information.

8. Proofread résumé.

9. Print résumé.

MEDICAL INSURANCE CODING/REIMBURSEMENT SPECIALIST

Mid-Atlantic Clinic, a 20-physician, multi-specialty group practice in Chicago, Illinois, has a need for a coding and reimbursement specialist. Knowledge of medical terminology, CPT and ICD-9-CM coding systems, Medicare regulations, third-party insurance reimbursement, and physician billing procedures required. Proficiency in the interpretation and coding of procedural and diagnostic codes is strongly preferred. Successful candidates must have excellent communication and problem-solving skills. This position offers a competitive salary and superior benefits. Please send resume to:

George B. Pason, Personnel Director
Mid-Atlantic Clinic
1230 South Main Street
Chicago, IL 60611

Fig. 20.1

ASSIGNMENT 20.4 COMPLETE A COVER LETTER

Performance Objective

Task: Compose a cover letter to accompany your résumé.

Conditions: Use one sheet of plain typing paper, a number 10 envelope, computer, printer, thesaurus, and English dictionary.

Standards: Time: ____________ minutes

Accuracy: ____________

(Note: The time element and accuracy criteria may be given by your instructor.)

Directions: Compose a cover letter introducing yourself, and create a rough draft. Consult the instructor for suggestions. Print the cover letter on plain bond paper in a form that can be mailed. Refer to the sample letter in Chapter 20 and Fig. 20.5 in the textbook as a guide to help organize your thoughts. Type the name and address of the employer on a number 10 envelope, and insert the letter with the résumé from Assignment 20.3.

ASSIGNMENT 20.5 COMPLETE A JOB APPLICATION FORM

Performance Objective

Task: Complete a job application form by using data from your résumé.

Conditions: Use an application form (Fig. 20.2), your résumé, and a computer.

Standards: Time: _______________ minutes

Accuracy: _______________

(Note: The time element and accuracy criteria may be given by your instructor.)

Directions: Assume that the employer asked you to come to his or her place of business to complete an application form and make an appointment for an interview. Using your data and résumé, complete an application form (see Fig. 20.2).

APPLICATION FOR POSITION/ Medical or Dental Office

AN EQUAL OPPORTUNITY EMPLOYER

(In answering questions, use extra blank sheet if necessary)

No employee, applicant, or candidate for promotion training or other advantage shall be discriminated against (or given preference) because of race, color, religion, sex, age, physical handicap, veteran status, or national origin.
PLEASE READ CAREFULLY AND WRITE OR PRINT ANSWERS TO ALL QUESTIONS. DO NOT TYPE.

Date of application

A. PERSONAL INFORMATION

Name- Last	First	Middle	Social Security No.	Area Code/Phone No. ( )
Present Address: -Street	(Apt. #)	City	State Zip	How long at this address?
Previous Address: -Street	City	State	Zip	Person to notify in case of Emergency or Accident - Name:
From:	To:			Address: Telephone:

B. EMPLOYMENT INFORMATION

For what position are you applying?	☐ Full-time ☐ Part-time ☐ Either	Date available for employment?:	Wage/Salary Expectations:
List hrs./days you prefer to work:	List any hrs./days you are not available: (Except for times required for religious practices or observances)		Can you work overtime, if necessary? ☐ Yes ☐ No
Are you employed now?: ☐ Yes ☐ No	If so, may we inquire of your present employer?: ☐ No ☐ Yes, If yes: Name of employer: Phone number: ( )		
Have you ever been bonded?: ☐ Yes ☐ No	If required for position, are you bondable? ☐ Yes ☐ No ☐ Uncertain	Have you applied for a position with this office before? ☐ No ☐ Yes, If yes, when?:	
Referred by/ or where did you hear of this job?:			
Can you, upon employment, submit verification of your legal right to work in the United States? ☐ Yes ☐ No Submit proof that you meet legal age requirement for employment? ☐ Yes ☐ No		Language(s) applicant speaks or writes (if use of a language other than English is relevant to the job for which applicant is applying):	

C. EDUCATIONAL HISTORY

Name and address of schools attended (Include current)	Dates From	Dates Thru	Highest grade/level completed	Diploma/degree(s) obtained/areas of study:
High school				
College				Degree/Major
Post graduate				Degree/Major
Other				Course/Diploma/License Certificate

Specific training, education, or experiences which will assist you in the job for which you have applied:

Future educational plans:

D. SPECIAL SKILLS

CHECK BELOW THE KINDS OF WORK YOU HAVE DONE:			
		☐ MEDICAL INSURANCE FORMS	☐ RECEPTIONIST
☐ BLOOD COUNTS	☐ DENTAL ASSISTANT	☐ MEDICAL TERMINOLOGY	☐ TELEPHONES
☐ BOOKKEEPING	☐ DENTAL HYGIENIST	☐ MEDICAL TRANSCRIPTION	☐ TYPING
☐ COLLECTIONS	☐ FILING	☐ NURSING	☐ STENOGRAPHY
☐ COMPOSING LETTERS	☐ INJECTIONS	☐ PHLEBOTOMY (Draw Blood)	☐ URINALYSIS
☐ COMPUTER INPUT	☐ INSTRUMENT STERILIZATION	☐ POSTING	☐ X-RAY
OFFICE EQUIPMENT USED: ☐ COMPUTER	☐ DICTATING EQUIPMENT	☐ WORD PROCESSOR	☐ OTHER:
Other kinds of tasks performed or skills that may be applicable to position:		Typing speed:	Shorthand speed:

RM NO. 72-110 ©1976 BIBBERO SYSTEMS INC. PETALUMA, CA (MB-CO) # 2-5 (REV. 10/92)
REORDER CALL 800-BIBBERO (800) 242-2376

(PLEASE COMPLETE OTHER SIDE)

Fig. 20.2

E. EMPLOYMENT RECORD

LIST MOST RECENT EMPLOYMENT FIRST — May we contact your previous Employer(s) for a reference? ☐ yes ☐ no

1) Employer — Work performed. Be specific.

Address — Street — City — State — Zip code

Phone number ( )

Type of business — Dates: From Mo. Yr. — To Mo. Yr.

Your position — Hourly rate/Salary: Starting — Final

Supervisor's name

Reason for leaving

2) Employer — Work performed. Be specific.

Address — Street — City — State — Zip code

Phone number ( )

Type of business — Dates: From Mo. Yr. — To Mo. Yr.

Your position — Hourly rate/Salary: Starting — Final

Supervisor's name

Reason for leaving

3) Employer — Work performed. Be specific.

Address — Street — City — State — Zip code

Phone number ( )

Type of business — Dates: From Mo. Yr. — To Mo. Yr.

Your position — Hourly rate/Salary: Starting — Final

Supervisor's name

Reason for leaving

F. REFERENCES: FRIENDS/ACQUAINTANCES NON-RELATED

1) Name — Address — Telephone Number (☐ Work ☐ Home) — Occupation — Years acquainted

2) Name — Address — Telephone Number (☐ Work ☐ Home) — Occupation — Years acquainted

Please feel free to add any information which you feel will help us consider you for employment.

READ THE FOLLOWING CAREFULLY, THEN SIGN AND DATE THE APPLICATION

I certify that all answers given by me on this application are true, correct and complete to the best of my knowledge. I acknowledge notice that the information contained in this application is subject to check. I agree that, if hired, my continued employment may be contingent upon the accuracy of that information. If employed, I further agree to comply with company/office rules and regulations.

Signature ______________________ Date: ____________

RM NO. 72-110 ©1976 BIBBERO SYSTEMS INC. PETALUMA, CA (MB-CO) # 6-7 (REV. 4/92) — TO REORDER CALL 800-BIBBERO (800) 242-2376

Fig. 20.2, cont'd

ASSIGNMENT 20.6 PREPARE A FOLLOW-UP THANK-YOU LETTER

Performance Objective

Task: Prepare a follow-up thank-you letter after the interview, sending it to the interviewer.

Conditions: Use one sheet of plain typing paper, a number 10 envelope, computer, printer, thesaurus, and English dictionary.

Standards: Time: ______________ minutes

Accuracy: ______________

(Note: The time element and accuracy criteria may be given by your instructor.)

Directions: After the interview, you decide to send a follow-up thank-you letter to the person who interviewed you. Compose a letter and address a number 10 envelope. Refer to Chapter 20 and Fig. 20.11 in the handook to help organize your thoughts.

ASSIGNMENT 20.7 VISIT WEBSITES FOR JOB OPPORTUNITIES

Performance Objective

Task: Access the internet and visit several websites.

Conditions: Use a computer with a printer and/or a pen or pencil to make notes.

Standards: Time: ______________ minutes

Accuracy: ______________

(Note: The time element and accuracy criteria may be given by your instructor.)

Directions: Visit at least five websites by using either a search engine (Yahoo, Google, Bing) or a job-search website. Some suggestions are:

www.healthcarejobs.org
www.indeed.com
www.juju.com
www.topusajobs.com
www.monster.com

Enter a keyword or job title, such as "medical billing specialist" or "medical coder." Enter your city and state to locate listings near you. Click on the search button. If you get some results, print the listings that appeal to you for sharing and discussing in class.

ASSIGNMENT 20.8 CRITICAL THINKING

Performance Objective

Task: Write a paragraph describing the benefits of becoming certified in this field.

Conditions: Use a computer with printer and/or a pen or pencil.

Standards: Time: ______________ minutes

Accuracy: ______________

(Note: The time element and accuracy criteria may be given by your instructor.)

Directions: Write a paragraph or two describing why you would like to become certified in this field, and incorporate a numbered list of benefits. Make sure grammar, punctuation, and spelling are correct.

Tests

TEST 1: PROCEDURE (E/M AND MEDICINE SECTIONS) AND DIAGNOSTIC PROCEDURE CODE TEST

Directions: Using a *Current Procedural Terminology* (CPT) code book insert the correct code numbers and modifiers for each service rendered. Give a brief description for each professional service rendered. An optional exercise is to abstract the pertinent data from each case, then use the *International Classification of Diseases*, Tenth Revision, Clinical Modifications (ICD-10-CM) code book to insert the diagnosis code.

Insert year of the CPT code book used:

____

Insert year of the ICD-10-CM code book used:

____

1. Dr. Input sees a new patient, Mrs. Post, in the office for acute abdominal distress. The physician spends approximately 1 hour obtaining a comprehensive history and physical examination with high-complexity decision making. Several diagnostic studies are ordered, and Mrs. Post is given an appointment to return in 1 week.

Description

______________________________ CPT # ________

______________________________ ICD-10-CM # ________

2. Mr. Nakahara, an established patient, sees Dr. Practon in the office on January 11 for a reevaluation of his type 2 diabetic condition. Dr. Practon takes a detailed history and performs a detailed examination. Decision making is moderately complex.

Description

______________________________ CPT # ________

______________________________ ICD-10-CM # ________

3. Dr. Cardi sees Mrs. Franklin for a follow-up office visit for her hypertension. A problem-focused history and examination of her cardiovascular system are obtained and reveal a blood pressure of 140/100. Decision making is straightforward, with medication being prescribed. The patient is advised to return in 2 weeks to have her blood pressure checked by the nurse. Mrs. Franklin returns 2 weeks later, and the nurse checks her blood pressure.

Description

____________________ CPT # ________

____________________ ICD-10-CM # ________

____________________ CPT # ________

____________________ ICD-10-CM # ________

4. Dr. Skeleton receives a call at 7 PM from Mrs. Snyder. Her husband, a patient of Dr. Skeleton's, has been very ill for 2 hours with profuse vomiting. Dr. Skeleton goes to their home to see Mr. Snyder and spends considerable time obtaining a detailed history and examination. The medical decision making is of a highly complex nature. The physician administers an injection of prochlorperazine (Compazine).

Description

____________________ CPT # ________

____________________ CPT # ________

____________________ ICD-10-CM # ________

5. Dr. Cutis sees an established patient, a registered nurse, for determination of pregnancy. A detailed history and examination are obtained, with moderate-complexity medical decision making. A Papanicolaou smear is taken, a blood sample is drawn, and the specimens are sent to an independent laboratory for a qualitative human chorionic gonadotropin (hCG) test. The patient also complains of something she has discovered under her armpit. On examination, there is a furuncle of the left axilla, which is incised and drained during this visit. The laboratory requires CPT coding on the laboratory requisition. List how these laboratory procedures would appear on the requisition sheet. The Papanicolaou smear is processed according to the Bethesda System and under physician supervision.

Professional Service Rendered by Dr. Cutis

____________________ CPT # ________

____________________ CPT # ________

____________________ CPT # ________

____________________ CPT # ________

____________________ ICD-10-CM # ________

____________________ ICD-10-CM # ________

Laboratory Service on Requisition Sheet

____________________ CPT # ________

____________________ CPT # ________

6. Dr. Antrum makes a house call on Betty Mason, an established patient, for a problem-focused history of acute otitis media. A problem-focused examination is performed, with straightforward medical decision making. While there, Dr. Antrum also sees Betty's younger sister, Sandra, whom she has seen previously in the office, for acute tonsillitis. A problem-focused history and examination are performed with low-complexity decision making. In addition to the examinations, Dr. Antrum gives both children injections of penicillin.

Professional Service Rendered to Betty

________________________________ CPT # ________

________________________________ CPT # ________

________________________________ ICD-10-CM # ________

Professional Service Rendered to Sandra

________________________________ CPT # ________

________________________________ CPT # ________

________________________________ ICD-10-CM # ________

7. Two weeks later, Dr. Antrum is called to the emergency department at College Hospital at 2 AM on Sunday to see Betty Mason for recurrent chronic otitis media with suppuration. A problem-focused history and examination are performed with straightforward decision making. Dr. Antrum administers a second injection of penicillin.

Description

________________________________ CPT # ________

________________________________ CPT # ________

________________________________ CPT # ________

________________________________ ICD-10-CM # ________

8. While at the hospital, Dr. Antrum is asked to see another patient in the emergency department, who is new to her. A problem-focused history is taken. She performs a problem-focused examination and straightforward decision making for an intermediate 3.5 cm laceration of the scalp. The laceration is sutured, and the patient is advised to come to the office in 4 days for a dressing change. Four days later, the patient comes into the office for a dressing change by the nurse.

Description

________________________________ CPT # ________

________________________________ CPT # ________

________________________________ ICD-10-CM # ________

9. Dr. Menter, a psychiatrist, sees the following patients in the hospital. Code each procedure.

Ms. Blake: consultation, expanded problem-focused history and examination and straightforward decision making; referred by Dr. Practon — CPT # ________

Mrs. Clark: group psychotherapy (50 min) — CPT # ________

Mrs. Samson: group psychotherapy (50 min) — CPT # ________

Mr. Shoemaker: group psychotherapy (50 min) — CPT # ________

Miss James: individual psychotherapy (25 min) — CPT # ________

10. Dr. Input, a gastroenterologist, sees Mrs. Chan in the hospital at the request of Dr. Practon for an esophageal ulcer. In addition to the detailed history and examination and the low-complexity decision making, Dr. Input performs a flexible, transoral esophagogastroduodenoscopy with washings. Two days later, he sees Mrs. Chan in a follow-up hospital visit and obtains a problem-focused interval history and examination with low-complexity decision making.

Description

________________________________ CPT # ________

________________________________ CPT # ________

________________________________ ICD-10-CM # ________

____

________________________________ CPT # ________

________________________________ ICD-10-CM # ________

11. Mrs. Galati, a new patient, goes to Dr. Cardi because of chest pain (moderate to severe), weakness, fatigue, and dizziness. Dr. Cardi takes a comprehensive history and performs a comprehensive examination, followed by a treadmill ECG with interpretation and report. He also performs a vital capacity test and dipstick urinalysis, and draws blood for triiodothyronine (T_3) testing and for analysis by sequential multiple analyzer computer (SMAC) (16 panel tests, including complete blood cell count [CBC]), which are sent to and billed by a laboratory. Medical decision making is of high complexity.

Description

________________________________ CPT # ________

________________________________ CPT # ________

________________________________ CPT # ________

________________________________ CPT # ________

________________________________ CPT # ________

________________________________ CPT # ________

________________________________ ICD-10-CM # ________

________________________________ ICD-10-CM # ________

________________________________ ICD-10-CM # ________

12. Jake Wonderhill has not had his eyes examined by Dr. Lenser for about 5 years. He is seen by Dr. Lenser, who performs the following ophthalmologic procedures in addition to a comprehensive eye examination: fluorescein angioscopy and electroretinography. Mr. Wonderhill receives a diagnosis of retinitis pigmentosa.

Description

____________________	CPT # ________
____________________	CPT # ________
____________________	CPT # ________
____________________	ICD-10-CM # ________

13. Dr. Practon is making rounds at the College Hospital and answers an urgent call on Third Floor East. He performs cardiopulmonary resuscitation on Mr. Sanchez for cardiac arrest and orders the patient taken to the critical care unit. Chest radiographs, laboratory work, blood gas measurements, and ECG are performed. The physician is detained 2 hours in constant attendance on the patient.

Description

____________________	CPT # ________
____________________	CPT # ________
____________________	CPT # ________
____________________	ICD-10-CM # ________

14. Mrs. Powers, a new patient, sees Dr. Skeleton for low sciatica. Dr. Skeleton takes a detailed history and performs a detailed examination of the patient's lower back and extremities. Medical decision making is of low complexity. Diathermy (30 minutes) is given. The next day the patient comes in for therapeutic exercises in the Hubbard tank (30 minutes).

Description

____________________	CPT # ________
____________________	CPT # ________
____________________	ICD-10-CM # ________
____________________	CPT # ________
____________________	ICD-10-CM # ________

15. a. Mrs. Garcia, a new patient, is seen by Dr. Caesar for occasional vaginal spotting (detailed history/examination and low-complexity decision making). The doctor determines that the bleeding is coming from the cervix and asks her to return in 3 days for cryocauterization of the cervix. During the initial examination, Mrs. Garcia asks for an evaluation for possible infertility. Dr. Caesar advises her to wait 2 to 3 weeks and make an appointment for two infertility tests.
    b. When the patient returns in 3 days for cryocauterization, the doctor also takes a wet mount for bacteria/fungi, which is sent to and billed by a laboratory.
    c. Three weeks later, an injection procedure for hysterosalpingography and endometrial biopsy are performed.

Description

a. ____________________ CPT # ________

____________________ ICD-10-CM # ________

b. ____________________ CPT # ________

____________________ CPT # ________

____________________ ICD-10-CM # ________

c. ____________________ CPT # ________

____________________ CPT # ________

____________________ ICD-10-CM # ________

Multiple Choice

After reading the boxed codes with descriptions, select the answer/answers that is/are best in each case.

59120	surgical treatment of ectopic pregnancy; tubal or ovarian, requiring salpingectomy and/or oophorectomy, abdominal or vaginal approach
59121	tubal or ovarian, without salpingectomy and/or oophorectomy
59130	abdominal pregnancy
59135	interstitial, uterine pregnancy requiring total hysterectomy
59136	interstitial, uterine pregnancy with partial resection of uterus
59140	cervical, with evacuation

16. In regard to this section of CPT codes, which of the following statements is true about codes 59120 through 59140? Mark all that apply.
    a. They refer to abdominal hysterotomy.
    b. They involve laparoscopic treatment of ectopic pregnancy.
    c. They refer to treatment of ectopic pregnancy by surgery.
    d. They involve tubal ligation.

17. In regard to this section of CPT codes, for treatment of a tubal ectopic pregnancy, necessitating oophorectomy, the code to select is
    a. 59121.
    b. 59120.
    c. 59135.
    d. 59136.
    e. 59130.

18. In regard to this section of CPT codes, for treatment of an ectopic pregnancy (interstitial, uterine) requiring a total hysterectomy, the code/codes to select is/are
    a. 59135.
    b. 59135 and 59120.
    c. 59120.
    d. 59130 and 59120.
    e. 59121.

TEST 2: PROCEDURE CODE WITH MODIFIERS AND DIAGNOSTIC CODE TEST

Directions: Match the description given in the right column with the procedure code/modifier combination in the left column. Write the letter in the blank.

Procedure With Modifier		Description
1. 99214-25	________	a. Dr. Practon assisted Dr. Caesar with a total abdominal hysterectomy and bilateral salpingo-oophorectomy.
2. 99204-57	________	b. Dr. Skeleton interprets a thoracolumbar x-ray film that was taken at College Hospital.
3. 58150-80	________	c. Mrs. Ulwelling saw Dr. Antrum for an office visit as a new patient, and she recommended that the patient undergo a laryngoscopy, with stripping of vocal cords to be done the following day.
4. 32440-55	________	d. Mrs. Gillenbach walked through a plate glass window and underwent a rhinoplasty, performed by Dr. Graff on February 16, 20xx. On February 26, 20xx, she came to see Dr. Graff for a consultation regarding reconstructive surgery on her right leg.
5. 72080-26	________	e. An established patient, Mrs. Mercado, is seen in a follow-up exam for type 2 diabetes. The patient asks Dr. Langerhans to look at some skin tags. The doctor examines them and says they need to be removed (11200). The evaluation and management service was detailed and of a moderate complexity.
6. 29425-58	________	f. Dr. Cutler performed a bilateral orchiopexy (inguinal approach) on baby Kozak.
7. 54640-50	________	g. Dr. Skeleton applied a short leg-walking cast to Mrs. Belchere's right leg 4 weeks after his initial treatment of her fractured tibia.
8. 99253-24	________	h. Dr. Cutler went on vacation, and Dr. Coccidioides took care of Mrs. Ash during the postoperative period after her total pneumonectomy.

Directions: Using a CPT code book, insert the correct code numbers and modifiers for each service rendered. Give a brief description for each professional service rendered.

9. Dr. Input performs a gastrojejunostomy for carcinoma in situ of the duodenum and calls in Dr. Scott to administer the anesthesia and Dr. Cutler to assist. This intraperitoneal surgery takes 2 hours, 30 minutes. The patient is otherwise normal and healthy. List the procedure and diagnostic code numbers with appropriate modifiers for each physician.

Professional Service Rendered by Dr. Input

____ CPT # ________

____ ICD-10-CM # ________

Professional Service Rendered by Dr. Scott

____ CPT # ________

____ ICD-10-CM # ________

Professional Service Rendered by Dr. Cutler

____ CPT # ________

____ ICD-10-CM # ________

10. Dr. Rumsey assists Dr. Cutler with a total colectomy (intraperitoneal procedure) with ileostomy. Dr. Scott is the anesthesiologist. Surgery takes 2 hours, 55 minutes. The patient has a secondary malignant neoplasm of the colon (severe systemic disease). List the procedure code numbers with appropriate modifiers and diagnostic code numbers for each physician.

Professional Service Rendered by Dr. Rumsey

____ CPT # ________

____ ICD-10-CM # ________

Professional Service Rendered by Dr. Scott

____ CPT # ________

____ ICD-10-CM # ________

Professional Service Rendered by Dr. Cutler

____ CPT # ________

____ ICD-10-CM # ________

11. Dr. Cutis removes a malignant tumor from a patient's back (1.5 cm) and does the local anesthesia herself.

Description

____ CPT # ________

____ ICD-10-CM # ________

12. Dr. Skeleton sees Mr. Richmond, a new patient worked into the office schedule on an emergency basis after a motor vehicle traffic accident with another car. Mr. Richmond has multiple lacerations of the face, arm, and chest and a fracture of the left tibia. The physician takes a comprehensive history and performs a comprehensive examination. Decision making is moderately complex. Dr. Skeleton orders bilateral radiographs of the tibia and fibula and two views of the chest and left wrist to be taken in his office. Then he closes the following lacerations: 2.6 cm, simple, face; 2.0 cm, intermediate, face; 7.5 cm, intermediate, right arm; 4.5 cm, intermediate, chest. All radiographs are negative except that of the left tibia. Dr. Skeleton performs a manipulative reduction of the left tibial shaft and applies a cast. Code this case as if you were actually listing the codes on the CMS-1500 claim form.

Description

____ CPT # ________ and ________

____ CPT # ________

____ CPT # ________

____ CPT # ________

____ CPT # ________

____ CPT # ________

____ CPT # ________

____ CPT # ________

____ CPT # ________

____ CPT # ________

____ ICD-10-CM # ________

____ ICD-10-CM # ________

____ ICD-10-CM # ________

____ ICD-10-CM # ________

____ ICD-10-CM # ________

Six weeks later, Dr. Skeleton sees the same patient for an office visit and obtains radiographs (two views) of the left tibia and fibula. Treatment involves application of a cast below the patient's left knee to the toes, including a walking heel.

Description

____ CPT # ________

____ CPT # ________

____ CPT # ________

____ ICD-10-CM # ________

13. Dr. Cutler performs an incisional biopsy of a patient's breast for a breast lump, which requires 40 minutes of anesthesia. Dr. Scott is the anesthesiologist. The patient is otherwise normal and healthy. List the procedure and diagnostic code numbers for each physician.

Professional Service Rendered by Dr. Cutler

____ CPT # ________

____ ICD-10-CM # ________

Professional Service Rendered by Dr. Scott

____ CPT # ________

____ ICD-10-CM # ________

14. Mrs. DeBeau is aware that Dr. Input will be out of town for 6 weeks; however, she decides to have him perform the recommended combined anterior-posterior colporrhaphy with enterocele repair for vaginal enterocele. Dr. Practon agrees to perform the follow-up care and assist. Dr. Scott is the anesthesiologist. The anesthesia time is 2 hours, 15 minutes. The patient is normal and healthy. List the procedure and diagnostic code numbers for each physician. Note: Emphasis for this problem should be placed on the choice of CPT modifiers.

Professional Service Rendered by Dr. Input

____ CPT # ________

____ ICD-10-CM # ________

Professional Service Rendered by Dr. Practon

______________________________ CPT # ________

______________________________ CPT modifier ________

______________________________ CPT modifier ________

______________________________ ICD-10-CM # ________

Professional Service Rendered by Dr. Scott

______________________________ CPT # ________

______________________________ ICD-10-CM # ________

15. Mr. Wong, a new patient, is seen in the College Hospital and undergoes a comprehensive history and physical examination (H&P) with moderately complex decision making. Dr. Coccidioides performs a bronchoscopy with biopsy. Results of the biopsy confirm the diagnosis: malignant neoplasm of upper left lobe of lung. The following day the physician performs a total pneumonectomy. Dr. Cutler assists on the total pneumonectomy (pulmonary resection), and Dr. Scott is the anesthesiologist. Surgery takes 3 hours, 45 minutes. The patient has mild systemic disease. List the procedure and diagnostic code numbers for each physician.

Professional Service Rendered by Dr. Coccidioides

______________________________ CPT # ________

______________________________ CPT # ________

______________________________ CPT # ________

______________________________ ICD-10-CM # ________

Professional Service Rendered by Dr. Cutler

______________________________ CPT # ________

______________________________ ICD-10-CM # ________

Professional Service Rendered by Dr. Scott

______________________________ CPT # ________

______________________________ ICD-10-CM # ________

When completing the CMS-1500 claim form for Dr. Scott, in which block would you list anesthesia minutes? ______________________________

TEST 3: PROCEDURE (RADIOLOGY AND PATHOLOGY SECTIONS) AND DIAGNOSTIC CODE TEST

Directions: Using a CPT code book, insert the correct procedure code numbers and modifiers and diagnostic codes for each service rendered. Give a brief description for each professional service rendered.

1. Mrs. Cahn sees Dr. Skeleton because of severe pain in her right shoulder. She is a new patient. Dr. Skeleton takes a detailed history and performs a detailed examination. A complete x-ray study of the right shoulder is done. Decision making is of low complexity. A diagnosis of bursitis is made, and an injection into the bursa is administered.

Description

______________________________ CPT # ________

______________________________ CPT # ________

______________________________ CPT # ________

______________________________ ICD-10-CM # ________

2. John Murphy comes into the Broxton Radiologic Group, Inc., for an extended radiation therapy consultation for prostatic cancer. The radiologist takes a detailed history and does a detailed examination. Decision making is of low complexity. The physician determines a simple treatment plan involving simple simulation-aided field settings. Basic dosimetry calculations are done, and the patient returns the following day and receives radiation therapy to a single treatment area (6 to 10 MeV).

Description

______________________________ CPT # ________

______________________________ CPT # ________

______________________________ CPT # ________

______________________________ CPT # ________

______________________________ CPT # ________

Diagnosis:

______________________________ ICD-10-CM # ________

3. Dr. Input refers Mrs. Horner to the Nuclear Medicine Department of the Broxton Radiologic Group, Inc., for a bone marrow imaging of the whole body, and imaging of the liver and spleen. List the procedure code numbers after each radiologic procedure to show how the radiology group would bill. Also, list the diagnosis of malignant neoplasm of the bone marrow.

Description

Total body bone marrow, imaging	CPT # ________
Radiopharmaceuticals, diagnostic (iodine I-123)	HCPCS # ________
Liver and spleen imaging	CPT # ________
Radiopharmaceuticals, diagnostic (iodine I-123)	HCPCS # ________

Diagnosis:

____ ICD-10-CM # ________

4. Dr. Input also refers Mrs. Horner to XYZ Laboratory for the following tests. List the procedure code numbers to indicate how the laboratory would bill.

Description

CBC, automated, and automated differential	CPT # ________
Urinalysis, automated with microscopy	CPT # ________
Urine culture (quantitative, colony count)	CPT # ________
Urine antibiotic sensitivity (microtiter)	CPT # ________

5. The general laboratory at College Hospital receives a surgical tissue specimen (ovarian biopsy) for gross and microscopic examination from a patient with Stein-Leventhal syndrome. List the procedure and diagnostic code numbers to indicate what the hospital pathology department would bill.

Description

____ CPT # ________

Diagnosis:

____ ICD-10-CM # ________

6. Dr. Langerhans refers Jerry Cramer to XYZ Laboratory for a lipid panel. He has a family history of cardiovascular disease. List the procedure and diagnostic code number or numbers to indicate how the laboratory would bill.

Description

____ CPT # ________

Diagnosis:

____ ICD-10-CM # ________

7. Dr. Caesar is an OB/GYN specialist who has her own ultrasound machine. Carmen Cardoza, age 45, is referred to Dr. Caesar for an obstetric consultation and an amniocentesis with ultrasonic guidance. The diagnosis is Rh incompatibility. The doctor performs a detailed history and physical examination, and decision making is of low complexity.

Description

____ CPT # _______

____ CPT # _______

Diagnosis:

____ ICD-10-CM # _______

8. Mr. Marcos's medical record indicates that a retrograde pyelogram followed by a percutaneous nephrostolithotomy, with basket extraction of a 1 cm stone, was performed by Dr. Ulibarri for nephrolithiasis.

Description

____ CPT # _______

____ CPT # _______

Diagnosis:

____ ICD-10-CM # _______

9. Broxton Radiologic Group, Inc., performs the following procedures on Mrs. Stephens at the request of Dr. Input. List the procedure code numbers after each radiologic procedure. On the laboratory slip, the following congenital diagnoses are listed: diverticulum of the stomach and colon; cystic lung. Locate the corresponding diagnostic codes.

Barium enema CPT # _______

Evaluation of upper gastrointestinal tract with small bowel CPT # _______

Complete chest x-ray CPT # _______

Diagnosis:

____ ICD # _______

Diagnosis:

____ ICD # _______

Diagnosis:

____ ICD # _______

10. Two weeks later, Mrs. Stephens is referred again for further radiologic studies for flank pain. List the procedure and diagnostic code numbers after each radiologic procedure.

    Intravenous pyelogram (IVP) with drip infusion CPT # ________

    Oral cholecystography CPT # ________

Diagnosis:

____ ICD # ________

TEST 4: COMPLETE A CMS-1500 CLAIM FORM

Performance Objective

Task: Complete a CMS-1500 claim form for a private case and post transactions to the patient's financial accounting record.

Conditions: Use the patient's record (Fig. 1) and financial statement (Fig. 2); one health insurance claim form; a computer or pen; procedural and diagnostic code books; and Appendix A in this *Workbook*.

Standards: Claim Productivity Management

Time: ____________ minutes

Accuracy: ____________

(Note: The time element and accuracy criteria may be given by your instructor.)

Directions:

1. Using NUCC guidelines, complete a CMS-1500 claim form and direct it to the private carrier. Refer to Jennifer T. Lacey's patient record for information and Appendix A in this *Workbook* to locate the fees to record on the claim, and post them to the financial statement. Date the claim August 15 of the current year. Dr. Caesar is accepting assignment, and the patient's signatures to release information to the insurance company and to have the payment forwarded directly to the physician are on file.

2. Use your CPT code book to determine the correct five-digit code numbers and modifiers for each professional service rendered. Use your HCPCS Level II code book for HCPCS procedure codes and modifiers. Use your ICD-10-CM coding manual to code each active diagnosis. Record the proper information on the financial record and claim form, and note the date that you billed the insurance company.

3. American Commercial Insurance Company sent a check (voucher number 5586) on November 17 in the amount of $880. The patient's responsibility is $220. Post the payment, write off (adjust) the remaining balance, and circle the amount billed to the patient.

PATIENT RECORD NO. T-4

LAST NAME: Lacey
FIRST NAME: Jennifer
MIDDLE NAME: T.
BIRTH DATE: 11-12-55
SEX: F
HOME PHONE: 555-549-0098

ADDRESS: 451 Roberts Street
CITY: Woodland Hills
STATE: XY
ZIP CODE: 12345

CELL PHONE: 555-443-9899
PAGER NO.: 555-549-0098
FAX NO.:
E-MAIL ADDRESS: lacey@wb.net

PATIENT'S SOC. SEC. NO.: 430-XX-7709
DRIVER'S LICENSE: Y0053498

PATIENT'S OCCUPATION: legal secretary
NAME OF COMPANY: Higgins and Higgins Attorneys at Law

ADDRESS OF EMPLOYER: 430 Second Avenue, Woodland Hills, XY 12345
PHONE: 555-540-6675

SPOUSE OR PARENT:
OCCUPATION:

EMPLOYER:
ADDRESS:
PHONE:

NAME OF INSURANCE: American Commercial Insurance Company, 5682 Bendix Blvd., Woodland Hills, XY 12345
INSURED OR SUBSCRIBER:

POLICY/CERTIFICATE NO.: 5789022
GROUP NO.: 444

REFERRED BY: Clarence Cutler, MD

Fig. 1

DATE	PROGRESS NOTES No. T-4
8-1-xx	New pt referred by Dr. Cutler, came into office for consultation and additional opinion.
	CC: Full feeling in stomach and low abdominal region.
	Irregular menstruation. Ultrasonic report showed
	leiomyomata uteri and rt ovarian mass; however, visualization of mass poor and type
	cannot be identified. Pap smear Class I. No personal or family hx of CA.
	Comprehensive hx and physical examination performed on healthy appearing white female.
	Wt: 136 lbs. BP 128/60. T 98.6 F. Palpated rt adnexal mass and
	enlarged uterus; vulva and cervix appear normal; LMP 7/16/XX.
	Medical decision making: mod complex
	Tx plan: Adv hospital admit and additional tests to R/O carcinoma.
	Tentatively scheduled abdominal hysterectomy with bilateral salpingo-oophorectomy.
	(M/MDM).
	BC/llf Bertha Caesar, MD
8-2-xx	Adm to College Hosp (C HX/PX M/MDM). Scheduled
	surgery at 7:00 A.M. tomorrow.
	BC/llf Bertha Caesar, MD
8-3-xx	Perf abdominal
	hysterectomy with bilateral salpingo-oophorectomy.
	BC/llf Bertha Caesar, MD
8-4-xx	HV (EPF HX/PX M/MDM) Path report revealed interstitial leiomyomata uteri and corpus
	luteum cyst of rt ovary. Pt C/O PO pain, otherwise doing well.
	BC/llf Bertha Caesar, MD
8-5-xx	HV (EPF HX/PX M/MDM). Pt ambulating well, pain decreased. Dressing changed, wound
	healing well.
	BC/llf Bertha Caesar, MD
8-6-xx	HV (PF HX/PX SF/MDM). Pain minimal. Pt ambulating without assistance.
	Removed staples, no redness or swelling. Pln DC tomorrow.
	BC/llf Bertha Caesar, MD
8-7-xx	Discharge to home; pt doing well. RTO next wk. Disability from 8-1 to 8-23-xx.
	BC/llf Bertha Caesar, MD

Fig. 1, cont'd

Acct. No. T-4

STATEMENT

COLLEGE CLINIC
4567 Broad Avenue
Woodland Hills, XY 12345-0001
Tel. 555-486-9002
Fax No. 555-487-8976

Jennifer T. Lacey
451 Roberts Street
Woodland Hills, XY 12345

Phone No. (H) (555) 549-0098 (W) (555) 540-6675 Birthdate 11-12-55

Insurance Co. American Commercial Insurance Company Policy/Group No. 5789022 / 444

DATE	REFERENCE	DESCRIPTION	CHARGES	CREDITS PYMNTS.	CREDITS ADJ.	BALANCE
20XX		BALANCE FORWARD →				
8-1-xx		Consult				
8-2-xx		Admit				
8-3-xx		TAH BSO				
8-4-xx		HV				
8-5-xx		HV				
8-6-xx		HV				
8-7-xx		Discharge				

PLEASE PAY LAST AMOUNT IN BALANCE COLUMN

THIS IS A COPY OF YOUR FINANCIAL ACCOUNT AS IT APPEARS ON OUR RECORDS

Fig. 2

TEST 5: COMPLETE A CMS-1500 CLAIM FORM

Performance Objective

Task: Complete a CMS-1500 claim form for a private case and post transactions to the patient's financial accounting record.

Conditions: Use the patient's record (Fig. 3) and financial statement (Fig. 4), one health insurance claim form, a computer or pen, procedural and diagnostic code books, and Appendixes A in this *Workbook*.

Standards: Claim Productivity Management

Time: ___________ minutes

Accuracy: ___________

(Note: The time element and accuracy criteria may be given by your instructor.)

Directions

1. Using NUCC guidelines, complete a CMS-1500 claim form and direct it to the private carrier. Refer to Hortense N. Hope's patient record for information and Appendix A in this *Workbook* to locate the fees to record on the claim, and post them to the financial statement. Date the claim July 31 of the current year. Dr. Practon is accepting assignment, and the patient's signatures to release information to the insurance company and to have the payment forwarded directly to the physician are on file.

2. Use your CPT code book to determine the correct five-digit code numbers and modifiers for each professional service rendered. Use your HCPCS Level II code book for HCPCS procedure codes and modifiers. Use your ICD-10-CM coding manual to code each active diagnosis.

3. Record the proper information on the financial record and claim form, and note the date that you billed the insurance company.

PATIENT RECORD NO. T-5

Hope	Hortense	N.	04-12-56	F	555-666-7821
LAST NAME	FIRST NAME	MIDDLE NAME	BIRTH DATE	SEX	HOME PHONE

247 Lantern Pike	Woodland Hills	XY	12345
ADDRESS	CITY	STATE	ZIP CODE

	555-323-1687	555-666-7821	hope@wb.net
CELL PHONE	PAGER NO.	FAX NO.	E-MAIL ADDRESS

321-XX-8809	N0058921
PATIENT'S SOC. SEC. NO.	DRIVER'S LICENSE

Clerk typist	R and S Manufacturing Company
PATIENT'S OCCUPATION	NAME OF COMPANY

2271 West 74 Street, Torres, XY 12349	555-466-5890
ADDRESS OF EMPLOYER	PHONE

Harry J. Hope	carpenter
SPOUSE OR PARENT	OCCUPATION

Jesse Construction Company,	3861 South Orange Street, Torres, XY 12349	555-765-2318
EMPLOYER	ADDRESS	PHONE

Ralston Insurance Company, 2611 Hanley Street, Woodland Hills, XY 12345	Hortense N. Hope
NAME OF INSURANCE	INSURED OR SUBSCRIBER

ATC321458809	T8471811A
POLICY/CERTIFICATE NO.	GROUP NO.

REFERRED BY: Harry J. Hope (husband)

DATE	PROGRESS NOTES
7-1-xx	New F pt comes in complaining of lt great toe pain. Incised, drained, and cleaned area
	around nail on lt great toe. Dx: onychia and paronychia. Started on antibiotic and adv to
	retn in 2 days for permanent excision of nail plate (EPF HX/PX SF/MDM).
	GP/llf Gerald Practon, MD
7-3-xx	Pt returns for nail excision. Injected procaine in lt great toe; removed entire toenail.
	Drs applied. PTR in 5 days for PO check.
	GP/llf Gerald Practon, MD
7-7-xx	PO check. Dressing changed, nail bed healing well. Pt to continue on AB until gone.
	Retn PRN (PF HX/PX SF/MDM).
	GP/llf Gerald Practon, MD

Fig. 3

Acct No. T-5

STATEMENT
Financial Account

COLLEGE CLINIC
4567 Broad Avenue
Woodland Hills, XY 12345-0001
Tel. 555-486-9002
Fax No. 555-487-8976

Hortense N. Hope
247 Lantern Pike
Woodland Hills, XY 12345

Phone No. (H) 555-666-7821 (W) 555-466-5890 Birthdate 4/12/56

Primary Insurance Co. Ralston Insurance Company Policy/Group No. ATC321458809 / T8471811A

Secondary Insurance Co. None Policy/Group No.

DATE	REFERENCE	DESCRIPTION	CHARGES	CREDITS PYMNTS.	CREDITS ADJ.	BALANCE
20xx		BALANCE FORWARD →				
7-1-xx		NP OV				
7-1-xx		I & D lt great toe				
7-3-xx		Excision lt great toenail				
7-7-xx		PO check				

PLEASE PAY LAST AMOUNT IN BALANCE COLUMN

THIS IS A COPY OF YOUR FINANCIAL ACCOUNT AS IT APPEARS ON OUR RECORDS

Fig. 4

TEST 6: COMPLETE A CLAIM FORM FOR A MEDICARE CASE

Performance Objective

Task: Complete a CMS-1500 claim form and post transactions to the patient's financial accounting record.

Conditions: Use the patient's record (Fig. 5) and financial statement (Fig. 6), one health insurance claim form, a computer or pen, procedural and diagnostic code books, and Appendix A in this *Workbook.*

Standards: Claim Productivity Management

Time: ____________ minutes

Accuracy: ____________

(Note: The time element and accuracy criteria may be given by your instructor.)

Directions

1. Using NUCC guidelines, complete a CMS-1500 claim form and direct it to your local Medicare Administrative Contractor. Refer to the CMS website to locate your local Medicare Administrative Contractor's address to mail the claim to. Refer to Frances F. Foote's patient record for information and Appendix A in this *Workbook* to locate the fees to record on the claim, and post them to the financial statement. Date the claim October 31 of the current year. Dr. Practon is a participating provider, and the patient's signatures to release information to the insurance company and to have the payment forwarded directly to the physician are on file.

2. Use your CPT code book to determine the correct five-digit code numbers and modifiers for each professional service rendered. Use your HCPCS Level II code book for HCPCS procedure codes and modifiers. Use your ICD-10-CM coding manual to code each active diagnosis.

3. Record the proper information on the patient's financial accounting record and claim form, and note the date that you billed the insurance company.

PATIENT RECORD NO. T-6

LAST NAME	FIRST NAME	MIDDLE NAME	BIRTH DATE	SEX	HOME PHONE
Foote	Frances	F.	08-10-32	F	555-678-0943

ADDRESS	CITY	STATE	ZIP CODE
984 North A Street	Woodland Hills	XY	12345

CELL PHONE	PAGER NO.	FAX NO.	E-MAIL ADDRESS
555-443-9908	555-320-7789	555-678-0943	foote@wb.net

PATIENT'S SOC. SEC. NO.	DRIVER'S LICENSE
578-XX-8924	B4309811

PATIENT'S OCCUPATION	NAME OF COMPANY
retired legal secretary	

ADDRESS OF EMPLOYER	PHONE

SPOUSE OR PARENT	OCCUPATION
Harry L. Foote	roofer

EMPLOYER	ADDRESS	PHONE
BDO Construction Company, 340 North 6th Street, Woodland Hills, XY 12345		555-478-9083

NAME OF INSURANCE	INSURED OR SUBSCRIBER
Medicare	self

POLICY/CERTIFICATE NO.	GROUP NO.
578-XX-8924A	

REFERRED BY: G. U. Curette, MD, 4780 Main Street, Ehrlich, XY 12350 Tel: 555-430-8788 NPI #34216600XX

DATE	PROGRESS NOTES
10-11-xx	NP pt referred by Dr. Curette with a CC of foot pain centering around rt great toe and
	sometimes shooting up her leg. PF history taken. PF exam revealed severe overgrowth
	of nail into surrounding tissues. AP and lat right foot x-rays taken & interpreted which
	indicate no fractures or arthritis. Pt has had a N workup for gout by Dr. Curette.
	DX: Severe onychocryptosis both margins of rt hallux. Adv to sched. OP surgery at
	College Hospital for wedge resection of skin of nail fold to repair ingrown nail.
	No disability from work (SF/MDM).
	NP/llf Nick Pedro, MD
10-13-xx	Pt admitted for OP surgery at College Hospital. Complete wedge resection performed for
	repair of rt hallux ingrown nail. Pt will stay off foot over the weekend and retn next wk for
	PO re ch.
	NP/llf Nick Pedro, MD
10-20-xx	PO visit (PF HX/PX SF/MDM). Rt hallux healing well. RTC as necessary.
	NP/llf Nick Pedro, MD

Fig. 5

Acct No. T-6

STATEMENT
Financial Account

COLLEGE CLINIC
4567 Broad Avenue
Woodland Hills, XY 12345-0001
Tel. 555-486-9002
Fax No. 555-487-8976

Frances F. Foote
984 North A Street
Woodland Hills, XY 12345

Phone No. (H) 555-678-0943 (W) ______ Birthdate 8/10/32

Primary Insurance Co. Medicare Policy/Group No. 578-XX-8924A

DATE	REFERENCE	DESCRIPTION	CHARGES	CREDITS		BALANCE
				PYMNTS.	ADJ.	
20xx		BALANCE FORWARD →				
10-11-xx		NP OV				
10-11-xx		X-rays				
10-13-xx		Wedge excision/skin of nail fold				
10-20-xx		PO				

PLEASE PAY LAST AMOUNT IN BALANCE COLUMN

THIS IS A COPY OF YOUR FINANCIAL ACCOUNT AS IT APPEARS ON OUR RECORDS

Fig. 6

TEST 7: COMPLETE A CLAIM FORM FOR A MEDICARE/MEDIGAP CASE

Performance Objective

Task: Complete two CMS-1500 claim forms for a Medicare/Medigap case and post transactions to the patient's financial accounting record.

Conditions: Use patient's record (Fig. 7) and financial statement (Fig. 8), two health insurance claim forms, a computer or pen, procedural and diagnostic code books, and Appendix A in this *Workbook*.

Standards: Claim Productivity Management

Time: ___________ minutes

Accuracy: ___________

(Note: The time element and accuracy criteria may be given by your instructor.)

Directions

1. Using NUCC guidelines, complete two CMS-1500 claim forms and direct them to your local Medicare Administrative Contractor. Refer to the CMS website to locate your local Medicare Administrative Contractor's address to mail the claim to. Refer to Charles B. Kamb's patient record for information and Appendix A to locate the fees to record on the claim, and post them to the financial statement. Be sure to include the Medigap information on the claim form so that it will be crossed over (sent to the Medigap insurance carrier) automatically. Date the claim June 30 of the current year. Dr. Practon is a participating provider with both Medicare and the Medigap program, and the patient's signatures to release information to the insurance companies and to have the payment forwarded directly to the physician are on file.

2. Use your CPT code book to determine the correct five-digit code numbers and modifiers for each professional service rendered. Use your HCPCS Level II code book for HCPCS procedure codes and modifiers. Use your ICD-10-CM coding manual to code each active diagnosis.

3. Record the proper information on the patient's financial accounting record and claim form, and note the date that you billed the insurance company.

PATIENT RECORD NO. T-7

LAST NAME	FIRST NAME	MIDDLE NAME	BIRTH DATE	SEX	HOME PHONE
Kamb	Charles	B.	01-26-27	M	555-467-2601

ADDRESS	CITY	STATE	ZIP CODE
2600 West Nautilus Street	Woodland Hills	XY	12345

CELL PHONE	PAGER NO.	FAX NO.	E-MAIL ADDRESS

PATIENT'S SOC. SEC. NO.	DRIVER'S LICENSE
454-XX-9569	M3200563

PATIENT'S OCCUPATION	NAME OF COMPANY
retired TV actor	Amer. Federation of TV & Radio Artists (AFTRA)

ADDRESS OF EMPLOYER	PHONE
30077 Ventura Boulevard, Woodland Hills, XY 12345	555-466-3331

SPOUSE OR PARENT	OCCUPATION
Jane C. Kamb	homemaker

EMPLOYER	ADDRESS	PHONE

NAME OF INSURANCE	INSURED OR SUBSCRIBER	
Medicare (Primary)	self	National Insurance Company (Medigap)

POLICY/CERTIFICATE NO.	GROUP NO.
454-XX-9569A	Medigap Policy No. 5789002

REFERRED BY: Mrs. O. S. Tomy (friend)

National PAYRID NAT234567

DATE	PROGRESS NOTES
6-1-xx	New pt comes into ofc to est new PCP in area; recently moved from Ohio. W obese M c/o
	nasal bleeding for two and a half months c̄ headaches and nasal congestion. Pt states he
	has had HBP for 1 yr. Taking med: Serpasil prescribed by dr in Ohio; does not know dosage.
	Took a C HX and performed a C PX which revealed post nasal hemorrhage. Coagulation
	time (Lee and White) and microhematocrit (spun) done in ofc are WNL. BP 180/100.
	Used nasal cautery and post nasal packs to control hemorrhage. Rx prophylactic antibiotic
	to guard against sinusitis NKA. Adv retn tomorrow, bring hypertensive medication.
	Pt signed authorization to request med records from dr in Ohio. D: Recurrent epistaxis
	due to nonspecific hypertension. No disability from work.
	GP/llf Gerald Practon, MD
6-2-xx	Pt retns and nasal hemorrhage is reevaluated (PF HX/PX SF/MDM). Postnasal packs
	removed and replaced. BP 182/98. Pt forgot medication for hypertension but states he is
	taking it 2 X d. Adv retn in 1 day, bring medication.
	GP/llf Gerald Practon, MD
6-3-xx	Pt retns and nasal hemorrhage is reevaluated (PF HX/PX SF/MDM). Postnasal packs
	removed. BP 178/100. Verified hypertensive medication. Pt to increase dosage to 4 X d.
	Adv retn in 5 days.
	GP/llf Gerald Practon, MD
6-8-xx	Pt retns and nasal hemorrhage is reevaluated (EPF HX/PX L/MDM). Prev medical records
	arrived and reviewed. BP 190/102. Pt referred to Dr. Perry Cardi (int) for future care of
	hypertension.
	GP/llf Gerald Practon, MD

Fig. 7

Acct No. T-7

STATEMENT
Financial Account

COLLEGE CLINIC
4567 Broad Avenue
Woodland Hills, XY 12345-0001
Tel. 555-486-9002
Fax No. 555-487-8976

Charles B. Kamb
2600 West Nautilus Street
Woodland Hills, XY 12345

Phone No. (H) 555-467-2601 (W) None/retired Birthdate 1-26-27

Primary Insurance Co. Medicare Policy/Group No. 454-XX-9569A

Secondary Insurance Co. National Insurance Company (Medigap) Policy/Group No. 5789002

DATE	REFERENCE	DESCRIPTION	CHARGES	CREDITS PYMNTS.	CREDITS ADJ.	BALANCE
20xx		BALANCE FORWARD →				
6-1-xx		NP OV				
6-1-xx		Coagulation time				
6-1-xx		Microhematocrit				
6-1-xx		Post nasal pack/cautery				
6-2-xx		OV				
6-2-xx		Subsequent nasal pack				
6-3-xx		OV				
6-8-xx		OV				

PLEASE PAY LAST AMOUNT IN BALANCE COLUMN

THIS IS A COPY OF YOUR FINANCIAL ACCOUNT AS IT APPEARS ON OUR RECORDS

Fig. 8

TEST 8: COMPLETE A CLAIM FORM FOR A MEDICAID CASE

Performance Objective

Task: Complete a CMS-1500 claim form for a Medicaid case and post transactions to the patient's financial accounting record.

Conditions: Use the patient's record (Fig. 9) and financial statement (Fig. 10), one health insurance claim form, a computer or pen, procedural and diagnostic code books, and Appendix A in this *Workbook*.

Standards: Claim Productivity Management

Time: ____________ minutes

Accuracy: ____________

(Note: The time element and accuracy criteria may be given by your instructor.)

Directions

1. Using NUCC guidelines, complete a CMS-1500 claim form and direct it to the Medicaid fiscal intermediary for your state. Refer to Louise K. Herman's patient record for information and Appendix A to locate the fees to record on the claim, and post them to the financial statement. Date the claim May 31 of the current year.
2. Use your CPT code book to determine the correct five-digit code numbers and modifiers for each professional service rendered. Use your HCPCS Level II code book for HCPCS procedure codes and modifiers. Use your ICD-10-CM coding manual to code each active diagnosis.
3. Record the proper information on the patient's financial accounting record and claim form and note the date that you billed the insurance company.
4. Post the payment of $350 (voucher number 4300), received from the Medicaid fiscal intermediary 40 days after claim submission, and write off (adjust) the balance of the account.

PATIENT RECORD NO. T-8

Herman	Louise	K.	11-04-60	F	555-266-9085
LAST NAME	FIRST NAME	MIDDLE NAME	BIRTH DATE	SEX	HOME PHONE

13453 Burbank Boulevard	Woodland Hills	XY	12345
ADDRESS	CITY	STATE	ZIP CODE

555-466-7003		555-266-9085	herman@wb.net
CELL PHONE	PAGER NO.	FAX NO.	E-MAIL ADDRESS

519-XX-0018	T0943995
PATIENT'S SOC. SEC. NO.	DRIVER'S LICENSE

unemployed budget analyst	
PATIENT'S OCCUPATION	NAME OF COMPANY

ADDRESS OF EMPLOYER	PHONE

Harold D. Herman	retired salesman
SPOUSE OR PARENT	OCCUPATION

EMPLOYER	ADDRESS	PHONE

Medicaid	self
NAME OF INSURANCE	INSURED OR SUBSCRIBER

0051936001X	
MEDICAID NO.	GROUP NO.

REFERRED BY: Raymond Skeleton, MD

DATE	PROGRESS NOTES
5-6-xx	NP pt referred by Dr. Skeleton. CC: Rectal bleeding. Took a comprehensive history and
	performed a comprehensive physical examination. Diagnostic anoscopy revealed
	bleeding int and ext hemorrhoids and 2 infected rectal polyps. Rx antibiotics. Retn in
	2 days for removal of hemorrhoids and polyps (M/MDM)
	RR/llf Rex Rumsey, MD
5-8-xx	Pt returned to office for simple internal/external hemorrhoidectomy. Rigid
	proctosigmoidoscopy also perf for removal of polyps using snare technique. Adv. sitz
	baths daily. Continue on AB until gone. Retn in 1 wk.
	RR/llf Rex Rumsey, MD
5-15-xx	DNS Telephoned pt and rescheduled.
	Mary Bright, CMA
5-17-xx	PO OV (EPF HX/PX LC/MDM). Pt progressing well. No pain, discomfort or bleeding.
	Discharged from care, retn PRN.
	RR/llf Rex Rumsey, MD

Fig. 9

Acct No. T-8

STATEMENT
Financial Account

COLLEGE CLINIC
4567 Broad Avenue
Woodland Hills, XY 12345-0001
Tel. 555-486-9002
Fax No. 555-487-8976

Louise K. Herman
13453 Burbank Boulevard
Woodland Hills, XY 12345

Phone No. (H) 555-266-9085 (W) ______ Birthdate 11/4/60

Primary Insurance Co. Medicaid Policy/Group No. 0051936001X

Secondary Insurance Co. ______ Policy/Group No. ______

DATE	REFERENCE	DESCRIPTION	CHARGES	CREDITS PYMNTS.	CREDITS ADJ.	BALANCE
20xx		BALANCE FORWARD →				
5-6-xx		NP OV				
5-6-xx		Dx anoscopy				
5-8-xx		Int/Ext Hemorrhoidectomy				
5-8-xx		Proctosigmoidoscopy with removal of polyps				
5-17-xx		PO OV				

PLEASE PAY LAST AMOUNT IN BALANCE COLUMN

THIS IS A COPY OF YOUR FINANCIAL ACCOUNT AS IT APPEARS ON OUR RECORDS

Fig. 10

TEST 9: COMPLETE A CLAIM FORM FOR A TRICARE CASE

Performance Objective

Task: Complete a CMS-1500 claim form for a TRICARE case and post transactions to the patient's financial accounting record.

Conditions: Use the patient's record (Fig. 11) and financial statement (Fig. 12), one health insurance claim form, a computer or pen, procedural and diagnostic code books, and Appendix A in this *Workbook*.

Standards: Claim Productivity Management

Time: ___________ minutes

Accuracy: ___________

(Note: The time element and accuracy criteria may be given by your instructor.)

Directions

1. Using NUCC guidelines, complete a CMS-1500 claim form and direct it to the TRICARE carrier for your area. Refer to Darlene M. Cash's patient record for information and Appendix A to locate the fees to record on the claim, and post them to the financial statement. Date the claim February 27 of the current year. Dr. Cutler is accepting assignment, and the patient's signatures to release information to the insurance company and to have the payment forwarded directly to the physician are on file.

2. Use your CPT code book to determine the correct five-digit code numbers and fees for each professional service rendered. Use your HCPCS Level II code book for HCPCS procedure codes and modifiers. Use your ICD-10-CM coding manual to code each active diagnosis.

3. Record the proper information on the patient's financial accounting record and claim form, and note the date that you billed the insurance company.

PATIENT RECORD NO. T-9

LAST NAME	FIRST NAME	MIDDLE NAME	BIRTH DATE	SEX	HOME PHONE
Cash	Darlene	M.	3-15-70	F	555-666-8901

ADDRESS	CITY	STATE	ZIP CODE
5729 Redwood Avenue	Woodland Hills	XY	12344

CELL PHONE	PAGER NO.	FAX NO.	E-MAIL ADDRESS
555-290-5400		555-666-8901	cash@wb.net

PATIENT'S SOC. SEC. NO.	DRIVER'S LICENSE
298-XX-6754	J3457789

PATIENT'S OCCUPATION	NAME OF COMPANY
teacher	City Unified School District

ADDRESS OF EMPLOYER	PHONE
Century High School, 2031 West Olympic Boulevard, Dorland, XY 12345	555-678-1076

SPOUSE OR PARENT	OCCUPATION
David F. Cash	Navy Petty Officer—Grade 8 (active status)

EMPLOYER	ADDRESS	PHONE
United States Navy	HHC, 2nd Batt, 26th Infantry, APO New York, NY, 10030	

NAME OF INSURANCE	INSURED OR SUBSCRIBER
TRICARE Standard	David Cash (DOB 4-22-70)

POLICY/CERTIFICATE NO.	GROUP NO.
767-XX-9080	

REFERRED BY: Hugh R. Foot, MD, 2010 Main St., Woodland Hills, XY 12345 NPI #61 25099XX

DATE	PROGRESS NOTES
1-4-xx	New pt, referred by Dr. Foot comes in complaining of head pain which began yesterday.
	Performed an EPF history and physical exam. Lt parietal area of skull slightly tender,
	some redness of scalp. Pain localized and not consistent with HA syndromes. Rest of
	exam N. Imp: head pain, undetermined nature, possible cyst. Apply hot compresses and
	observe. Take Ibuprofen for pain prn (200 mg up to 2 q. 4 h). Retn in 1 wk, no disability
	from work (SF/MDM).
	CC/llf Clarence Cutler, MD
1-11-xx	Pt retns and states that the hot compresses have helped but is concerned with some
	swelling in area. On exam noticed slt elevation of skin in lt parietal area of scalp, no
	warmth over area. Slt pain on palpation. Exam otherwise neg. Imp: Subcutaneous nodule.
	Continue with same tx plan: Hot compresses daily and Ibuprofen prn. Retn in 2 to 3 wks
	if not resolved (PF HX/PX SF/MDM).
	CC/llf Clarence Cutler, MD
2-3-xx	Pt retns for reexamination of parietal skull. Elevation of skin still persisting. It has now
	come to a head, is warm to the touch, and consistent with an inflammatory cystic lesion.
	A decision is made to excise the benign lesion. Scalp cyst, 1.5 cm removed under
	procaine block with knife dissection; closed wound with six #000 black silk sutures.
	Adv to retn 1 wk for removal of sutures (EPF HX/PX LC/MDM).
	CC/llf Clarence Cutler, MD
2-10-xx	Pt presents for suture removal. Sutures removed and slight oozing occurs in midsection
	of wound. Wound dressed and pt advised to apply antibacterial cream daily. Retn in 4 to
	5 days for final check (PF HX/PX SF/MDM).
	CC/llf Clarence Cutler, MD
2-15-xx	Pt presents for PO check of head wound. Parietal area healed well. RTO prn
	(PF HX/PX SF/MDM).
	CC/llf Clarence Cutler, MD

Fig. 11

Acct No. T-9

STATEMENT
Financial Account

COLLEGE CLINIC
4567 Broad Avenue
Woodland Hills, XY 12345-0001
Tel. 555-486-9002
Fax No. 555-487-8976

Darlene M. Cash
5729 Redwood Avenue
Woodland Hills, XY 12345

Phone No. (H) 555-666-8901 (W) 555-678-1076 Birthdate 3/15/70

Primary Insurance Co. TRICARE Standard Policy/Group No. 767-XX-9080

Secondary Insurance Co. ______ Policy/Group No. ______

DATE	REFERENCE	DESCRIPTION	CHARGES	CREDITS PYMNTS.	CREDITS ADJ.	BALANCE
20xx		BALANCE FORWARD →				
1-4-xx		NP OV				
1-11-xx		OV				
2-3-xx		OV				
2-3-xx		Excision inflammatory cystic scalp lesion				
2-10-xx		OV				
2-15-xx		OV				

PLEASE PAY LAST AMOUNT IN BALANCE COLUMN

THIS IS A COPY OF YOUR FINANCIAL ACCOUNT AS IT APPEARS ON OUR RECORDS

Fig. 12

TEST 10: COMPLETE TWO CLAIM FORMS FOR A PRIVATE PLAN

Performance Objective

Task: Complete two CMS-1500 claim forms for a private case and post transactions to the patient's financial accounting record.

Conditions: Use the patient's record (Fig. 13) and financial statement (Fig. 14), two health insurance claim forms, a computer or pen, procedural and diagnostic code books, and Appendix A in this *Workbook*.

Standards: Claim Productivity Management

Time: ____________ minutes

Accuracy: ____________

(Note: The time element and accuracy criteria may be given by your instructor.)

Directions

1. Using NUCC guidelines, complete two CMS-1500 claim forms and direct them to the private carrier. Refer to Gertrude C. Hamilton's patient record for information and Appendix A in this *Workbook* to locate the fees to record on the claim, and post them to the financial statement. Date the first claim August 15 and the second one October 15. Dr. Cardi is accepting assignment, and the patient's signatures to release information to the insurance company and to have the payment forwarded directly to the physician are on file.

2. Use your CPT code book to determine the correct five-digit code numbers and modifiers for each professional service rendered. Use your HCPCS Level II code book for HCPCS procedure codes and modifiers. Use your ICD-10-CM coding manual to code each active diagnosis. Frequently, surgeons wait to receive the pathology report before entering a final diagnosis on the claim form. In this case, the claim was submitted before the pathology report was received.

3. Record the proper information on the financial record and claim form, and note the date that you billed the insurance company.

4. Mrs. Hamilton makes a payment of $200, check number 5362, on her account on October 26. Post the proper entry for this transaction.

PATIENT RECORD NO. T-10

LAST NAME	Hamilton
FIRST NAME	Gertrude
MIDDLE NAME	C.
BIRTH DATE	03-06-57
SEX	F
HOME PHONE	555-798-3321
ADDRESS	5320 Phillips Street
CITY	Woodland Hills
STATE	XY
ZIP CODE	12345
CELL PHONE	555-399-4990
PAGER NO.	555-312-6677
FAX NO.	555-798-3321
E-MAIL ADDRESS	hamilton@wb.net
PATIENT'S SOC. SEC. NO.	540-XX-7677
DRIVER'S LICENSE	D9043557
PATIENT'S OCCUPATION	retired secretary
NAME OF COMPANY	
ADDRESS OF EMPLOYER	
PHONE	
SPOUSE OR PARENT	deceased
OCCUPATION	
EMPLOYER	
ADDRESS	
PHONE	
NAME OF INSURANCE	Colonial Health Insurance, 1011 Main Street, Woodland Hills, XY 12345
INSURED OR SUBSCRIBER	self
POLICY/CERTIFICATE NO.	540XX7677
GROUP NO.	4566 (through previous employment)

REFERRED BY: Gerald Practon, MD, 4567 Broad Avenue, Woodland Hills, XY 12345

Fig. 13

DATE	PROGRESS NOTES No. T-10
7-29-xx	Dr. Practon asked me to consult on this 57-year-old pt adm to College Hosp today.
	Duplex carotid ultrasonography indicates bilateral carotid stenosis. C/HX: Suffered CVA lt
	hemisphere 1 yr prior to adm. Marked rt arm & leg weakness c̄ weakness of rt face and
	slurring of speech. C/PE revealed lt carotid bruit, II/IV, & right carotid bruit, II/IV.
	Performed hand-held Doppler vascular study on bilateral carotids which indicated
	decreased blood flow. Adv brain scan and lt carotid thromboendarterectomy; rt carotid
	thromboendarterectomy at a later date H/MDM.
	PC/llf Perry Cardi, MD
7-30-xx	HV (EPF HX/PX MC/MDM). Dr. Practon asked me to take over pt's care. Pt had brain scan
	done today, ECG, and lab work.
	PC/llf Perry Cardi, MD
7-31-xx	HV (EPF HX/PX MC/MDM). Brain scan indicates prior CVA; no new findings. ECG, normal
	sinus rhythm with occasional premature ventricular contractions. Lab work WNL.
	Discussed test results with Mrs. Hamilton.
	PC/llf Perry Cardi, MD
8-1-xx	HV (PF HX/PX LC/MDM). Decision made for surgery, to be scheduled tomorrow.
	PC/llf Perry Cardi, MD
8-2-xx	Pt taken to the operative suite. Performed lt carotid thromboendarterectomy by neck
	incision (see op report). Surgery went as planned, pt in recovery.
	PC/llf Perry Cardi, MD
8-3-xx	HV (PF HX/PX SF/MDM). Operative site appears normal. Pt resting comfortably.
	PC/llf Perry Cardi, MD
8-4-xx	DC from hosp. Pt to be seen in ofc in 1 week.
	PC/llf Perry Cardi, MD
8-12-xx	PO OV (D HX/PX M/MDM). Discussed outcome of surgery. Pt making satisfactory
	progress. Adv rt carotid thromboendarterectomy. Pt would like it done as soon as possible;
	next month if there is an operative time. Scheduled surgery for September 16, 20XX at
	College Hospital.
	PC/llf Perry Cardi, MD
9-16-xx	Adm to College Hospital. Performed a D history, D physical examination, and SF medical
	decision making. Rt carotid thromboendarterectomy performed by neck incision.
	DX: Rt carotid stenosis.
	PC/llf Perry Cardi, MD
9-17-xx	HV (PF HX/PX SF/MDM). Pt stable and doing well. Operative site looks good. Plan for
	discharge tomorrow.
	PC/llf Perry Cardi, MD
9-18-xx	DC from hosp to home. RTC 1 wk.
	PC/llf Perry Cardi, MD
9-25-xx	PO visit (PF HX/PX SF/MDM). Pt making satisfactory recovery. Her neighbor will monitor
	BP daily. Retn 1 month.
	PC/llf Perry Cardi, MD

Fig. 13, cont'd

STATEMENT

Acct No. T-10

COLLEGE CLINIC
4567 Broad Avenue
Woodland Hills, XY 12345-0001
Tel. 555-486-9002
Fax No. 555-487-8976

Gertrude C. Hamilton
5320 Phillips Street
Woodland Hills, XY 12345

Phone No. (H) (555) 798-3321 (W) ______ Birthdate 03-06-57

Insurance Co Colonial Health Insurance Policy/Group No. 540Xx7677 / 4566

	REFERENCE	DESCRIPTION	CHARGES	CREDITS PYMNTS.	CREDITS ADJ.	BALANCE
20xx					BALANCE FORWARD →	
7-29-xx		Inpatient consult				
7-30-xx		HV				
7-31-xx		HV				
8-1-xx		HV				
8-2-xx		L carotid thromboendarterectomy				
8-3-xx		HV				
8-4-xx		Discharge				
8-12-xx		PO OV				
9-16-xx		Admit				
9-16-xx		R carotid thromboendarterectomy				
9-17-xx		HV				
9-18-xx		Discharge				
9-25-xx		PO OV				

PLEASE PAY LAST AMOUNT IN BALANCE COLUMN

THIS IS A COPY OF YOUR FINANCIAL ACCOUNT AS IT APPEARS ON OUR RECORDS

Fig. 14

A College Clinic Office Policies and Mock Fee Schedule

College Clinic

In this simulation, you are employed as an insurance billing specialist for a group of medical doctors, other allied health specialists, and podiatrists. Each clinic is configured in its own way. The College Clinic has staff physicians who are employed, receive monthly pay checks, and are given Wage and Tax Statements (Form W-2) at the end of the tax year. These doctors are on the staff of a nearby hospital, College Hospital.

Medical practices can have different configurations. For example, individuals or groups can be incorporated. Physicians can be independent contractors, running their own practices outside of the clinic; receive payment by the job and not a salary; and receive a Form 1099 at the end of the tax year.

Reference information to complete insurance claim forms for each assignment follows. Claim forms are to be submitted for the group unless a case involves a physician working as an independent contractor.

Office address:
College Clinic
4567 Broad Avenue
Woodland Hills, XY 12345-0001
Telephone: 555-486-9002
FAX: 555-487-8976
Clinic e-mail: cclinic@cmail.net
Staff e-mail: insert physician's last name followed by a period (.) then cclinic@cmail.net
(example: Pedro Atrics, MD, would have an e-mail address of atrics.cclinic@cmail.net
Group practice, National Provider Identifier (NPI): 3664021CC
Medicare durable medical equipment (DME) supplier number: 3400760001
Group tax ID #: XX12210XX

Hospital address:
College Hospital
4500 Broad Avenue
Woodland Hills, XY 12345-0001
Telephone: 555-487-6789
FAX: 555-486-8900
Hospital NPI: X950731067

College Clinic Staff

Patient records in this *Workbook* include the doctors' names, specialties, subspecialties, and physicians' identification numbers of the College Clinic staff. They are shown in Table 1.

Table 1. College Clinic Staff

Name	Specialty (Abbreviation)	Social Security No.[a]	State License No.	EIN No. or Federal Tax Identification No.	Medicare CMS-Assigned National Provider Identifier (NPI)[b]
Concha Antrum, MD	Otolaryngologist (OTO) or Ear, Nose, and Throat Specialist (ENT)	082–XX–1707	C 01602X	74–10640XX	12458977XX
Pedro Atrics, MD	Pediatrician (PD)	134–XX–7600	D 06012X	71–32061XX	37640017XX
Bertha Caesar, MD	Obstetrician and Gynecologist (OBG)	230–XX–6700	A 01817X	72–57130XX	43056757XX
Perry Cardi, MD	Internist (I) Subspecialty: Cardiovascular Disease (CD)	557–XX–9980	C 02140X	70–64217XX	67805027XX
Brady Coccidioides, MD	Internist (I) Subspecialty: Pulmonary Disease (PUD)	670–XX–0874	C 04821X	75–67321XX	64211067XX
Vera Cutis, MD	Dermatologist (D)	409–XX–8620	C 06002X	71–80561XX	70568717XX
Clarence Cutler, MD	General Surgeon (GS)	410–XX–5630	B 07600X	71–57372XX	43050047XX
Max Glutens, RPT	Physical Therapist (PT)	507–XX–4300	87610X	79–36500XX	65132277XX
Cosmo Graff, MD	Plastic Surgeon (PS)	452–XX–9899	C 08104X	74–60789XX	50307117XX
Malvern Grumose, MD	Pathologist (Path)	470–XX–2301	A 01602X	72–73651XX	
Gaston Input, MD	Internist (I) Subspecialty: Gastroenterologist (GE)	211–XX–6734	C 08001X	75–67210XX	32783127XX
Adam Langerhans, MD	Endocrinologist	447–XX–6720	C 06051X	60–57831XX	47680657XX
Cornell Lenser, MD	Ophthalmologist (OPH)	322–XX–8963	C 06046X	61–78941XX	54037217XX
Michael Menter, MD	Psychiatrist (P)	210–XX–5302	C 07140X	73–66577XX	67301237XX
Astro Parkinson, MD	Neurosurgeon (NS)	210–XX–8533	C 02600X	75–44530XX	46789377XX
Nick Pedro, DPM	Podiatrist	233–XX–4300	E 08340X	62–74109XX	54022287XX
Gerald Practon, MD	General Practitioner (GP) or Family Practitioner (FP)	123–XX–6789	C 01402X	70–34597XX	46278897XX
Walter Radon, MD	Radiologist (R)	344–XX–6540	C 05001X	95–46137XX	40037227XX
Rex Rumsey, MD	Proctologist (Proct)	337–XX–9743	C 03042X	95–32601XX	01999047XX
Sensitive E. Scott, MD	Anesthesiologist (Anes)	220–XX–5655	C 02041X	72–54203XX	99999267XX
Raymond Skeleton, MD	Orthopedist (ORS, Orthop)	432–XX–4589	C 04561X	74–65412XX	12678547XX
Gene Ulibarri, MD	Urologist (U)	990–XX–3245	C 06430X	77–86531XX	25678831XX

[a]Social Security numbers are shown in the table because each individual is issued one and this is a realistic picture because they would be on file.
[b]Providers began using the NPI on May 23, 2007, except for small health plans, whose compliance date was May 23, 2008.

Abbreviations and Symbols

Abbreviations and symbols may appear on patient records, prescriptions, hospital charts, and patient ledger cards. Abbreviation styles differ, but the current trend is to omit periods in capital letter abbreviations except for doctors' academic degrees. Following is a list of abbreviations and symbols used in this *Workbook* and their meanings.

Abbreviations

A allergy
AB antibiotics
Abdom abdomen
abt about
a.c. before meals
Adj[a] adjustment
adm admit; admission; admitted
adv advise(d)
aet at the age of
agit shake or stir
$AgNO_3$ silver nitrate
ALL allergy
AM, a.m. ante meridiem (time—before noon)
ant anterior
ante before
AP anterior-posterior; anteroposterior
approx approximate
appt appointment
apt apartment
ASA acetylsalicylic acid (aspirin)
ASAP as soon as possible
ASCVD arteriosclerotic cardiovascular disease
ASHD arteriosclerotic heart disease
asst assistant
auto automated, automobile
AV atrioventricular
Ba barium (enema)
Bal/fwd[a] balance forward
BE barium enema
B/F[a] balance forward; brought forward
b.i.d. two times daily
BM bowel movement
BMR basal metabolic rate
BP blood pressure
Brev Brevital sodium
BX, bx biopsy
C cervical (vertebrae); comprehensive (history/examination)
Ca, CA cancer, carcinoma
c/a[a] cash on account
CABG coronary artery bypass graft
CAT computed axial tomography
cau Caucasian
CBC complete blood count
CBS chronic brain syndrome
cc cubic centimeter
CC chief complaint
chr chronic
ck[a] check
cm centimeter
CO, c/o complains of; care of
compl, comp complete; comprehensive
Con, CON, Cons consultation
Cont continue
CPX complete physical examination
C&R compromise and release
Cr[a] credit
C&S culture and sensitivity
cs, CS[a] cash on account
C-section cesarean section
CT computed or computerized tomography
CVA cardiovascular accident; cerebrovascular accident
CXR chest radiograph
cysto cystoscopy
D, d diagnosis; detailed (history/examination); day(s)
D&C dilatation and curettage
dc discontinue
DC discharge
DDS Doctor of Dental Surgery
def[a] charge deferred
Del delivery; obstetrics and gynecology
Dg diagnosis
dia diameter
diag diagnosis; diagnostic
dil dilate (stretch, expand)
Disch discharge
DM diabetes mellitus
DNA does not apply
DNS did not show
DPM Doctor of Podiatric Medicine
DPT diphtheria, pertussis, and tetanus
Dr Doctor
Dr[a] debit
DRG diagnosis-related group
Drs dressing
DUB dysfunctional uterine bleeding
Dx diagnosis
E emergency
EC[a] error corrected
ECG, EKG electrocardiogram; electrocardiograph
echo echocardiogram; echocardiography
ED emergency department
EDC estimated date of confinement
EEG electroencephalograph

[a]Bookkeeping abbreviation.

EENT	eye, ear, nose, and throat
EGD	esophagogastroduodenoscopy
EKG, ECG	electrocardiogram; electrocardiograph
E/M	Evaluation and Management (*Current Procedural Terminology* code)
EMG	electromyogram
EPF	expanded problem-focused (history/examination)
epith	epithelial
ER	emergency room
Er, ER[a]	error corrected
ESR	erythrocyte sedimentation rate
est	established (patient); estimated
Ex, exam	examination
exc	excision
Ex MO[a]	express money order
ext	external
24F, 28F	French (size of catheter)
F	female
FBS	fasting blood sugar
FH	family history
ft	foot, feet
FU	follow-up (examination)
fwd[a]	forward
Fx	fracture
gb, GB	gallbladder
GGE	generalized glandular enlargement
GI	gastrointestinal
Grav, grav	gravida, a pregnant woman; used with Roman numerals (I, II, III) to indicate the number of pregnancies
GU	genitourinary
H	hospital call
HA	headache
HBP	high blood pressure
HC	hospital call or consultation; high-complexity (decision making)
HCD	house call (day)
HCN	house call (night)
Hct	hematocrit
HCVD	hypertensive cardiovascular disease
Hgb	hemoglobin
hist	history
hosp	hospital
H&P	history and physical (examination)
hr, hrs	hour, hours
h.s.	before bedtime
HS	hospital surgery
Ht	height
HV	hospital visit
HX, hx	history
HX PX	history and physical examination
I	injection
IC	initial consultation
I&D	incision and drainage
I/f[a]	in full
IM	intramuscular (injection)
imp, imp.	impression (diagnosis)
incl.	include; including
inflam	inflammation
init	initial (office visit)
inj, INJ	injection
ins, INS[a]	insurance
int	internal
intermed	intermediate (office visit)
interpret	interpretation
IUD	intrauterine device
IV	intravenous (injection)
IVP	intravenous pyelogram
K 35	Kolman (instrument used in urology)
KUB	kidneys, ureters, and bladder
L	left; laboratory
lab, LAB	laboratory
lat	lateral; pertaining to the side
lbs	pounds
LC	low-complexity (decision making)
LMP	last menstrual period
LS	lumbosacral
lt	left
ltd	limited (office visit)
L & W	living and well
M	medication; married
MC	moderate-complexity (decision making)
MDM	medical decision making
med	medicine
mg	milligram(s)
mg/dL	milligrams per deciliter
MI	myocardial infarction
micro	microscopy
mL, ml	milliliter
mo	month(s)
MO[a]	money order
N	negative
NA	not applicable
NAD	no appreciable disease
NC, N/C[a]	no charge
NEC	not elsewhere classifiable
neg	negative
NKA	no known allergies
NOS	not otherwise specified
NP	new patient
NYD	not yet diagnosed
OB, Ob-Gyn	obstetrics and gynecology
OC	office call
occ	occasional
OD	right eye

[a]Bookkeeping abbreviation.

ofc	office
OP	outpatient
Op, op	operation
OR	operating room
orig	original
OS	office surgery; left eye
OV	office visit
oz	ounce
PA	posterior-anterior; posteroanterior
Pap	Papanicolaou (smear, stain, test)
Para I	woman having borne one child
PC	present complaint
p.c.	after meals
PCP	primary care physician
PD	permanent disability
Pd, PD[a]	professional discount
PE	physical examination
perf	performed
PF	problem-focused (history/examination)
PFT	pulmonary function test
PH	past history
Ph ex	physical examination
phys	physical
PID	pelvic inflammatory disease
PM, p.m.	post meridiem (time—after noon)
PND	postnasal drip
PO, P Op	postoperative
p.o.	by mouth (per os)
post	posterior
postop	postoperative
PPD	purified protein derivative (such as in tuberculin test)
preop	preoperative
prep	prepared
PRN, p.r.n.	as necessary (pro re nata)
Proc	procedure
Prog	prognosis
P & S	permanent and stationary
PSA	prostate-specific antigen (blood test to determine cancer in prostate gland)
Pt, pt	patient
PT	physical therapy
PTR	patient to return
PVC	premature ventricular contraction
PVT ck[a]	private check received
PX	physical examination
q	every
qd	one time daily, every day
qh	every hour
q.i.d.	four times daily
QNS	quantity not sufficient
qod	every other day
R	right; residence call; report
RBC, rbc	red blood cell (count)
rec	recommend
rec'd	received
re ch	recheck
re-exam	reexamination
Reg	regular
ret, retn, rtn	return
rev	review
RHD	rheumatic heart disease
RN	registered nurse
R/O	rule out
ROA[a]	received on account
RPT	registered physical therapist
rt	right
RTC	return to clinic
RTO	return to office
RTW	return to work
RX, Rx, Rx	prescribe; prescription; any medication or treatment ordered
S	surgery
SC	subcutaneous
sched.	scheduled
SD	state disability
SE	special examination
SF	straightforward (decision making)
Sig	directions on prescription
SLR	straight leg raising
slt	slight
Smr	smear
SOB	shortness of breath
Sp gr	specific gravity
SQ	subcutaneous (injection)
STAT	immediately
strep	*Streptococcus*
surg	surgery
Sx	symptom(s)
T	temperature
T&A	tonsillectomy and adenoidectomy
Tb, tb	tuberculosis
TD	temporary disability
tech	technician
temp	temperature
tet. tox.	tetanus toxoid
t.i.d.	three times daily
TPR	temperature, pulse, and respiration
Tr, trt	treatment
TURB	transurethral resection of bladder
TURP	transurethral resection of prostate
TX	treatment
u	units
UA, ua	urinalysis
UCHD	usual childhood diseases
UCR	usual, customary, and reasonable (fees)

[a]Bookkeeping abbreviation.

UGI	upper gastrointestinal
UPJ	ureteropelvic junction or joint
UR	urinalysis
URI	upper respiratory infection
Urn	urinalysis
UTI	urinary tract infection
W	work; white
WBC, wbc	white blood cell (count); well baby care
WC	workers' compensation
wk	week; work
wks	weeks
WNL	within normal limits
Wr	Wassermann reaction (test for syphilis)
Wt, wt	weight
X	xray, x-ray(s), times (e.g., 3X means three times)
XR	xray, x-ray(s)
yr(s)	year(s)

Symbols	
+	positive
#	pound(s)
c̄, /c	with
s̄, /s	without
c̄c, c̄/c	with correction (eye glasses)
s̄c, s̄/c	without correction (eye glasses)
-	negative
0̄	negative
!, +	positive
(L)	left
(R)	right
♂	male
♀	female
–[a]	charge already made
⊖[a]	no balance due
√[a]	posted
($0.00) [a]	credit

Laboratory Abbreviations

ABG	arterial blood gas(es)
AcG	factor V (AcG or proaccelerin); a factor in coagulation that converts prothrombin to thrombin
ACTH	adrenocorticotropic hormone
A/C ratio	albumin-coagulin ratio
AFB	acid-fast bacilli
AHB	alpha-hydroxybutyric (dehydrogenase)
AHG	antihemophilic globulin; antihemolytic globulin (factor)
ALA	aminolevulinic acid
ALT	alanine aminotransferase (*see* SGPT)
AMP	adenosine monophosphate
APT test	aluminum-precipitated toxoid test
AST	aspartate aminotransferase (*see* SGOT)
ATP	adenosine triphosphate
BSP	bromosulfophthalein (bromsulphalein; sodium sulfobromophthalein) (test)
BUN	blood urea nitrogen
CBC	complete blood count
CNS	central nervous system
CO	carbon monoxide
CPB	competitive protein binding: plasma
CPK	creatine phosphokinase
CSF	cerebrospinal fluid
D hemoglobin	hemoglobin fractionation by electrophoresis for hemoglobin D
DAP	direct agglutination pregnancy (Gravindex and DAP)
DEAE	diethylaminoethanol
DHT	dihydrotestosterone
diff	differential
DNA	deoxyribonucleic acid
DRT	test for syphilis
EACA	epsilon-aminocaproic acid (a fibrinolysin)
EMIT	enzyme-multiplied immunoassay technique (for drugs)
ENA	extractable nuclear antigen

[a]Bookkeeping abbreviation.

esr, ESR	erythrocyte sedimentation (sed) rate
FDP	fibrin degradation products
FIGLU	formiminoglutamic acid
FRAT	free radical assay technique (for drugs)
FSH	follicle-stimulating hormone
FSP	fibrinogen split products
FTA	fluorescent-absorbed treponema antibodies
Gc, Gm, Inv	immunoglobulin typing
GG, gamma G, A, D, G, M	gamma-globulin (immunoglobulin fractionation by electrophoresis)
GG, gamma G E, RIA	immunization E fractionation by radioimmunoassay
GGT	gamma-glutamyl transpeptidase
GLC	gas liquid chromatography
GMP	guanosine monophosphate
GTT	glucose tolerance test
G6PD	glucose-6-phosphate dehydrogenase
HAA	hepatitis-associated agent (antigen)
HBD, HBDH	hydroxybutyrate dehydrogenase
HCT	hematocrit
hemoglobin, electrophoresis	letters of the alphabet used for different types or factors of hemoglobins (includes A_2, S, C, etc.)
Hgb	hemoglobin, qualitative
HGH	human growth hormone
HI	hemagglutination inhibition
HIA	hemagglutination inhibition antibody
HIAA	hydroxyindoleacetic acid (urine), 24-hour specimen
HIV	human immunodeficiency virus
HLA	human leukocyte antigen (tissue typing)
HPL	human placental lactogen
HTLV-III	antibody detection; confirmatory test
HVA	homovanillic acid
ICSH	interstitial cell-stimulating hormone
IFA	intrinsic factor, antibody (fluorescent screen)
IgA, IgE, IgG, IgM	immunoglobulins: quantitative by gel diffusion
INH	isonicotinic hydrazide, isoniazid
LAP	leucine aminopeptidase
LATS	long-acting thyroid-stimulating (hormone)
LDH	lactic dehydrogenase
LE Prep	lupus erythematosus cell preparation
L.E. factor	antinuclear antibody
LH	luteinizing hormone
LSD	lysergic acid diethylamide
L/S ratio	lecithin-sphingomyelin ratio
MC *(Streptococcus)*	antibody titer
MIC	minimum inhibitory concentration
NBT	nitro-blue tetrazolium (test)
OCT	ornithine carbamoyltransferase
PAH	para-aminohippuric acid
PBI	protein-bound iodine
pCO_2	arterial carbon dioxide pressure (or tension)
PCP	phencyclidine piperidine
pcv	packed cell volume
pH	symbol for expression of concentration of hydrogen ions (degree of acidity)
PHA	phenylalanine

PIT	prothrombin inhibition test
PKU	phenylketonuria—a metabolic disease affecting mental development
PO_2	oxygen pressure
P&P	prothrombin-proconvertin
PSP	phenolsulfonphthalein
PT	prothrombin time
PTA	plasma thromboplastin antecedent
PTC	plasma thromboplastin component; phenylthiocarbamide
PTT	prothrombin time; partial thromboplastin time (plasma or whole blood)
RBC, rbc	red blood cells (count)
RIA	radioimmunoassay
RISA	radioiodinated human serum albumin
RIST	radioimmunosorbent test
RPR	rapid plasma reagin (test)
RT_3U	resin triiodothyronine uptake
S-D	strength-duration (curve)
SGOT	serum glutamic oxaloacetic transaminase (*see* AST)
SGPT	serum glutamic pyruvic transaminase (*see* ALT)
STS	serologic test for syphilis
T_3	triiodothyronine (uptake)
TB	tubercle bacillus, tuberculosis
TBG	thyroxine-binding globulin
T&B differentiation, lymphocytes	thymus-dependent lymphs and bursa-dependent lymphs
THC	tetrahydrocannabinol (marijuana)
TIBC	total iron-binding capacity, chemical
TLC screen	thin-layer chromatography screen
TRP	tubular reabsorption of phosphates
UA	urinalysis
VDRL	Venereal Disease Research Laboratory (agglutination test for syphilis)
VMA	vanillylmandelic acid
WBC, wbc	white blood cells (count)

Mock Fee Schedule

Refer to the Mock Fee Schedule (Table 2) to complete the financial accounting statements (ledgers) and claim forms in this *Workbook*. The fees listed are hypothetical and are intended only for use in completing the questions. For the cases that are private, Medicaid, TRICARE, and workers' compensation, use the amounts in the column labeled Mock Fees. For Medicare cases, refer to the three columns pertaining to Medicare and use the amounts in the column labeled Limiting Charge. Follow these instructions unless your instructor wishes you to round out the amounts on the fee schedule to the next dollar.

In a real medical practice, some offices round out the amounts to the next dollar unless the physician is nonparticipating with Medicare, and then according to Medicare regulations, the provider can only bill the exact limiting amount on nonassigned claims. Other offices may have two fee schedules. Schedule B is for Medicare participating physicians, and amounts are listed in dollars and cents. Schedule A is used for other plans, and the amounts are rounded to the next dollar. However, if a fee schedule is sent by the insurance plan, then the medical practice may use the dollars and cents provided.

When completing the insurance claim forms, use the latest edition of *Current Procedural Terminology* (CPT), the professional code book published by the American Medical Association, to find the correct code numbers and modifiers for the services rendered. The Mock Fee Schedule (Table 2) is arranged in the same sequence as the six CPT code book sections (i.e., Evaluation and Management; Anesthesia; Surgery; Radiology, Nuclear Medicine, and Diagnostic Ultrasound; Pathology and Laboratory; and Medicine).

Table 2. Mock Fee Schedule

Code No.	Description	Mock Fees	Medicare[a] Participating	Medicare[a] Nonparticipating	Medicare[a] Limiting Charge	Follow-Up Days
EVALUATION AND MANAGEMENT[b]						
Office						
New Patient						
99201	Level 1 Problem Focused	33.25	30.43	28.91	33.25	
99202	Level 2 Expanded Prob Foc	51.91	47.52	45.14	51.91	
99203	Level 3 Detailed	70.92	64.92	61.67	70.92	
99204	Level 4 Comprehensive	106.11	97.13	92.27	106.11	
99205	Level 5 Comprehensive	132.28	121.08	115.03	132.28	
Established Patient						
99211	Level 1 Nurse Visit	16.07	14.70	13.97	16.07	
99212	Level 2 Problem Focused	28.55	26.14	24.83	28.55	
99213	Level 3 Expanded Prob Foc	40.20	36.80	34.96	40.20	
99214	Level 4 Comprehensive	61.51	56.31	53.79	61.51	
99215	Level 5 Comprehensive	96.97	88.76	84.32	96.97	
Hospital						
Observation Services (new or established patient)						
99217	Observation Care Dischg	66.88	61.22	58.16	66.88	
99218	Dhx/exam SF/LC MDM	74.22	67.94	64.54	74.22	
99219	Chx/exam MC MDM	117.75	107.78	102.39	117.75	
99220	Chx/exam HC MDM	147.48	134.99	128.24	147.48	
Inpatient Services (new or established patient)						
99221	30 min Dhx, Dpx, SF or low MDM	73.00	66.84	63.48	73.00	
99222	50 min Comp/Comp/Moderate	120.80	110.57	105.04	120.80	
99223	70 min Comp/Comp/High MDM	152.98	140.03	133.03	152.98	
Subsequent Hospital Care						
99231	15 min PF, PF, SF MDM	37.74	34.55	32.82	37.74	
99232	25 min EPF, EPF, Moderate	50.85	48.31	55.56		

[a]Some services and procedures may not be considered a benefit under the Medicare program and when listed on a claim form, no reimbursement may be received. However, it is important to include these codes when billing because Medicare policies may change without an individual knowing of a new benefit. For this reason, some of the services shown in this Mock Fee Schedule do not have any amounts listed under the three Medicare columns.

[b]Mock fees for laboratory tests presented in this schedule may not be representative of fees in your region because of the variety of capitation and managed care contracts, as well as discount policies made by laboratories. At the time of this edition, Medicare guidelines may or may not pay for automatic multichannel tests where a large number of tests are performed per panel. Some cases require documentation and a related diagnostic code for each test performed. Provider must have the CLIA level of licensure to bill for tests, and test results must be documented.

Continued

Table 2. Mock Fee Schedule—cont'd

Code No.	Description	Mock Fees	Medicare[a] Participating	Medicare[a] Nonparticipating	Medicare[a] Limiting Charge	Follow-Up Days
99233	35 min D, D, HC MDM	76.97	70.45	66.93	76.97	
99238	Discharge <30 min	65.26	59.74	56.75	65.26	
99239	Discharge >30 min					
Consultations						
Office (new or established patient)						
99241	Level 1 PF, PF, SF	51.93				
99242	Level 2 EPF, EPF, SF	80.24				
99243	Level 3 D, D, LC MDM	103.51				
99244	Level 4 C, C, Moderate MDM	145.05				
99245	Level 5 C, C, HC MDM	195.45				
Inpatient (new or established patient)						
99251	Level 1 PF, PF, SF	53.29				
99252	Level 2 EPF, EPF, SF	80.56				
99253	Level 3 D, D, LC MDM	106.10				
99254	Level 4 C, C, Moderate MDM	145.26				
99255	Level 5 C, C, HC MDM	196.55				
Emergency Department (new/established patient)						
99281	PF hx/exam SF MDM	24.32	22.26	21.15	24.32	
99282	EPF hx/exam LC MDM	37.02	33.88	32.19	37.02	
99283	EPF hx/exam MC MDM	66.23	60.62	57.59	66.23	
99284	D hx/exam MC MDM	100.71	92.18	87.57	100.71	
99285	C hx/exam HC MDM	158.86	145.41	138.14	158.86	
Critical Care Services						
99291	First hour	208.91	191.22	181.66	208.91	
99292	Each addl. 30 min	102.02	92.46	87.84	102.02	
Neonatal Intensive Care						
99468	Initial	892.74	817.16	776.30	892.74	
99469	Subsequent unstable case	418.73	383.27	364.11	418.73	
Initial Nursing Facility						
99304	25 min (Low Severity)	64.11	58.68	55.75	64.11	
99305	35 min (Moderate Severity)	90.55	82.88	78.74	90.55	
99306	45 min (High Severity)	136.76	125.18	118.92	136.76	
Subsequent Nursing Facility Care						
99307	PF hx/exam SF DM	37.95	34.74	33.00	37.95	
99308	15 min EPF hx/exam LC DM	55.11	50.44	47.92	55.11	
99309	25 min D hx/exam MC DM	69.61	63.72	60.53	69.61	
99310	35 min C hx/exam HC DM	84.73	77.00	73.14	84.73	
Domiciliary, Rest Home, Custodial Care						
New Patient						
99324	PF hx/exam SF DM	46.10	42.20	40.09	46.10	
99325	EPF hx/exam LC DM	65.02	59.53	56.54	65.02	
99326	D hx/exam MC DM	86.18	78.88	74.94	86.18	
99327	C hx/exam MC DM	107.34	98.23	93.34	107.34	
99328	C hx/exam HC DM	128.50	117.58	111.74	128.50	
Established Patient						
99334	PF hx/exam SF MDM	37.31	34.15	32.44	37.31	
99335	EPF hx/exam LC MDM	49.22	45.05	42.80	49.22	
99336	D hx/exam Moderate MDM	60.61	55.47	52.70	60.61	
99337	C hx/exam M-H DM	72.00	65.89	62.60	72.00	

[a]Some services and procedures may not be considered a benefit under the Medicare program and when listed on a claim form, no reimbursement may be received. However, it is important to include these codes when billing because Medicare policies may change without an individual knowing of a new benefit. For this reason, some of the services shown in this Mock Fee Schedule do not have any amounts listed under the three Medicare columns.

Table 2. Mock Fee Schedule—cont'd

Code No.	Description	Mock Fees	Medicare[a] Participating	Medicare[a] Nonparticipating	Medicare[a] Limiting Charge	Follow-Up Days
Home Services						
New Patient						
99341	PF hx/exam SF DM	70.32	64.37	61.15	70.32	
99342	EPF hx/exam LC DM	91.85	84.07	79.87	91.85	
99343	D hx/exam MC DM	120.24	110.06	104.56	120.24	
99344	C hx/exam MC DM	148.63	136.05	129.25	148.63	
99345	C hx/exam HC DM	177.02	162.04	153.50	177.02	
Established Patient						
99347	PF hx/exam SF DM	54.83	50.19	47.68	54.83	
99348	EPF hx/exam LC DM	70.06	64.13	60.92	70.06	
99349	D hx/exam MC DM	88.33	80.85	76.81	88.33	
99350	C hx/exam M-H DM	106.60	97.57	92.70	106.60	
Prolonged Services With Direct (Face-to-Face) Patient Contact (Report in Addition to the Designated E/M Service at Any Level)						
Outpatient						
99354	First hour	96.97	88.76	84.32	96.97	
99355	Each addl. 30 min	96.97	88.76	84.32	96.97	
Inpatient						
99356	First hour	96.42	88.25	83.84	96.42	
99357	Each addl. 30 min	96.42	88.25	83.84	96.42	
Prolonged Services Without Direct Contact						
99358	First hour	90.00				
99359	Each addl. 30 min	90.00				
Physician Standby Service						
99360	Each 30 min	95.00				
Case Management Services						
Team Conferences						
99366		85.00				
99367-99368		105.00				
Telephone Calls						
99441	5–10 min	30.00				
99442	11–20 min	40.00				
99443	21–30 min	60.00				
Care Plan Oversight Services						
99375	30 min or more/month	93.40	85.49	81.22	93.40	
Preventive Medicine						
New Patient						
99381	Infant younger than 1 year	50.00				
99382	1–4 years	50.00				
99383	5–11 years	45.00				
99384	12–17 years	45.00				
99385	18–39 years	50.00				
99386	40–64 years	50.00				
99387	65 years and older	55.00				
Established Patient						
99391	Infant younger than year	35.00				
99392	1–4 years	35.00				

[a]Some services and procedures may not be considered a benefit under the Medicare program and when listed on a claim form, no reimbursement may be received. However, it is important to include these codes when billing because Medicare policies may change without an individual knowing of a new benefit. For this reason, some of the services shown in this Mock Fee Schedule do not have any amounts listed under the three Medicare columns.

Continued

Table 2. Mock Fee Schedule—cont'd						
			Medicare[a]			
Code No.	Description	Mock Fees	Participating	Nonparticipating	Limiting Charge	Follow-Up Days
99393	5–11 years	30.00				
99394	12–17 years	30.00				
99395	18–39 years	35.00				
99396	40–64 years	35.00				
99397	65 years and older	40.00				
Counseling (new/est pt)						
Individual						
99401	15 min	35.00				
99402	30 min	50.00				
99403	45 min	65.00				
99404	60 min	80.00				
Group						
99411	30 min	30.00				
99412	60 min	50.00				
Other Preventive Medicine Services						
99420	Health hazard appraisal	50.00				
99429	Unlisted preventive med service	Variable				
Newborn Care						
99460	Birthing room delivery	102.50	93.50	88.83	102.15	
99461	Other than birthing room	110.16	100.83	95.79	110.16	
99462	Subsequent hospital care	54.02	49.44	46.97	54.02	
99465	Newborn resuscitation	255.98	234.30	222.59	255.98	
Anesthesiology						
Anesthesiology fees are presented here for CPT codes. However, each case would require a fee for time, e.g., every 15 minutes would be worth $55. This fee is determined according to the relative value system, calculated, and added into the anesthesia (CPT) fee. Some anesthetists may list a surgical code using an anesthesia modifier on a subsequent line for carriers that do not acknowledge anesthesia codes.						
99100	Anes for pt younger than 1 year or older than 70 years	55.00				
99116	Anes complicated use total hypothermia	275.00				
99135	Anes complicated use hypotension	275.00				
99140	Anes complicated emer cond	110.00				
Physician Status Modifier Codes						
P-1	Normal healthy patient	00.00				
P-2	Patient with mild systemic disease	00.00				
P-3	Patient with severe systemic disease	55.00				
P-4	Patient with severe systemic disease that is a constant threat to life	110.00				
P-5	Moribund pt not expected to survive without operation	165.00				
P-6	Declared brain-dead pt, organs being removed for donor	00.00				

[a]Some services and procedures may not be considered a benefit under the Medicare program and when listed on a claim form, no reimbursement may be received. However, it is important to include these codes when billing because Medicare policies may change without an individual knowing of a new benefit. For this reason, some of the services shown in this Mock Fee Schedule do not have any amounts listed under the three Medicare columns.

Table 2. Mock Fee Schedule—cont'd						
			Medicare[a]			
Code No.	Description	Mock Fees	Participating	Nonparticipating	Limiting Charge	Follow-Up Days
Head						
00160	Anes nose/sinus (NEC)	275.00				
00172	Anes repair cleft palate	165.00				
Thorax						
00400	Anes for proc ant integumentary system of chest, incl SC tissue	165.00				
00402	Anes breast reconstruction	275.00				
00546	Anes pulmonary resection with thoracoplasty	275.00				
00600	Anes cervical spine and cord	550.00				
Lower Abdomen						
00800	Anes for proc lower ant abdominal wall	165.00				
00840	Anes intraperitoneal proc lower abdomen: NOS	330.00				
00842	Amniocentesis	220.00				
00914	Anes TURP	275.00				
00942	Anes colporrhaphy, colpotomy, colpectomy	220.00				
Upper Leg						
01210	Anes open proc hip joint; NOS	330.00				
01214	Total hip replacement	440.00				
Upper Arm and Elbow						
01740	Anes open proc humerus/elbow; NOS	220.00				
01758	Exc cyst/tumor humerus	275.00				
Radiologic Procedures						
01922	Anes CAT scan	385.00				
Miscellaneous Procedure(s)						
01999	Unlisted anes proc	Variable				
Neurology						
95812	Electroencephalogram	129.32	118.37	112.45	129.32	
95819	Electroencephalogram—awake	126.81	116.07	110.27	126.81	
95860	Electromyography, 1 extremity	88.83	81.31	77.24	88.83	
95864	Electromyography, 4 extremities	239.99	219.67	208.69	239.99	
96101	Psychological testing (per hour)	80.95	74.10	70.39	80.95	
Physical Medicine						
97024	Diathermy	14.27	13.06	12.41	14.27	
97036	Hubbard tank, each 15 min	24.77	22.67	21.54	24.77	
97110	Therapeutic proc, one or more areas, each 15 min	23.89	21.86	20.77	23.89	
97140	Manual therapy (manipulation, traction), one or more regions, each 15 min	16.93	15.49	14.72	16.93	
Special Services and Reports						
99000	Handling of specimen (transfer from Dr.'s office to lab)	5.00				
99024	Postoperative visit (bundled)	No charge				

[a]Some services and procedures may not be considered a benefit under the Medicare program and when listed on a claim form, no reimbursement may be received. However, it is important to include these codes when billing because Medicare policies may change without an individual knowing of a new benefit. For this reason, some of the services shown in this Mock Fee Schedule do not have any amounts listed under the three Medicare columns.

Continued

Table 2. Mock Fee Schedule—cont'd

Code No.	Description	Mock Fees	Medicare[a] Participating	Medicare[a] Nonparticipating	Medicare[a] Limiting Charge	Follow-Up Days
99050	Services provided, in the office at times other than regularly scheduled office hours or days when office is normally closed (e.g., holidays, Saturday or Sunday) in addition to basic service	25.00				
99053	Services between 10:00 PM and 8:00 AM in addition to basic service (24 hr facility)	35.00				
99056	Services normally provided in office requested by pt in location other than office in addition to basic service	20.00				
99058	Office services provided on an emergency basis, which causes disruption of other sched svcs.					
99070	Supplies and materials (itemize drugs and materials provided)	10.00				
99080	Special reports: insurance forms					
	Review of data to clarify pt's status	20.00				
	WC reports	50.00				
	WC extensive review report	250.00				
10060	I & D furuncle, onychia, paronychia; single	75.92	69.49	66.02	75.92	10
11042	Débridement; skin, partial thickness	79.32	75.60	68.97	79.32	10
11044	Débridement; skin, subcu. muscle, bone	269.28	246.48	234.16	269.28	10
11100	Biopsy of skin, SC tissue &/or mucous membrane; 1 lesion	65.43	59.89	56.90	65.43	10
11200	Exc, skin tags; up to 15	55.68	50.97	45.42	55.68	10
11401	Exc, benign lesion, 0.6–1.0 cm trunk, arms, legs	95.62	87.53	83.15	96.62	10
11402	1.1–2.0 cm	121.52	111.23	105.67	121.52	10
11403	2.1–3.0 cm	151.82	138.97	132.02	151.82	10
11420	Exc, benign lesion, 0.5 cm or less scalp, neck, hands, feet, genitalia	75.44	69.05	65.60	75.44	10
11422	Exc, benign lesion scalp, neck, hands, feet, or genitalia; 1.1–2.0 cm	131.35	120.23	114.22	131.35	10
11441	Exc, benign lesion face, ears, eyelids, nose, lips, or mucous membrane	119.08	109.00	103.55	119.08	10
11602	Exc, malignant lesion, trunk, arms, or legs; 1.1–2.0 cm dia	195.06	178.55	169.62	195.06	10
11719	Trimming of nondystrophic nails, any number	30.58	27.82	26.33	30.58	0
11720	Débridement of nails, any method, 1–5	32.58	29.82	28.33	32.58	0
11721	6 or more	32.58	29.82	28.33	32.58	0
11730	Avulsion nail plate, partial or complete, simple repair; single	76.91	70.40	66.88	76.91	0
11750	Exc, nail or nail matrix, partial or complete	193.45	177.07	168.22	193.45	10

[a]Some services and procedures may not be considered a benefit under the Medicare program and when listed on a claim form, no reimbursement may be received. However, it is important to include these codes when billing because Medicare policies may change without an individual knowing of a new benefit. For this reason, some of the services shown in this Mock Fee Schedule do not have any amounts listed under the three Medicare columns.

Table 2. Mock Fee Schedule—cont'd

Code No.	Description	Mock Fees	Medicare[a] Participating	Medicare[a] Nonparticipating	Medicare[a] Limiting Charge	Medicare[a] Follow-Up Days
11765	Wedge excision of nail fold	57.95	53.04	50.39	57.95	10
12001	Simple repair (scalp, neck, axillae, ext genitalia, trunk, or extremities incl. hands & feet); 2.5 cm or less	91.17	83.45	79.28	91.17	10
12011	Simple repair (face, ears, eyelids, nose, lips, or mucous membranes); 2.5 cm or less	101.44	92.85	88.21	101.44	10
12013	2.6–5.0 cm	123.98	113.48	107.81	123.98	10
12032	Repair, scalp, axillae, trunk (intermediate)	169.73	155.36	147.59	169.73	10
12034	Repair, intermediate, wounds (scalp, axillae, trunk, or extremities) excl hands or feet; 7.6–12.5 cm	214.20	196.06	186.26	214.20	10
12051	Repair, intermediate, layer closure of wounds (face, ears, eyelids, nose, lips, or mucous membranes); 2.5 cm or less	167.60	153.41	145.74	167.60	10
17000	Cauterization, 1 lesion	52.56	48.11	45.70	52.56	10
17003	Second through 14 lesions, each	15.21	17.77	16.88	5.21	
17004	Destruction (laser surgery), 15 or more lesions					10
19020	Mastotomy, drainage/exploration deep abscess	237.36	217.26	206.40	237.36	90
19100	Biopsy, breast, needle	96.17	88.03	83.63	96.17	0
19101	Biopsy, breast, incisional	281.51	257.67	244.79	281.51	10
20610	Arthrocentesis, aspiration or injection major joint (shoulder, hip, knee, or bursa)	52.33	47.89	45.50	52.33	0
21330	Nasal fracture, open treatment complicated	599.46	548.71	521.27	599.46	90
24066	Biopsy, deep, soft tissue, upper arm, elbow	383.34	350.88	333.34	383.34	90
27455	Osteotomy, proximal tibia	1248.03	1142.36	1085.24	1248.03	90
27500	Treatment closed femoral shaft fracture without manipulation	554.90	507.92	482.52	554.90	90
27530	Treatment closed tibial fracture, proximal, without manipulation	344.24	315.09	299.34	344.24	90
27750	Treatment closed tibial shaft fracture, without manipulation	400.94	366.99	348.64	400.94	90
27752	With manipulation	531.63	486.62	462.29	531.63	90
29280	Strapping of hand or finger	35.13	31.36	29.79	35.13	0
29345	Appl long leg cast (thigh to toes)	123.23	112.80	107.16	123.23	0
29355	Walker or ambulatory type	133.75	122.42	116.30	133.75	0
29425	Appl short leg walking cast	102.10	93.45	88.78	102.10	0
30110	Excision, simple nasal polyp	145.21	132.92	126.27	145.21	10
30520	Septoplasty	660.88	604.93	574.68	660.88	90
30903	Control nasal hemorrhage; unilateral	118.17	108.17	102.76	118.17	0

[a]Some services and procedures may not be considered a benefit under the Medicare program and when listed on a claim form, no reimbursement may be received. However, it is important to include these codes when billing because Medicare policies may change without an individual knowing of a new benefit. For this reason, some of the services shown in this Mock Fee Schedule do not have any amounts listed under the three Medicare columns.

Continued

Table 2. Mock Fee Schedule—cont'd

Code No.	Description	Mock Fees	Medicare[a] Participating	Nonparticipating	Limiting Charge	Follow-Up Days
30905	Control nasal hemorrhage, posterior with posterior nasal packs and/or cautery; initial	190.57	174.43	165.71	190.57	0
30906	Subsequent	173.01	158.36	150.44	173.01	
31540	Laryngoscopy with excision of tumor and/or stripping of vocal cords	488.95	447.55	425.17	488.95	0
31541	With operating microscope	428.33	392.06	372.46	428.33	0
31575	Laryngoscopy, flexible fiberoptic; diagnostic	138.48	126.76	120.42	138.48	0
31625	Bronchoscopy with biopsy	312.87	286.38	272.06	312.87	0
32310	Pleurectomy	1234.79	1130.24	1073.73	1234.79	90
32440	Pneumonectomy, total	1972.10	1805.13	1714.87	1972.10	90
33020	Pericardiotomy	1289.25	1180.09	1121.09	1289.25	90
33206	Insertion of pacemaker; atrial	728.42	666.75	633.41	728.42	90
33208	Atrial and ventricular	751.57	687.89	653.50	751.57	90
35301	Thromboendarterectomy, with or without patch graft; carotid, vertebral, subclavian, by neck incision	1585.02	1450.82	1378.28	1585.02	90
36005	Intravenous injection for contrast venography	59.18	54.17	51.46	59.18	0
36248	Catheter placement (selective) arterial system, 2nd, 3rd order and beyond	68.54	62.74	59.60	68.54	0
36415	Routine venipuncture for collection of specimen(s)	10.00				
38101	Splenectomy, partial	994.44	910.24	864.73	994.44	90
38220	Bone marrow; aspiration only	73.52	67.29	63.93	73.52	NA
38221	Biopsy, needle or trocar	90.65	82.98	78.83	90.65	NA
38510	Biopsy/excision deep cervical node/s	327.42	299.69	284.71	327.42	10
39540	Hernia repair	1436.50	1314.87	1249.13	1436.50	90
42820	T&A under age 12 years	341.63	312.71	297.07	341.63	90
42821	T&A over age 12 years	410.73	375.96	357.16	410.73	90
43200	Upper GI endoscopy, simple primary exam	201.86	184.77	175.53	201.86	0
43235	Upper GI endoscopy incl. esophagus, stomach, duodenum, or jejunum; complex	238.92	218.69	207.76	238.92	0
43239	Esophagogastro-duodenoscopy, with biopsy, single or multiple	238.92	218.69	207.76	238.92	0
43255	With control of bleeding, any method	281.51	257.67	244.79	281.51	0
43453	Dilation esophagus	254.52	232.97	221.32	254.52	0
43754	Gastric intubation	87.41	80.01	76.01	87.41	
43820	Gastrojejunostomy	971.86	889.58	845.10	971.86	90
44150	Colectomy, total, abdominal	1757.81	108.98	1528.53	1757.81	90
44320	Colostomy or skin level cecostomy	966.25	884.44	840.22	966.25	90
44950	Appendectomy	568.36	520.24	494.23	568.36	90
45308	Proctosigmoidoscopy; removal of polyp	135.34	123.88	117.69	135.34	0
45315	Multiple polyps	185.12	169.44	160.97	185.12	0

[a]Some services and procedures may not be considered a benefit under the Medicare program and when listed on a claim form, no reimbursement may be received. However, it is important to include these codes when billing because Medicare policies may change without an individual knowing of a new benefit. For this reason, some of the services shown in this Mock Fee Schedule do not have any amounts listed under the three Medicare columns.

Table 2. Mock Fee Schedule—cont'd

Code No.	Description	Mock Fees	Medicare[a] Participating	Medicare[a] Nonparticipating	Medicare[a] Limiting Charge	Follow-Up Days
45330	Sigmoidoscopy (flexible), diagnostic (with or without biopsy or collection of specimen by brushing or washing)	95.92	87.80	83.41	95.92	0
45333	Sigmoidoscopy (flexible) with removal of polyps	183.99	168.41	159.99	183.99	0
45380	Colonoscopy with biopsy	382.35	349.98	332.48	382.35	0
46255	Hemorrhoidectomy int & ext, simple	503.57	460.94	437.89	503.57	90
46258	Hemorrhoidectomy with fistulectomy	636.02	582.17	553.06	636.02	90
46600	Anoscopy; diagnostic	32.86	30.07	28.57	32.86	0
46614	With control of hemorrhage	182.10	166.68	158.35	182.10	0
46700	Anoplasty, for stricture, adult	657.39	601.73	571.64	657.39	90
47562	Cholecystectomy; laparoscopic	714.99	654.45	621.73	714.99	90
47600	Cholecystectomy; abdominal excision	937.74	858.35	815.43	937.74	90
49505	Inguinal hernia repair, age 5 or over	551.07	504.41	479.19	551.07	90
49520	Repair, inguinal hernia, any age; reducible	671.89	615.00	584.25	671.89	90
50080	Nephrostolithotomy, percutaneous	1323.93	1211.83	1151.24	1323.93	90
50780	Ureteroneocystostomy	1561.23	1429.84	1357.59	1561.23	90
51900	Closure of vesicovaginal fistula, abdominal approach	1196.82	1095.48	1040.71	1196.82	90
52000	Cystourethroscopy	167.05	152.90	145.26	167.05	0
52601	Transurethral resection of prostate	1193.53	1092.47	1037.85	1193.53	90
53040	Drainage of deep periurethral abscess	379.48	347.35	329.98	379.48	90
53060	Drainage of Skene's gland	147.45	134.97	128.22	147.45	10
53230	Excision, female diverticulum (urethral)	859.69	786.91	747.56	859.69	90
53240	Marsupialization of urethral diverticulum, M or F	520.11	476.07	452.27	520.11	90
53270	Excision of Skene's gland(s)	184.39	168.78	160.34	184.39	10
53620	Dilation, urethra, male	100.73	92.20	87.59	100.73	0
53660	Dilation urethra, female	48.32	44.23	42.02	48.32	0
54150	Circumcision	111.78	102.32	97.20	111.78	10
54520	Orchiectomy, simple	523.92	479.56	455.58	523.92	90
55700	Biopsy of prostate, needle or punch	156.22	142.99	135.84	156.22	0
55801	Prostatectomy, perineal subtotal	1466.56	1342.39	1275.27	1466.56	90
57265	Colporrhaphy AP with enterocele repair	902.24	825.85	784.56	902.24	90
57452	Colposcopy	84.18	77.05	73.20	84.18	0
57510	Cauterization of cervix, electro or thermal	115.15	105.40	100.13	115.15	10
57520	Conization of cervix with or without D&C, with or without repair	387.08	354.30	336.59	387.08	90
58100	Endometrial biopsy	71.88	65.79	62.50	71.88	0
58120	D&C, diagnostic and/or therapeutic (non-OB)	272.83	249.73	237.24	272.83	10
58150	TAH w/without salpingo-oophorectomy	1167.72	1068.85	1015.41	1167.72	90
58200	Total hysterectomy, extended, corpus	1707.24	1562.69	1484.56	1707.24	90

[a]Some services and procedures may not be considered a benefit under the Medicare program and when listed on a claim form, no reimbursement may be received. However, it is important to include these codes when billing because Medicare policies may change without an individual knowing of a new benefit. For this reason, some of the services shown in this Mock Fee Schedule do not have any amounts listed under the three Medicare columns.

Continued

Table 2. Mock Fee Schedule—cont'd

Code No.	Description	Mock Fees	Medicare[a] Participating	Medicare[a] Nonparticipating	Medicare[a] Limiting Charge	Medicare[a] Follow-Up Days
58210	Radical abdominal hysterectomy with bilateral total pelvic lymphadenectomy	2160.78	1977.83	1878.94	2160.78	90
	completed surgically	357.39	327.13	310.77	357.39	90
58300	Insertion of intrauterine device	100.00	93.45	88.78	100.00	0
58340	Hysterosalpingography, inj proc for	73.06	66.87	63.53	73.06	0
58720	Salpingo-oophorectomy, complete or partial, unilateral or bilateral surgical treatment of ectopic pregnancy	732.40	670.39	636.87	732.40	90
59120	Ectopic pregnancy requiring salpingectomy and/or oophorectomy	789.26	722.43	686.31	789.26	90
59121	Without salpingectomy and/or oophorectomy	638.84	584.75	555.51	638.84	90
59130	Abdominal pregnancy	699.12	639.93	607.93	699.12	90
59135	Total hysterectomy, interstitial, uterine pregnancy	1154.16	1056.44	1003.62	1154.16	90
59136	Partial uterine resection, interstitial uterine pregnancy	1154.16	1056.44	1003.62	1154.16	90
59140	Cervical, with evacuation	489.68	448.22	425.81	489.68	90
59160	Curettage postpartum hemorrhage (separate proc)	293.46	268.61	255.18	293.46	10
59400	OB care—routine, incl. antepartum/postpartum care	1864.30	1706.45	1621.13	1864.30	N/A
59510	C-section including antepartum and postpartum care	2102.33	1924.33	1828.11	2102.33	N/A
59515	C-section, postpartum care only	1469.80	1345.36	1278.09	1469.80	N/A
59812	Treatment of incompl. abortion, any trimester	357.39	327.13	310.77	357.39	90
61314	Craniotomy infratentorial	2548.09	2332.35	2215.73	2548.09	90
62270	Spinal puncture, lumbar; diagnostic	77.52	70.96	67.41	77.52	0
65091	Evisceration of eye, without implant	708.22	648.25	615.84	708.22	90
65205	Removal of foreign body, ext eye	56.02	51.27	48.71	56.02	0
65222	Removal of foreign body, corneal, with slit lamp	73.81	67.56	64.18	73.81	0
69420	Myringotomy	97.76	89.48	85.01	97.76	10
RADIOLOGY, NUCLEAR MEDICINE, AND DIAGNOSTIC ULTRASOUND						
70120	X-ray mastoids, less than 3 views per side	38.96	35.66	33.88	38.96	
70130	Complete, min., 3 views per side	56.07	51.33	48.76	56.07	
71010	Chest x-ray, 1 view	31.95	29.24	27.78	31.95	
71045	Chest x-ray, single view	31.95	29.24	27.78	31.95	
71046	Chest x-ray, 2 views	40.97	37.50	35.63	40.97	
71048	Chest x-ray, 4 or more views	54.02	49.44	46.97	54.02	
72100	X-ray spine, LS; 2 or 3 views	43.23	39.57	37.59	43.23	
72114	Complete, incl. bending views	74.97	68.62	65.19	74.97	
73100	X-ray wrist, 2 views	31.61	28.94	27.49	31.61	
73501	Hip x-ray, unilateral 1 view	31.56	28.88	27.44	31.56	

[a]Some services and procedures may not be considered a benefit under the Medicare program and when listed on a claim form, no reimbursement may be received. However, it is important to include these codes when billing because Medicare policies may change without an individual knowing of a new benefit. For this reason, some of the services shown in this Mock Fee Schedule do not have any amounts listed under the three Medicare columns.

Table 2. Mock Fee Schedule—cont'd

Code No.	Description	Mock Fees	Medicare[a] Participating	Nonparticipating	Limiting Charge	Follow-Up Days
73502	Hip x-ray, unilateral 2–3 views	37.94	34.73	32.99	37.94	
73590	X-ray tibia & fibula, 2 views	33.35	30.53	29.00	33.35	
73620	Radiologic exam, foot; 2 views	31.61	28.94	27.49	31.61	
73650	X-ray calcaneus, 2 views	30.71	28.11	26.70	30.71	
74241	Radiologic exam, upper gastrointestinal tract; with/without delayed films with KUB	108.93	99.71	94.72	108.93	
74245	With small bowel, serial films	161.70	148.01	140.61	161.70	
74270	Barium enema	118.47	108.44	103.02	118.47	
74290	Cholecystography, oral contrast	52.59	48.14	45.73	52.59	
74400	Urography (pyelography), intravenous, with or without KUB	104.78	95.90	91.11	104.78	
74410	Urography, infusion	116.76	106.87	101.53	116.76	
74420	Urography, retrograde	138.89	127.13	120.77	138.89	
76805	Ultrasound, pregnant uterus, or real time; complete, first gestation	154.18	141.13	134.07	154.18	
76810	Ultrasound, pregnant uterus, complete: each additional gestation, after first trimester	306.54	280.59	266.56	306.54	
76946	Ultrasonic guidance for amniocentesis	91.22	83.49	79.32	91.22	
77065	Diagnostic mammography; unilateral	62.57	57.27	54.41	62.57	
77066	Diagnostic mammography; bilateral	82.83	75.82	72.03	82.83	
77300	Radiation dosimetry	97.58	89.32	84.85	97.58	
77307	Teletherapy, isodose plan, complex	213.59	195.51	185.73	213.59	
78104	Bone marrow imaging, whole body	230.56	211.04	200.49	230.56	
78215	Liver and spleen imaging	160.44	146.85	139.51	160.44	
78800	Tumor localization, limited area	191.53	175.32	166.55	191.53	
PATHOLOGY AND LABORATORY[1]						
ORGAN OR DISEASE-ORIENTED PANELS						
80048	Basic metabolic panel	15.00	14.60	13.87	16.64	
80050	General health panel	20.00	19.20	15.99	21.87	
80051	Electrolyte panel	20.00	19.20	15.99	21.87	
80053	Comprehensive metabolic panel	25.00	20.99	19.94	23.93	
80055	Obstetric panel	25.00	20.99	19.94	23.93	
80061	Lipid panel	30.00	28.60	25.97	32.16	
80074	Acute hepatitis panel	27.00	25.00	20.88	24.88	
80076	Hepatic function panel	27.00	25.00	20.88	24.98	
81000	Urinalysis, nonautomated, with microscopy	8.00	7.44	5.98	8.84	
81001	Urinalysis, automated, with microscopy	8.00	7.44	5.98	8.84	
81002	Urinalysis, nonautomated without microscopy	8.00	7.44	5.98	8.84	
81015	Urinalysis, microscopy only	8.00	7.44	5.98	8.84	
82270	Blood, occult; feces screening 1–3	4.05	3.56	3.31	4.05	
82565	Creatinine; blood	10.00	9.80	8.88	12.03	
82947	Glucose; quantitative	15.00				

[a]Some services and procedures may not be considered a benefit under the Medicare program and when listed on a claim form, no reimbursement may be received. However, it is important to include these codes when billing because Medicare policies may change without an individual knowing of a new benefit. For this reason, some of the services shown in this Mock Fee Schedule do not have any amounts listed under the three Medicare columns.

Continued

Table 2. Mock Fee Schedule—cont'd						
			Medicare[a]			
Code No.	Description	Mock Fees	Participating	Nonparticipating	Limiting Charge	Follow-Up Days
82951	Glucose tolerance test, 3 spec	40.00	41.00	36.80	45.16	
82952	Each add spec beyond 3	30.00	28.60	25.97	32.16	
83020	Hemoglobin, electrophoresis	25.00	20.00	19.94	23.93	
83700	Lipoprotein, blood; electrophoretic separation	25.00	20.00	19.94	23.93	
84478	Triglycerides, blood	20.00	19.20	15.999	21.87	
84480	Triiodothyronine (T-3)	20.00	19.20	15.99	21.87	
84520	Urea nitrogen, blood (BUN); quantitative	25.00	20.99	19.94	23.93	
84550	Uric acid, blood chemical	20.00	19.20	15.99	21.87	
84702	Gonadotropin, chorionic; quantitative	20.00	19.20	15.99	21.87	
84703	Gonadotropin, chorionic; qualitative	20.00	19.20	15.99	21.87	
85013	Microhematocrit (spun)	20.00	19.20	15.99	21.87	
85025	Complete blood count (hemogram), platelet count, automated, differential WBC count	25.00	20.00	19.94	23.93	
85032	Manual cell count (erythrocyte, leukocyte, or platelet) each	20.00	19.20	15.99	21.87	
85345	Coagulation time; Lee & White	20.00	19.20	15.99	21.87	
86038	Antinuclear antibodies	25.00	20.00	19.94	23.93	
86580	Skin test; TB, intradermal	11.34	10.38	9.86	11.34	
87081	Culture, bacterial, screening for single organisms	25.00	20.00	19.94	23.93	
87181	Sensitivity studies, antibiotic; per antibiotic	20.00	19.20	15.99	21.87	
87184	Disk method, per plate (12 disks or less)	20.00	19.20	15.99	21.87	
87210	Smear, primary source, wet mount with simple stain, for bacteria, fungi, ova, and/or parasites	35.00	48.35	45.93	55.12	
88150	Papanicolaou, cytopath	35.00	48.35	45.93	55.12	
88302	Surgical pathology, gross & micro exam (skin, fingers, nerve, testis)	24.14	22.09	20.99	24.14	
88305	Bone marrow, interpret	77.69	71.12	67.56	77.69	
MEDICINE PROCEDURES						
Immunization Injections						
90700	Diphtheria, tetanus, pertussis	34.00				
90703	Tetanus toxoid	28.00				
90712	Poliovirus vaccine, oral	28.00				
Therapeutic Injections						
96372	Therapeutic prophylactic or Dx injection; IM or SC	5.22	4.37	4.15	5.22	
96374	Intravenous push, single or initial substance/drug	21.33	19.53	18.55	21.33	
96379	Intravenous therapeutic prophylactic, or diagnostic	21.33	19.53	18.55	21.33	
Psychiatry						
90832	Individual psychotherapy 20–30 min	60.25	55.15	52.39	60.25	
90853	Group therapy	29.22	26.75	25.41	29.22	

[a]Some services and procedures may not be considered a benefit under the Medicare program and when listed on a claim form, no reimbursement may be received. However, it is important to include these codes when billing because Medicare policies may change without an individual knowing of a new benefit. For this reason, some of the services shown in this Mock Fee Schedule do not have any amounts listed under the three Medicare columns.

Table 2. Mock Fee Schedule—cont'd						
			Medicare[a]			
Code No.	Description	Mock Fees	Participating	Nonparticipating	Limiting Charge	Follow-Up Days
Hemodialysis						
90935	Single phys evaluation	117.23	107.31	101.94	117.23	
90937	Repeat evaluation	206.24	188.78	179.34	206.24	
Gastroenterology						
91010	Esophageal incubation	69.82	63.91	60.71	69.82	
Ophthalmologic Services						
92004	Comprehensive eye exam	90.86	83.17	79.01	90.86	
92100	Tonometry	47.31	43.31	41.14	47.31	
92230	Fluorescein angioscopy	55.49	50.79	48.25	55.49	
92275	Electroretinography	81.17	74.29	70.58	81.17	
92531	Spontaneous nystagmus	26.00				
Audiologic Function Tests						
92557	Comprehensive audiometry	54.33	49.73	47.24	54.33	
92596	Ear measurements	26.81	24.54	23.31	26.81	
Cardiovascular Therapeutic Services						
93000	Electrocardiogram (ECG)	34.26	31.36	29.79	34.26	
93015	Treadmill ECG	140.71	128.80	122.36	140.71	
93040	Rhythm ECG, 1–3 leads	18.47	16.90	16.06	18.47	
93306	Doppler echocardiography	250.73	229.50	218.03	250.73	
93307	Echocardiography without Doppler	114.60	104.90	99.65	114.60	
Pulmonary						
94010	Spirometry	38.57	35.31	33.54	38.57	
94060	Spirometry before and after bronchodilator	71.67	65.60	62.32	71.67	
94150	Vital capacity, total	13.82	12.65	12.02	13.82	
Allergy and Clinical Immunology						
95024	Intradermal tests; immediate reaction	6.58	6.02	5.72	6.85	
95028	Intradermal tests; delayed reaction	9.32	8.85	10.18	9.32	
95044	Patch tests	8.83	8.08	7.68	8.83	
95115	Treatment for allergy, single inj.	17.20	15.75	14.96	17.20	
95117	2 or more inj.	22.17	20.29	19.28	22.17	
95165	Allergen immunotherapy, single or multiple antigens, multiple-dose vials (professional svcs for preparation supervision)		6.50	6.18	7.11	
Neurology						
95812	Electroencephalogram, 41–60 min	129.32	118.37	112.45	129.32	
95819	Electroencephalogram—awake and	126.81	116.07	110.27	126.81	
95860	Electromyography, 1 extremity	88.83	81.31	77.24	88.83	
96101	Psychological testing (per hour)	80.95	74.10	70.39	80.95	
Physical Medicine						
97024	Diathermy	14.27	13.06	12.41	14.27	
97036	Hubbard tank, each 15 min	24.77	22.67	21.54	24.77	
97110	Physical therapy, initial 30 min	23.89	21.86	20.77	23.89	
97140	Manual therapy (manipulation, traction), one or more regions, each 15 min	16.93	15.49	14.72	16.93	

[a]Some services and procedures may not be considered a benefit under the Medicare program and when listed on a claim form, no reimbursement may be received. However, it is important to include these codes when billing because Medicare policies may change without an individual knowing of a new benefit. For this reason, some of the services shown in this Mock Fee Schedule do not have any amounts listed under the three Medicare columns.

Continued

Table 2. Mock Fee Schedule—cont'd						
			Medicare[a]			
Code No.	Description	Mock Fees	Participating	Nonparticipating	Limiting Charge	Follow-Up Days
Chiropractic Manipulative Treatment						
98940	Chiropractic manipulative treatment; spinal 1–2 regions	75.00				
Special Services and Reports						
99000	Handling of specimen (transfer from Dr.'s office to lab)	5.00				
99050	Services provided after office hours, or on Sundays and holidays in addition to basic service in the office	25.00				
99053	Services between 10 PM and 8 AM in addition to basic service	35.00				
99056	Services normally provided in office requested by pt in location other than office	20.00				
99058	Office services provided on an emergency basis	65.00				
99070	Supplies and materials (itemize drugs and materials provided)	25.00				
99080	Special reports:					
	Insurance forms	10.00				
	Review of data to clarify pt's status	20.00				
	WC reports	50.00				
	WC extensive review report	250.00				

[a]Some services and procedures may not be considered a benefit under the Medicare program and when listed on a claim form, no reimbursement may be received. However, it is important to include these codes when billing because Medicare policies may change without an individual knowing of a new benefit. For this reason, some of the services shown in this Mock Fee Schedule do not have any amounts listed under the three Medicare columns.

[b]Data for the surgical follow-up days from St. Anthony's CPT '96 Companion: A Guide to Medicare Billing.